THE HOSPITAL RESEARCH AND EDUCATIONAL TRUST

Being a Nursing Assistant

Third Edition

Rose Schniedman
Susan Lambert
Barbara Wander

The Robert J. Brady Publishing Company, Bowie, Maryland
A Prentice-Hall Publishing and Communications Company

ACKNOWLEDGMENTS

This edition of *Being a Nursing Assistant* was prepared by Rose B. Schniedman, M.S.Ed., R.N.; Susan M. Lambert, M.A.Ed.; and Barbara R. Wander, B.S.N., R.N. Mrs. Schniedman directed the training of nursing assistants for community hospitals in the Miami area for more than 16 years and is now coordinator of nursing education for a hospital in southern Florida. Mrs. Lambert is an educational curriculum consultant specializing in adult and vocational education. Mrs. Wander is a maternal and infant care patient educator in a teaching hospital in north-central Florida. The Trust gratefully acknowledges their wisdom, their perseverance, and, above all, their dedication as authors of this book.

The professional guidance and expertise of Dianne V. Spenner of the Hospital Research and Educational Trust, Paula K. Aldrich, Production Editor, of the Robert J. Brady Co. and Bernard J. Vervin, Assistant Art Director, of the Robert J. Brady Co., ensured that this edition maintained the quality and upheld the reputation of the previous editions.

Deeply appreciated are the contributions of the reviewers and colleagues in the fields of nursing service, education, and epidemiology whose comments, suggestions, and criticism aided greatly in determining the content of this edition of *Being A Nursing Assistant*. By sharing their knowledge and experience so generously, they ensured the accuracy and quality of this book.

Being a Nursing Assistant.

Published for Hospital Research and Educational Trust by the Robert J. Brady Co.,
Bowie, Maryland 20715.

Library of Congress Cataloging in Publication Data

Schniedman, Rose B.
  Being a nursing assistant.
  Previous ed.: Being a nursing aide/Hospital Research and Educational Trust. 2nd ed. c1978.
  Includes index.
  1. Nurses' aides.   2. Care of the sick. I. Lambert, Susan.   II. Wander, Barbara.   III. Being a nursing aide.   IV. Title.   [DNLM: 1. Nurses' aides. WY 193 S361b]
RT84.S35   1981   610.73'7   81-10113 AACR2
ISBN 0-89303-027-9 (Brady)   ISBN 0-87914-055-0 HRET

Prentice-Hall International, Inc., London
Prentice-Hall of Australia, Pty., Ltd., Sydney
Prentice-Hall of India Private Limited, New Delhi
Prentice-Hall of Japan, Inc., Tokyo
Prentice-Hall of Southeast Asia Pte. Ltd., Singapore
Whitehall Books, Limited, Petone, New Zealand

Printed in the United States of America

82 83 84 85 86 87 88 89 90 91 92   10 9 8 7 6 5 4 3 2 1

DEDICATION

To Della, who motivated and inspired us, with all our love, respect, and admiration

To Marty, Alan, and Barry, who sustain us with their love

To Carrie and Joey, who are our future, whom we all love

CONTENTS

PREFACE

This edition of *Being a Nursing Assistant* has been re-organized and updated both to meet the needs of the student, and also to keep pace with the newest applicable advances in nursing care. The name of this manual was changed to reflect the position title now most commonly used in health care institutions throughout the country.

The course of instruction has certain features built in that make this student text unique. This edition does much more than add small bits of new information. As educators dedicated to research, the authors have prepared this manual to establish a logical plan of action for the nursing assistant. The text is designed to lead the student through each nursing task that may be assigned. Each task, or procedure, outlines precisely the necessary steps involved in every nursing assistant function.

In addition to the increased scope and depth of the nursing procedures, the following are the most prominent revisions to this text:

- New chapter on extended care for:
  Incontinent patients
  Diabetic patients
  Orthopedic patients
  Ostomy patients
  Seizure patients
- New chapter on home health care, which includes:
  Introduction to home health care
  Geriatric home care
  Newborn and infant home care
  Household management
- Range-of-motion exercises
- Application of sling bandages
- Complete description of nutrient classes and food sources
- Updated, detailed job description
- Expanded medical and hospital abbreviations
- Expanded list of words to remember
- Expanded section on safety
- Expanded description of oxygen therapy

Along with these revisions and additions, the authors have worked to preserve the clarity of the text through constant evaluation, deliberation, and comprehensive involvement in nursing practice.

INTRODUCTION

Welcome to being a nursing assistant. You are beginning a new career in the field of health care. Delivering health care is a very special job, one you can take much pride in. You will be helping people and making your community a better place to live.

You are or will be working in a health care institution. Such institutions are hospitals, nursing homes, clinics, and other places where sick and injured people are treated and cared for. The most important person in the health care institution is the patient. All health care personnel are there to meet the needs of the patients.

This book has been written to help you do well in your training and on the job. Your instructor will guide your training during class lectures, practice sessions, and clinical experiences. Your instructor will teach you the methods and policies that are required in your state and in the institution in which you will be working. The reason for this is that methods and policies vary from state to state and from health care institution to health care institution. If your instructor demonstrates a procedure differently than it is explained in this book, follow your instructor's method.

Health care delivery is a growing field of rapid changes and improvements. A textbook cannot be changed as quickly or as often as new insights, techniques, or equipment are adopted by modern health care institutions. Your instructor keeps informed of these changes and is your best source of current information. Should you have any questions about two sources saying different things, ask your instructor. If this text takes one approach to a situation and your instructor takes a different one, follow your instructor. Your instructor is an expert in health care delivery and is the authority for your course.

On the job, you will be working under the supervision of the head nurse or team leader. They are not necessarily the same person, although they might be. We use the terms head nurse or team leader throughout this book to refer to the person who supervises you and keeps record of your performance. During your training, if you do not understand a procedure, ask your instructor for help. On the job, ask your head nurse or team leader if you need help. If you are not sure of yourself, tell her. It is far better to get help than to do something wrong.

Use this book. Read through the procedures until you remember every step. Try to meet every objective in each section of every chapter. Like a dictionary, this text is a learning tool and a reference book. Use it in class for taking notes. Look at it whenever you have a chance. Use this book at home for studying and reading before class. Use it during your work to review procedures you may not be sure of. Check the illustrations, charts, and lists. They will help to make things clear. Keep working on your vocabulary. Use the *Words To Remember* section in Chapter 20 to find the meaning for words you do not fully understand or that are unfamiliar to you.

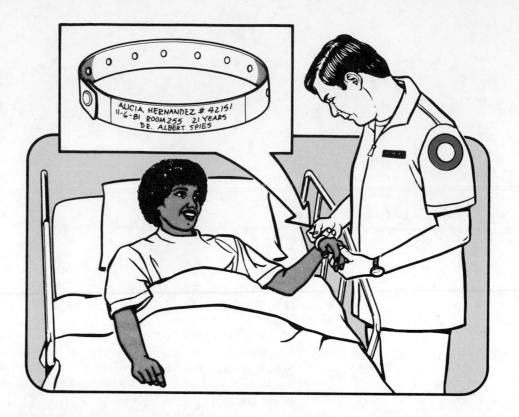

Sample Procedure

1. Assemble your equipment.
2. Wash your hands.
3. Identify the patient by checking the identification bracelet.
4. Ask visitors to step out of the room.
5. Tell the patient what you are going to do. For example, "I am going to measure your vital signs."
6. Pull the curtain around the bed for privacy.
7. The procedure, each step of which is numbered in order of performance.
8. Discard disposable equipment in the proper containers.
9. Clean the standard equipment and put in its proper place.
10. Make the patient comfortable.
11. Wash your hands.
12. Report to your head nurse or team leader:
    - That you have completed the procedure.
    - The time and date the procedure was done.
    - The pertinent facts concerning the procedure.
    - The results of the procedure.
    - Area of the patient's body where the procedure was done, if appropriate.
    - The patient's reaction and tolerance of the procedure.
    - Your observations of anything unusual.

HOW TO USE THIS MANUAL
EFFECTIVELY

Contents

All of the chapters, sections of each chapter, and the procedures are listed in the Contents. Use it to find the page number of any procedure you might want to review.

Sections

Most chapters are divided into sections to give you a smaller amount of material to learn at one time. This is designed to make it easier for you to study, to understand the lesson, and to learn the many nursing tasks that are involved in your job.

Objectives: What You Will Learn

Each section begins with a list of objectives. These objectives should serve as realistic goals for you to reach. Objectives tell you what you should be able to do by the end of each section. Objectives are your destination, things you can expect to accomplish.

The objectives give you a specific goal, a particular action you need to be able to perform. These are actions or behaviors which can be observed by you and by others. For example, the best way for you and your instructor to see if you understand how to make an occupied bed is for you to actually perform the procedure, to make an occupied bed.

Read each section, keeping the list of objectives in mind. You can use the objectives as self-tests. When you finish reading a section, go back and reread the objectives. See if you are able to perform each objective in the list. Study any pages that deal with the objective you could not meet.

When you have completed each section you should be able to define, explain, apply or demonstrate the material covered in that section.

Key Ideas

Under the heading of key ideas you will find the reasons behind each procedure you will be doing. Knowing why you are doing something will help you to prepare for and carry out the procedures in the best possible way. Pay careful attention to all the illustrations, charts, and lists in every section. These are all designed to make it easier for you to remember the important information.

Often there are basic principles, ideas, and methods that must be remembered for the overall care of a patient. As an example, you will always treat the patient with courtesy, kindness, and sympathy. Such a principle or rule does not make up a full procedure. In some situations the order in which the tasks are done does not matter. For example, you will check the patient unit (the room) to make sure that everything needed is there. Tasks like this do not follow a definite numerical order. Therefore, they are not true procedures. They are called Rules To Follow.

Procedures

A task is an assigned duty, something you are expected to do. In this manual, each nursing task has been divided into a logical, orderly series (sequence) of actions or steps. The full set of steps is a procedure. In health care institutions, procedures are done according to a set method. Nursing procedures will be somewhat different in different health care institutions. The underlying principles or ideas are always the same, but the wording, sequence, or style for a task may be different. Be sure you know the methods, the policies, and the style of the institution where you are working. Usually, the way things are done will be very similar to the series of steps given in this manual for a procedure.

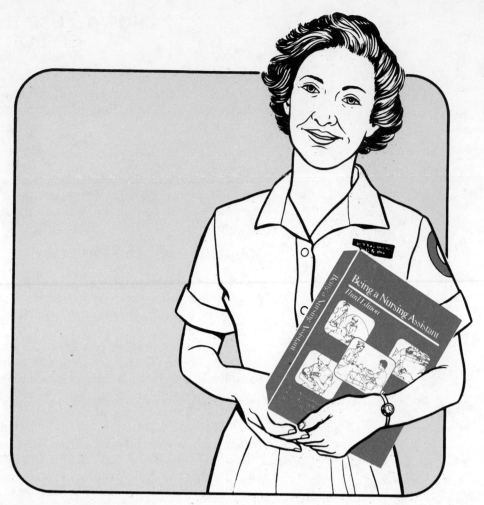

Words To Remember

New words are tools for communication. In your work as a nursing assistant, you will be introduced to medical terminology. You should increase your vocabulary as much as you can so you always understand what the head nurse or team leader tells you. Besides, it is a personal achievement. Learning new words can help to make you more confident.

When you are reporting to your supervisor, head nurse, or team leader, you must make yourself clearly understood. It is important that you accurately communicate information about the patient and his or her situation or condition. Chapter 20 and Words to Remember will help you understand the meaning of many words used in the health care institution. Use the list throughout this course and on the job.

What You Have Learned

Each chapter has a summary at the end. Reading this will remind you of what you have learned. You can quickly review the chapter's main ideas and how they affect your job as a nursing assistant.

Notes Column

Use the blank space on each page to make notes. Or underline the important information on each page. Writing things down will help you to remember them. Keep a pencil in hand as you study. Jot down key words and "thought clues." They will come back to you later when you need them. As your instructor goes over each procedure with you, he or she will explain things that may be done differently in your health care institution. Taking notes is a good way to record those differences.

1 INTRODUCTION TO BEING A NURSING ASSISTANT

SECTION 1: THE HEALTH CARE INSTITUTION

OBJECTIVES: WHAT YOU WILL LEARN

When you have completed this section, you will be able to:

- Explain the purpose and organization of health care institutions.
- Describe three ways of organizing the nursing health care team.
- Identify the nursing health care team.
- Explain the difference between the registered nurse and the licensed practical nurse, between the nursing assistant and the ward clerk.

FIVE BASIC FUNCTIONS AND PURPOSES OF HEALTH CARE INSTITUTIONS:

1. TO PROVIDE CARE FOR ILL AND/OR INJURED

2. TO PREVENT DISEASE

3. TO PROMOTE INDIVIDUAL AND COMMUNITY HEALTH

4. TO PROVIDE FACILITIES FOR THE EDUCATION OF HEALTH WORKERS

5. TO PROMOTE RESEARCH IN THE SCIENCES OF MEDICINE AND NURSING

KEY IDEAS: THE HEALTH CARE INSTITUTION

We will use the term HEALTH CARE INSTITUTION to mean hospital, nursing home for extended care, or clinic.

The Nursing Assistant: Part of a Team

As a nursing assistant, you are a member of a health care team. Everyone on the team must understand teamwork. Teamwork means that everyone knows what he is supposed to do and does it to the best of his ability with a spirit of cooperation.

You will be working under the supervision of a professional nurse. Also,

1

ORGANIZATION OF HEALTH CARE INSTITUTIONS

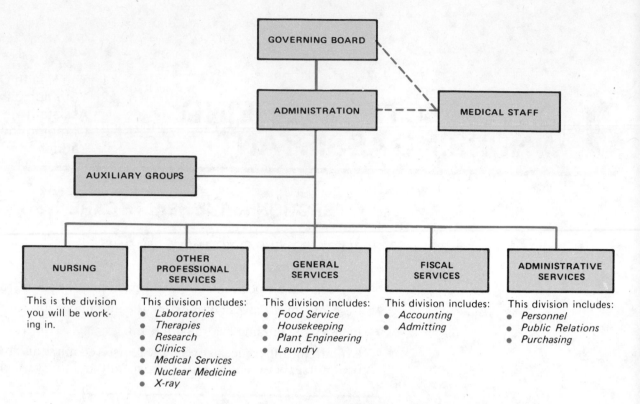

AUXILIARY GROUPS

NURSING	OTHER PROFESSIONAL SERVICES	GENERAL SERVICES	FISCAL SERVICES	ADMINISTRATIVE SERVICES
This is the division you will be working in.	This division includes: • *Laboratories* • *Therapies* • *Research* • *Clinics* • *Medical Services* • *Nuclear Medicine* • *X-ray*	This division includes: • *Food Service* • *Housekeeping* • *Plant Engineering* • *Laundry*	This division includes: • *Accounting* • *Admitting*	This division includes: • *Personnel* • *Public Relations* • *Purchasing*

ORGANIZATION OF THE HEALTH CARE TEAM

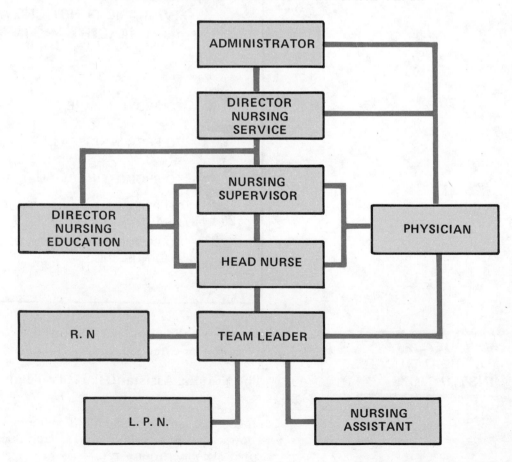

you will be working cooperatively with other members of the nursing service staff. Remember that the nurse recognizes the nursing assistant as a valuable worker, as a member of the team. Look to your head nurse or team leader as a friend who will help you to learn and understand your job.

THE NURSING HEALTH CARE TEAM IN YOUR INSTITUTION MAY BE ORGANIZED IN ONE OF SEVERAL WAYS:

- *Functional Nursing*: The head nurse assigns and directs all patient care responsibilities for the nursing staff. This system is sometimes called "direct assignment."

- *Team Nursing:* The head nurse is sometimes called the resource nurse. She divides her staff into teams. Each team has a leader. The head nurse assigns a group of patients to each team. The team leader then makes out patient care assignments for members of her team. Team members may be registered nurses (RN), licensed practical nurses (LPN), or nursing assistants (NA). The team leader is teacher, adviser, and helper to all of her team members. This system is *TASK ORIENTED*. This means that nursing care is arranged according to what must be done.

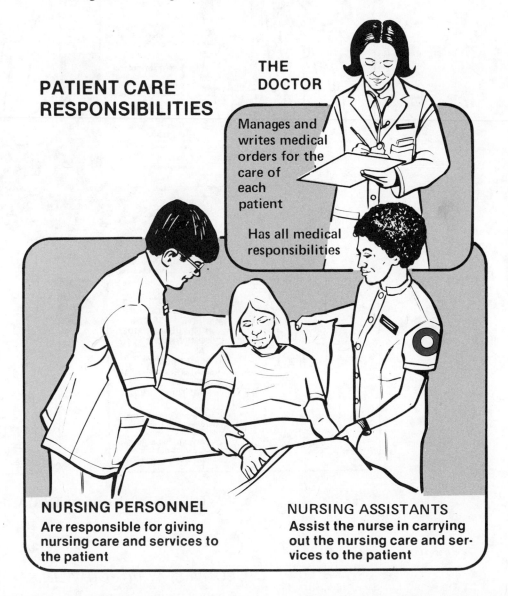

PATIENT CARE RESPONSIBILITIES

THE DOCTOR

Manages and writes medical orders for the care of each patient

Has all medical responsibilities

NURSING PERSONNEL
Are responsible for giving nursing care and services to the patient

NURSING ASSISTANTS
Assist the nurse in carrying out the nursing care and services to the patient

- *Primary Nursing:* Primary nursing is a method of patient care delivery in which the professional nurse is responsible and accountable for the entire nursing care of the patient. She is responsible for assessing the patient's needs and for planning, implementing, and evaluating the patient's nursing care. The purpose is to ensure that the professional nurse works directly with the patient. In addition, her responsibilities include family teaching, patient education, discharge planning, and recruiting community agencies to assist the patient after discharge. This system is *PATIENT ORIENTED*. This means that the nursing care is arranged according to the total needs of the individual patient sometimes called "Total Nursing Care".

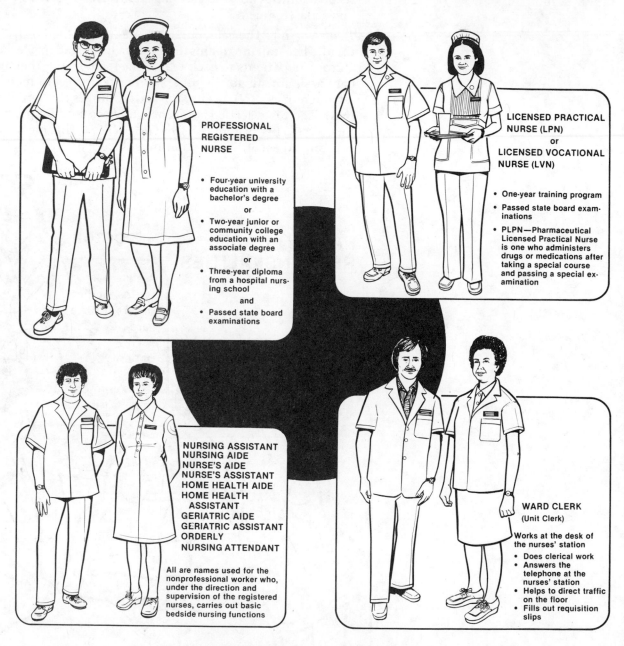

PROFESSIONAL REGISTERED NURSE

- Four-year university education with a bachelor's degree
  or
- Two-year junior or community college education with an associate degree
  or
- Three-year diploma from a hospital nursing school
  and
- Passed state board examinations

LICENSED PRACTICAL NURSE (LPN)
or
LICENSED VOCATIONAL NURSE (LVN)

- One-year training program
- Passed state board examinations
- PLPN—Pharmaceutical Licensed Practical Nurse is one who administers drugs or medications after taking a special course and passing a special examination

**NURSING ASSISTANT
NURSING AIDE
NURSE'S AIDE
NURSE'S ASSISTANT
HOME HEALTH AIDE
HOME HEALTH ASSISTANT
GERIATRIC AIDE
GERIATRIC ASSISTANT
ORDERLY
NURSING ATTENDANT**

All are names used for the nonprofessional worker who, under the direction and supervision of the registered nurses, carries out basic bedside nursing functions

WARD CLERK
(Unit Clerk)

Works at the desk of the nurses' station

- Does clerical work
- Answers the telephone at the nurses' station
- Helps to direct traffic on the floor
- Fills out requisition slips

THE NURSING HEALTH CARE TEAM

SECTION 2: YOUR JOB AS A NURSING ASSISTANT

OBJECTIVES: WHAT YOU WILL LEARN

When you have completed this section you will be able to:

- List the nursing tasks you will be doing on the job.
- Display qualities that are desirable in good nursing assistants.

The Nursing Assistant: An Important Person

Being a nursing assistant is not just another job. There are so many things to learn, so many things to do. Yours is a serious occupation. Making mistakes can cause extra pain and suffering for patients, even death. Doing a good job is something to be proud of. You will be helping sick people and making their stay in the health care institution easier.

During your training and while you are at work, always think about the patient as a person. Try to imagine what it is like to have his or her problems. As much as possible, try to develop a feeling for the patients, a sensitivity to their needs. Sympathy and understanding by those caring for a patient are part of the treatment. Sometimes these are as important as medicine in helping the patient to get well.

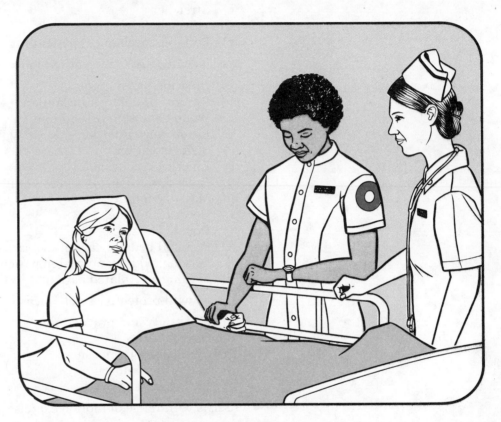

You will be working under the supervision of the head nurse or team leader. They are not necessarily the same person, although they might be. We will use the term head nurse or team leader to refer to the person who supervises you and keeps track of your performance. If you do not know how to do a procedure, ask your head nurse or team leader for help. If you are not sure of yourself, tell her. It is better to get help than to do something wrong.

What You Will Do in Your Job

The fundamental nursing tasks and procedures you, the nursing assistant, will be accountable for in your work will be found on the job description given to you by your health care institution or agency. Job descriptions vary from institution to institution and agency to agency. These job descriptions are written to meet the needs of each employer, as stated in their nursing philosophy, objectives, or policies.

Listed here are basic tasks and procedures that you will be able to perform and demonstrate when you have completed this manual. Remember, everything you do as a nursing assistant will be under the supervision of a registered nurse.

- Objective reporting of activities/observations.
- Performance of aseptic handwashing technique.
- Performance of bed-making techniques:
    a) Empty fan-folded bed/empty closed bed
    b) Occupied bed
    c) Operating room/stretcher bed
    d) Use of bed-cradle
    e) Use of bed-rails/side rails
- Assists with lifting, moving, turning, and transporting patients:
    a) Chair
    b) Out of/into bed
    c) Stretcher
    d) Wheelchair
    e) Portable mechanical patient lift
- Assists with care of the patient in isolation:
    a) Isolation precautions
    b) Reverse protective precautions
    c) Wound and skin precautions
    d) Respiratory isolation
    e) Strict isolation
    f) Enteric precautions
    g) Enter and leave an isolation unit
    h) Mask technique
    i) Gown technique
    j) Double bagging
    k) Personal bedside care of the patient in isolation
    l) Serving food to an isolated patient
    m) Feeding an isolated patient
- Assists with protective/safety measures:
    a) Fire safety and prevention
    b) Oxygen safety
    c) General safety measures
    d) Safety for children
    e) Electrical safety
- Assists with range of motion exercises.
- Determines the patient's height and weight.
- Assists with the care and environment of the patient's unit.
- Assists in the care of equipment and supplies.
- Assists with positioning the patient.
- Performs personal bedside care of the patient:
    a) Routine mouth care
    b) Oral hygiene
    c) Care of dentures
    d) Oral hygiene and mouth care for the unconscious patient
    e) Special mouth care
    f) Complete bed bath
    g) Partial bed bath
    h) Tub bath
    i) Shower
    j) Back rub
    k) Changing the patient's gown
    l) Hair care/combing/shampooing
    m) Shaving the patient's beard

- Assists with excretory functions:

  a) Assists with bedpan
  b) Assists with urinal
  c) Assists with bedside commode

- Assists with measuring intake and output:

  a) Fluid balance
  b) Measuring fluid intake
  c) Forcing fluids
  d) Restricting fluids
  e) Measuring fluid output
  f) Emptying and measuring contents of urine from indwelling urinary drainage container

- Assist with food:

  a) Preparing the patient for a meal
  b) Serving a meal
  c) Feeding the patient
  d) Serving between meal nourishments
  e) Passing drinking water

- Assists with specimen collection:

  a) Collecting routine urine specimen
  b) Collecting routine urine specimen from an infant
  c) Collecting a mid-stream clean-catch
  d) Collecting a 24-hour urine specimen
  e) Collecting a sputum specimen
  f) Collecting a stool specimen

- Assists with straining the urine.

- Assists with rectal treatments:

  a) Administers the cleansing enema
  b) Administers the ready-to-use cleansing enema
  c) Administers the oil retention enema
  d) Administers the Harris flush/return flow enema
  e) Assists with the rectal tube
  f) Assists with rectal suppositories

- Performs perineal care.

- Gives daily indwelling catheter care.

- Performs nonsterile (clean) vaginal irrigation/douche.

- Cares for the artificial eye.

- Assists with determination of vital signs:

  a) Measures oral temperature using both Fahrenheit and Centigrade scale
  b) Measures rectal temperature using both Fahrenheit and Centigrade scale
  c) Measures axillary temperature using both Fahrenheit and Centigrade scale
  d) Measures radial pulse
  e) Measures apical/radial pulse deficit
  f) Measures respiration
  g) Measures blood pressure using mercury or aneroid equipment

- Assists with admission, discharge, and transfer procedures.

- Assists with preparing the patient for physical examination.

- Changes the gown of a patient with an intravenous.

- Assists with observations of an intravenous.
- Assists with pre-operative preparation of the patient
  - a) Shaving the skin
  - b) Dentures
  - c) Clothing
  - d) Pre-op check list
- Assists with postoperative care and observation of the patient.
- Assists with deep breathing postoperative exercises.
- Assists with the application of elastic bandages, binders, and anti-embolism stockings.
- Assists with the application of a triangle sling bandage.
- Assists with non-sterile warm and cold applications both moist and dry:
  - a) Application and observation of warm compress
  - b) Application and observation of cold compress
  - c) Application and observation of warm soak
  - d) Application and observation of cold soak
  - e) Application and observation of warm water bottles
  - f) Application and observation of cold ice bag, cap, or collar
  - g) Application and observation of perineal heat lamp
  - h) Application and observation of aquamatic K-pad
  - i) Application and observation of sitz bath
  - j) Application and observation of alcohol sponge baths
- Assists with the care of the incontinent patient:
  - a) Assists in the prevention of decubitus ulcers
  - b) Assists with special back care and skin care
  - c) Assists with care of areas with potential skin breakdown
- Assists with the care of the diabetic patient:
  - a) Performs urine test for sugar: the Clinitest and Clinistix
  - b) Performs urine test for acetone: the Acetest and Ketostix
  - c) Assists with collection of a fresh urine specimen
- Assists with the care of the orthopedic patient:
  - a) Assists with turning the patient on a manually operated turning frame
  - b) Assists with the patient in the electric circular double frame bed
  - c) Assists with the care of the patient in traction
  - d) Assists with the care of the patient in a plaster cast
- Assists with the care of the ostomy patient.
- Assists with the care of a home-bound patient.
- Assists with the care of the geriatric patient in the home.
- Assists with the care of a seizure patient.
  - a) Employs seizure precautions
  - b) Creates a safe environment for the seizure patient
- Assists with the care of the bedridden patient in the home.
- Assists with the care of an infant in the home:
  - a) Preparing formula
  - b) Feeding the infant
  - c) Burping the infant
  - d) Caring for the umbilical cord of the infant
  - e) Bathing the infant
  - f) Assisting with safety for the infant
- Assists with the household management.

- Assists with the activities of daily living in the home.
- Assists with the care of the dying patient.
- Assists with postmortem care.

You have decided that you want to be the best nursing assistant you can be. You want to do the best possible job. What kind of person makes a good nursing assistant? Certain traits, attitudes, and habits are often seen regularly in people who have been successful in their work in the health care institution, especially on the nursing team. Some of these traits are built into one's personality—you have had them all along. Others can be learned through practice and become part of one's changed (improved) personality.

Go through this list and see where you stand. Review those qualities you already have. Then check out those you think you could learn and actually make a part of yourself. You are an excellent nursing assistant if:

- You are a person who can be trusted and depended on
- You relate easily to new people
- You make friends quickly
- You enjoy working with people
- You get along well with others
- You are sensitive to the feelings of others
- You are considerate and tactful
- You want to help people
- You try to be gracious and polite at all times
- You get satisfaction out of being of service to others
- You show sympathy and patience with others
- You try always to keep your temper under control
- You believe that you are doing important work
- You want to improve your performance
- You like to learn new things
- You never let your private life interfere with your work
- When the work is heavy and everyone is tense, you try a little harder
- Remember that you are helping those who are unable to help themselves. Your head, your heart, and your hands should be strong, willing, and capable.

Dependability

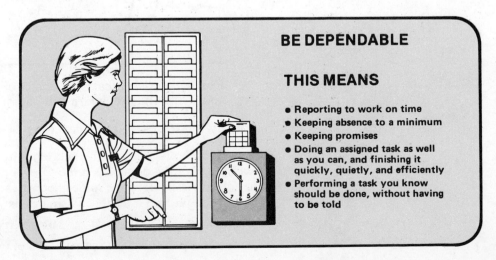

BE DEPENDABLE

THIS MEANS

- Reporting to work on time
- Keeping absence to a minimum
- Keeping promises
- Doing an assigned task as well as you can, and finishing it quickly, quietly, and efficiently
- Performing a task you know should be done, without having to be told

Your health care institution is organized to function efficiently when a certain number of people are on the job. If you are not there, a patient could be deprived of the care he needs. Also, your absence may cause your fellow workers to have an overload of work. It is essential that you arrive promptly every day unless you are ill. If you are sick, call the nursing office at the appropriate time.

Dependability means more than coming to work on time every day. It means that the head nurse or team leader who asks you to do something can rely on you to do it at the proper time and in the proper way.

Accuracy

Accuracy is part of being dependable. In a health care institution you are concerned with human lives. What might appear to you to be a tiny mistake or oversight could delay the recovery of a patient.

It is vitally important for you to follow your head nurse's or team leader's instructions exactly. Be accurate when you are recording a temperature. Be careful in making a bed. Stay alert when you answer the patient's call light. Try never to make mistakes; however, should a mistake occur, report this to your head nurse or team leader immediately. If you do not understand something, ask again. Always remember: "There is a reason for every step in the routine of the health care institution."

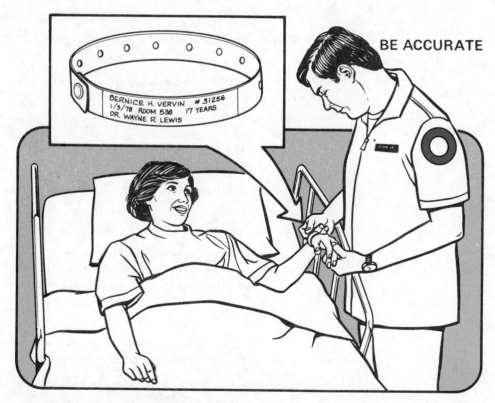

Check the identification bracelet or band before every procedure, to be sure the procedure will be done on the right patient.

Following Rules and Instructions

Everybody follows instructions and goes by rules. Otherwise, the job would never get done. Even the top people in the health care institution have to follow rules. Here are some good rules to remember in your work. These can help to make you a better nursing assistant.

- Be accurate to the best of your ability.
- Follow carefully the instructions of your head nurse or team leader.

- If you do not understand something, ask your head nurse or team leader.
- There are good reasons for every rule and every procedure in the health care institution. Be aware of them all.
- Report accidents or errors immediately to the head nurse or team leader.
- Keep confidences to yourself, except when it might be dangerous to a patient. For example, a patient tells you she is not taking her medicine. Report this to your head nurse or team leader.
- Do not waste supplies or equipment.
- Be ready to adjust quickly to new situations.
- Try to get things done on time. Use a systematic work schedule.

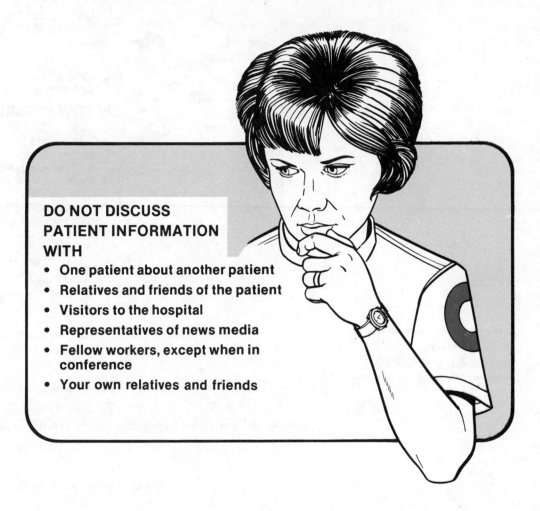

DO NOT DISCUSS PATIENT INFORMATION WITH
- **One patient about another patient**
- **Relatives and friends of the patient**
- **Visitors to the hospital**
- **Representatives of news media**
- **Fellow workers, except when in conference**
- **Your own relatives and friends**

KEY IDEAS: STAFF RELATIONSHIPS

You will find your fellow workers and other health care personnel more agreeable and helpful if you treat them properly. Some good practices are:

- Report to the head nurse or team leader whenever you leave the unit for any purpose and at the end of your shift. Report to her again when you return.
- Take all questions you may have about patients and their care to your head nurse or team leader.
- Tell your head nurse or team leader about personal problems that you feel might be interfering with your work.
- Do not talk about your personal problems with other staff members.
- Do not discuss your personal problems with patients.

- Follow all instructions given to you by your head nurse or team leader. If you are confused about any of your assignments, discuss them with the head nurse or team leader.
- Report all complaints from patients and visitors to the head nurse or team leader. Never ignore complaints, no matter how silly or unreasonable they may seem to you.
- Perform all of your duties in a spirit of cooperation and follow orders willingly.

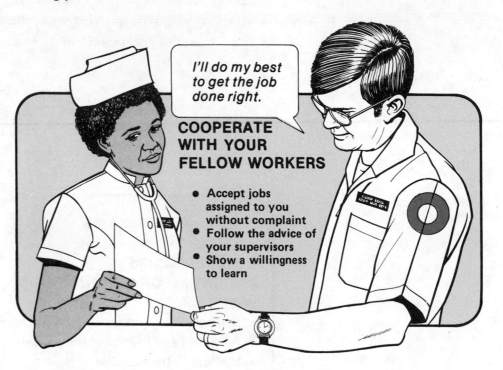

KEY IDEAS: ETHICAL BEHAVIOR

Ethical behavior means keeping your promises and doing what you ought to do. As a nursing assistant you should observe the following code for ethical behavior:

- Be conscientious in the performance of your duties. This means do the best you can.
- Be generous in helping your patients and your fellow workers.
- Carry out faithfully the instructions you are given by your head nurse or team leader.
- Respect the right of all patients to have beliefs and opinions that might be different from yours.
- Let the patient know that it is your pleasure, not just your job, to assist him.
- Try to demonstrate that you are sincere in your involvement in the care of a human being. Always show that the patient's well-being is of the utmost importance to you.

KEY IDEAS: LEGAL ASPECTS

Laws concerning patients and workers in health care institutions were written to protect both the patient and the worker. As a nursing assistant, you need to understand how the law affects you and the patients you care for. Patients are entitled to respect for their human rights. They must be kept safe and must be cared for properly.

Negligence. The words negligence and malpractice are often used interchangeably, as if they were the same thing. Officially, **negligence** is the commission of an act or failure to perform an act where the respective performance or nonperformance would deviate from that act which should have been done by a reasonably prudent person under the same or similar conditions. **Malpractice** is negligence when applied to the performance of a professional. Examples are:

- If the nursing assistant fails to fasten the safety strap over a patient on a stretcher and as a result the patient falls, the nursing assistant is guilty of negligence.
- When a nursing assistant performs procedures not included in her job description or for which she has not been trained, or performs any procedure incorrectly, she is guilty of negligence.
- When a nursing assistant serves a regular diet to a diabetic patient, she is guilty of negligence.
- Any nursing assistant who neglects to wash her hands after contact with a patient is guilty of negligence.

KEY IDEAS: PERSONAL HYGIENE AND APPEARANCE

All members of the nursing team are teachers by the example they set. They influence each other to become better in their jobs. The practice of good personal hygiene as used in a hospital environment becomes a teaching tool. Here are things to remember about personal cleanliness and your appearance.

- Dress properly and neatly. Follow the dress code of the health care institution where you work.
- Use good personal hygiene.
- Bathe daily.
- Use an unscented deodorant.
- Keep your mouth and teeth clean and in good condition.
- Keep your hair clean and neatly combed.
- Keep your nails short and clean.
- Wear conservative makeup.
- Try to be completely free of odor. Do not use perfume or scented sprays.
- Have a physical checkup every year.
- Eat a well-balanced diet every day.
- Get plenty of sleep. Be alert when you come to work.
- Keep your body fit; do daily exercises.
- Wear clean clothes every day.
- Wear comfortable low-heeled shoes with nonskid soles and heels.
- Polish your shoes every day. Be sure the laces are clean.
- Repair rips and hems, and replace missing buttons on your clothing.
- Never wear jewelry such as earrings, bracelets, or pendants.
- Wear a white sweater if you are cold.
- Always wear your name pin and institutional badge.
- Always wear a wristwatch with a second hand.
- Always carry a pen and a pad of paper.

KEY IDEAS: INCIDENTS

An **incident** is an event that does not fit the routine operation of the health care institution or the routine care of the patients. It may be an accident or something that might cause one. For example, a staff person stumbles into a patient in a wheelchair because someone spilled liquid and failed to wipe it

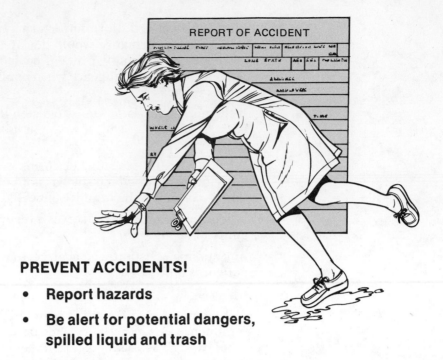

PREVENT ACCIDENTS!

- **Report hazards**
- **Be alert for potential dangers, spilled liquid and trash**

up. Such incidents can affect the patients, visitors, and members of the institution's staff.

Types of incidents are:

- Patient, visitor, or employee accidents.
- Thefts from patients, visitors, or employees.
- Thefts of hospital property.
- Accidents occurring on outlying hospital property, such as sidewalks, parking lots, or entrances.

Whenever an incident occurs, a report must be made. Report any incident you observe. Also report any bad conditions you think might lead to an incident. Reporting is very important to the safety program of the health care institution and for the protection of all health care workers. For the institution to be prepared for the possible liability suits or damage claims, all the facts related to such incidents must be known.

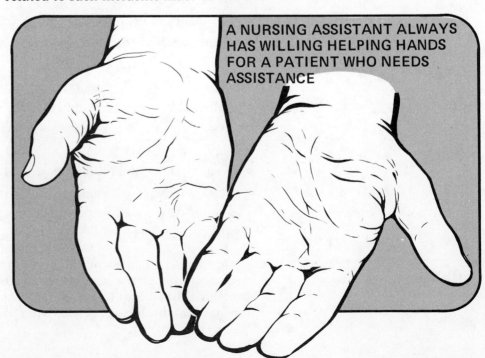

A NURSING ASSISTANT ALWAYS HAS WILLING HELPING HANDS FOR A PATIENT WHO NEEDS ASSISTANCE

SECTION 3: CLIMBING THE CAREER LADDER

OBJECTIVES: WHAT YOU WILL LEARN

When you have completed this section, you will be able to:

- Explain the function of the inservice, staff development, and nursing education department in your health care institution.
- Plan your career by using the career ladder.

**KEY IDEAS:
CONTINUING TO LEARN**

Continue your education! To keep up with new developments in the medical field, all health care workers are expected to take refresher courses and study new medical developments that affect their employment all their working lives. As you continue to learn, your job will become more rewarding personally and professionally. You and your employer, the health care institution, will be happy and grateful that you decided to be a nursing assistant.

You can continue to learn while you are on the job. You can expand your knowledge of nursing care procedures. You can find better ways to do your work. You can learn more about other aspects of health care. All this can make you a more effective nursing assistant. This means you will become more secure in your job.

DEPARTMENT OF INSERVICE STAFF DEVELOPMENT AND NURSING EDUCATION

The department of inservice staff development and nursing education is individualized to meet the needs of the health care institution it serves. In some institutions it is called inservice education, in others it is called staff development, and in still others it is called nursing education. In very large teaching health care institutions, the three types of education are separated; however, in the small rural institutions it is one department. As a result, no two departments of nursing education are exactly the same. Basically it includes inservice education, continuing education, staff development, and patient education. These departments are designed to act as resources for all employees in the department of nursing for continuing the life-long educational process to which nursing practitioners are dedicated. They orient new employees, develop internship programs for graduate nurses, demonstrate the use of new equipment and new techniques, update the nurses' skills following the procedures and policies of the health care institution, and they constantly seek new methods for improving health care delivery for the patients through the development of the nursing staff. In the states where continuing education units are needed for re-licensure, they provide the necessary learning experiences.

If you enjoy your work as a nursing assistant, you may be interested in advancement where you are employed. Maybe you would like to be a registered nurse or a licensed practical nurse. The career ladder shown here can give you a pattern to guide you in planning your advancement. The pattern can be changed to meet your needs and goals. Skills, time, hard work, and careful planning are needed to climb to the top of the ladder.

If you do not have a high school diploma, that should be your first goal. Adult education programs at local high schools offer basic education programs that lead to a high school equivalency diploma. Community colleges offer the prerequisite courses necessary to move up to a program for the licensed practical nurse or registered nurse level. They have counselors to advise you along the way. The director of nursing education in your health care institution is the person to ask about planning your career ladder.

CAREER LADDER

Attend graduate school for a doctorate (PhD) in nursing
↑
Attend graduate school for a master of science (MS) in nursing
↑
Work for one year as a registered professional nurse
↑
Attend a university to get a bachelor of science (BS) in nursing
↑
Work for one year as a registered nurse
↑
Become a registered nurse (RN) in an associate degree program or diploma school
↑
Work for one year as a licensed practical nurse
↑
Become a licensed practical nurse (LPN)
↑
Work for one year as a nursing assistant
↑
Become a nursing assistant

If you do not have a high school diploma, that should be your first goal. Adult education programs at local high schools offer basic education programs that lead to a high school equivalency diploma. Community colleges offer the prerequisite courses necessary to move up to a program for the licensed practical nurse or registered nurse level. They have counselors to advise you along the way. The director of nursing education in your health care institution is the person to ask about planning your career ladder.

WHAT YOU HAVE LEARNED

You are now a part of the nursing health care team. Be sympathetic and understanding toward the patients. Remember that the health care facility exists only for the care and the treatment of the patient. The patient's welfare comes first. Keep this in mind as you do your work with dependability and accuracy.

Remember who you are. You are in a serious learning process. As you develop skills, as you grow in experience, you will have more and more self-confidence. As you become more sure of yourself, the work will get easier.

If you find your work as a nursing assistant enjoyable and rewarding, the career ladder can guide you to develop a pattern (plan) for advancement and further education.

You have started to climb the career ladder. You have taken the first step. You are ready to be a productive and effective nursing assistant.

2 COMMUNICATION AND THE PATIENT

SECTION 1: THE PATIENTS YOU WILL CARE FOR

OBJECTIVES: WHAT YOU WILL LEARN

When you have completed this section, you will be able to:

- Describe the five major kinds of patients.
- Describe the common characteristics and needs of each group of patients.
- Describe the patient care departments in the health care institution.

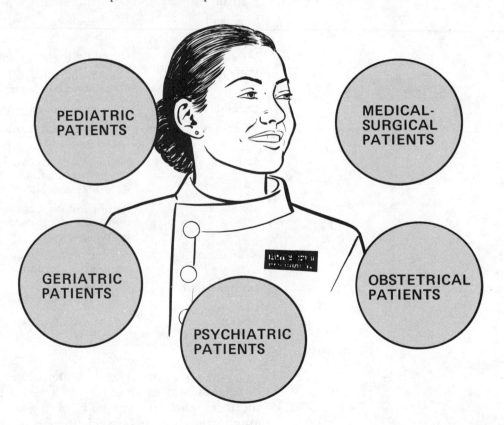

**KEY IDEAS:
THE PATIENTS YOU
WILL CARE FOR**

Patients who have similar illnesses or medical conditions often have similar needs and require similar treatments. Therefore it is convenient to place each group on a separate floor or area of the health care institution. In most hospitals there are five major groups of patients:

- Medical/Surgical
- Obstetrical
- Pediatric

- Geriatric
- Psychiatric

Medical/Surgical Patients

Medical-surgical patients are those who have an acute or chronic illness that is treated with medication or surgery.

Acute Illness: Comes on suddenly and runs its course within a few days. Examples are appendicitis and pneumonia.

Chronic Illness: Continues over years or a lifetime. Examples are arthritis and diabetes.

Classification of Disease. Diseases, conditions, infections, and illnesses all can be chronic or acute. These categories often overlap. They are based on the cause of the disease, the body system that has been affected, or the way the disease has been acquired.

Types of Disease Classified by Cause

Type (cause)	Meaning	Disease (examples)
Aging	Degeneration of all the body systems	Hardening of the arteries Arteriosclerosis
Birth injury	Occurring at birth	Cerebral palsy
Chemical	Foreign substance interfering with normal processes	Alcoholic cirrhosis of the liver
Congenital	Occurring during pregnancy	Cleft palate
Deficiency	Lacking the right foods or nutrients and/or hormones	Scurvy (lack of vitamin C)
Hereditary	Passed on through genes	Sickle-cell anemia
Infectious	Communicable—caused by microorganisms	Measles, chickenpox, mumps
Mechanical blocks	Formation of an obstruction of body wastes, fluids, or natural chemicals	Gallstones, kidney stones, blood clots
Metabolic	Failing to produce or break down substances needed for normal processes	Diabetes (lack of insulin)
Neoplastic	Abnormal growth of tissue— tumors (benign or malignant)	Fibroids (benign) Cancer (malignant)
Occupational	Peculiar to a job	Lead poisoning (painter) Black lung disease (miner)
Trauma	Injury, usually physical	Fracture, broken bone

Surgical patients need an operation because of an illness or injury. It may be necessary to repair or remove a part of the body. Some surgery may change the form of a person's body or the way it functions. For example, when amputation is necessary, a body part is removed (for example, an arm or leg). Of course this changes the person's body form. Another example of surgery is a colostomy, which changes the way the body functions. This operation creates a new outlet for the large intestine. It is made in the wall of the abdomen. The person's feces are discharged through this outlet instead of through the rectum and anus.

A surgical patient usually has to get used to (or adapt to) changes in the form of his or her body or in the way the body functions.

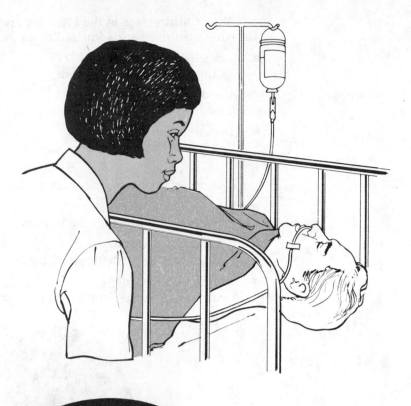

SURGICAL PATIENTS... CAN BE DIVIDED INTO 3 GROUPS:

1 PREOPERATIVE . . . BEFORE THE OPERATION

2 THOSE IN THE PROCESS OF HAVING AN OPERATION

3 POSTOPERATIVE . . . AFTER THE OPERATION

Pediatric Patients

Pediatric patients are children. In most hospitals, anyone under age 16 is called a pediatric patient. These patients may be grouped in several ways. For example, pediatric patients are sometimes grouped according to age. That is because children of different ages need different kinds and amounts of care. Children may also be grouped according to the medical condition they have.

Importance of the Family. A child is still a member of a family, even when he or she is in the hospital. The child may have only one parent, but there is always someone (or several persons) to care for the child in his home. These persons represent his family. The small child's mother is usually the family member closest to him. Often the mother, or both parents, will want to stay with the sick child in the hospital. Many hospitals and pediatric patient care units have a policy of allowing parents to stay with their child and even encourage them to do so.

This may be the first time the child has been away from home. He may be frightened or he may view hospitalization as punishment. These patients need to be held, touched, and talked to in order to be comforted and reassured.

Why Children are in the Health Care Institution. Some of the conditions for which children are admitted to the health care institution are:

- Congenital defects
  Examples: Harelip, club foot

- Accidents
  Examples: Falls, poisoning

- Tumors
  Examples: Cysts, cancerous growths

- Long-term or chronic conditions
  Examples: Diabetes, rheumatic heart disease

- Infectious diseases
  Examples: Pneumonia, meningitis

- Emotional disturbances
  Examples: Severe depression, acute anxiety

- Nutritional disorders
  Examples: Rickets, iron-deficiency anemia

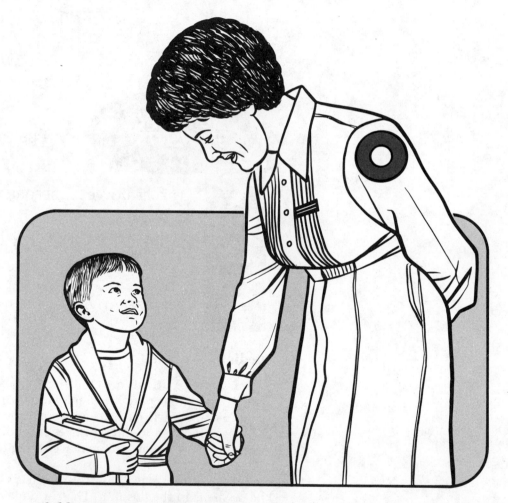

Children May be Grouped by Age

- *Premature babies* are babies who are born before the completion of the 37 week of gestation (pregnancy) or three weeks less than full term, as the normal period is 40 weeks, and/or are under 2500 gm. or 5.5 pounds in weight.

- *Newborn babies* (neonates) are full-term babies from birth until the age of one month.

- *Infants* are babies from one month to one year old.

- *Toddlers* are children from one to three years old.
- *Preschoolers* are children from three to five years of age.
- *School-age children* are children from six to twelve years of age.
- *Teenagers* are children from twelve to eighteen years of age.

Geriatric Patients

The geriatric patient should be treated with the same respect, dignity, consideration, and tender loving care as any patient of any age. Aging is a gradual process. It takes place all during life. One person at 70 may be "old" and ready to retire. Another person of the same age is neither "old" nor ready to retire.

Each person develops, matures, and deteriorates at his own rate, not by the calendar. It is not unusual to see an aged person who has an alert, active mind but who has some condition that prevents his body from functioning as it once did. An example is the person who likes to read, but now is developing cataracts that restrict his vision. Another person of the same age might be active, energetic, and able to work productively for several more years, without any problems with his eyes.

Possible Body Changes in Some Geriatric Patients. Please Note: These Changes May or May Not Occur in a Particular Patient.

- Hair may change color.
- Skin may become dry and wrinkled.
- Vision may decrease and they may wear glasses.
- Hearing may decrease and they may use a hearing aid.
- Joints may be stiff at times.
- Bones may be more brittle and the person may be unsteady on his feet, so fractures are common.
- There may be an increased chance for chronic disease.
- Appetite may decrease.
- There may be changes in the frequency of urination.

Psychiatric Patients

Psychiatric patients are those who have a mental illness, which means there is a disturbance in the person's feelings and emotions. Mental illness may cause changes in the way a person talks and acts. Sometimes mentally ill people change so much that they can no longer care for themselves properly. Sometimes they are dangerous to themselves and others and need to be restrained. Mental illness is treatable.

Until recent years, most psychiatric patients were kept in separate health care institutions. However, today, more and more general hospitals have special patient care units for psychiatric patients. In these units most psychiatric patients are in bed only when they sleep. They are up, around, and dressed all day. They are not handicapped by physical illness or the effects of surgery.

Examples of psychiatric patients are:

- Persons who are extremely depressed, agitated, or fearful.
- Persons who are confused about people, events, and their surroundings.
- Persons who think that everyone is against them.

Obstetrical Patients

Obstetrical patients are women having babies. These women are different from all other kinds of patients. This is because pregnancy without complications is a normal, natural event. Sometimes obstetrical patients do have complications. Complications happen either because of the pregnancy itself or because of a disease that is not related to the pregnancy. For example, complications can affect a pregnant woman who has diabetes.

Specialty Areas in the Health Care Institution

Labor and Delivery Rooms. Most hospitals have labor and delivery rooms. These are areas where women who are in labor or who are delivering babies are cared for. The labor and delivery patient care unit is a part of the obstetrical department. There is also an obstetrical recovery room where women who have just delivered a baby will stay for a short time. New mothers need a special place to rest until they recover from any anesthesia they might have received during the delivery.

Newborn Nursery. A newborn nursery is a patient care unit where full-term babies are cared for. Full-term means that the mother carried the baby for the full normal nine months of pregnancy. Newborn nurseries are part of the obstetrical department.

Premature Nursery. Babies are sometimes born early, that is, before the full nine months are over. They are called premature babies. A premature nursery is a patient care unit for premature babies. This nursery is also a part of the obstetrical department. Premature babies are almost always smaller than full-term babies. They are usually kept in incubators for the first few days or weeks of their lives. The incubator is a special crib that makes it possible for a premature baby to get the extra warmth, humidity and oxygen it needs.

Intensive Care-Critical Care Unit. An intensive/critical care unit is for patients who are critically ill. These patients are usually in bed, and require complete care. Nurses are always present. These patients need much closer observation and more nursing care than other patients.

Coronary Care Unit. A coronary care unit is for patients who have had a severe heart attack or heart surgery. In some hospitals the coronary care unit is part of the intensive care unit.

Postoperative Recovery Room. A postoperative recovery room is where patients who have had surgery are cared for until they recover from anesthesia. Life-saving equipment is kept ready at all times in the surgical recovery room.

Emergency Department. An emergency patient care unit is a place for people who need emergency treatment. A crisis intervention center is usually part of the emergency department. Emergency patients are those who have suddenly become ill. Others have had an accident. Others think they need medical attention and cannot reach their own doctor.

Patients found in emergency departments include:

- A child who has swallowed the contents of a bottle of aspirin.
- A person who has been injured in a car accident.
- A person having an epileptic convulsion.
- A person who has been badly cut.
- A child with a high fever.
- A rape victim.
- An assault victim.
- A person having a heart attack.

SECTION 2: COMMUNICATION

OBJECTIVES: WHAT YOU WILL LEARN

When you have completed this section, you will be able to:

- Maintain a courteous and professional manner toward patients, visitors, and co-workers.
- Keep your emotions under control while on the job.
- Deal with patients and visitors in a sympathetic and tactful manner.
- Show interest and concern about the patient's welfare.
- Answer the patient's signal promptly.
- Use communication skills effectively.

KEY IDEAS: COMMUNICATION

Relating to people means making a connection between yourself and another human being. The relations between yourself and patients, visitors, parents, and fellow workers depend on your approach to them. If you have a kind, courteous, tactful, sympathetic, and open manner, you will find it easier to form positive connections. Relationships depend upon receiving as well as giving, so listening attentively is as important as what you say. Communication skills will be necessary to your success as a nursing assistant.

Being successful as a nursing assistant depends partly on understanding the various responsibilities of the job.

Patients must have help to recover. You are the person who provides most of the personal bedside assistance. Every time you bathe or turn a patient in his bed, you are helping him toward his recovery and discharge.

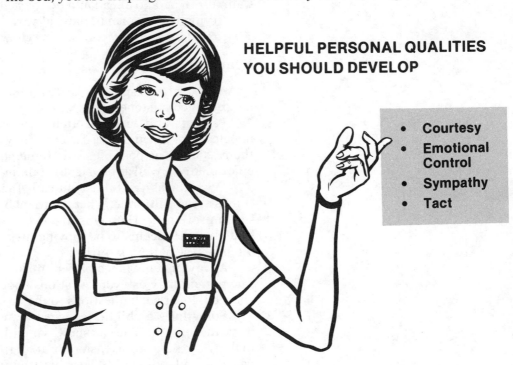

HELPFUL PERSONAL QUALITIES YOU SHOULD DEVELOP

- Courtesy
- Emotional Control
- Sympathy
- Tact

Courtesy

Behaving courteously means putting the needs of the other person before your own. It means cooperating, sharing, and giving. Being polite and considerate of others shows them that you care about them. Think about how you would feel if you were in their place and you will understand how far a cheerful word and a smile can go.

Emotional Control

Sometimes a patient, another staff member, or a visitor can upset you so much you get angry. You may feel like making a rude or nasty remark. Don't do it. Stop and think! The patient and his visitors may be worried, nervous or tense. Fellow workers may be under extra stress because of a problem at home or on the job. Try to be understanding and the anger will fade.

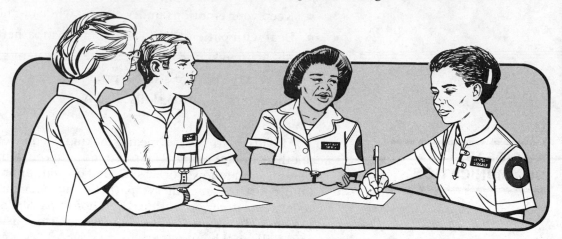

Learn to take criticism and accept suggestions without feeling you're being attacked. Try to avoid becoming defensive. Your supervisor may criticize you or tell you to do something. You may feel like saying "That is not my job" or "Why do you pick on me?" Stop, think, and examine your attitude. Calm down and go ahead and do the right thing.

Crying is the normal, natural way for children to express their feelings. Try to understand why a child is crying. Do not let it irritate you.

Sympathy and Tact

A sick patient's problems are all-important to him. Try to be understanding. Be a good listener, even when you would rather leave.

Patients and visitors often relieve their feelings of helplessness and hopelessness through words. They may try to take it out on you. Bear with them as much as possible. Also, remember that the patient may be suffering emotionally as well as physically; talking may relieve his emotional suffering.

Try to be as tactful as you can. Tact means doing and saying the right things at the right time. When a patient begins to recover, tell him that you can see improvement. He seems to move more easily. He appears to be standing straighter. He seems to be moving his arm or leg better. Remarks like these often lift the patient's spirits.

Always listen when a patient makes a complaint or brings up a problem. The patient may ask you questions about his doctor or when he will be discharged. Refer such questions to the head nurse or team leader.

Sometimes a child cries when his visiting parents are getting ready to leave the hospital. You can show sympathy to both the child and his parents by making the separation easier for all of them. Pick up the child (if permitted), pat him, and soothe him. Turn his attention to something other than the pain of being separated from his parents.

Never tell a child that you are going to take his temperature or blood pressure. He may think you are going to take something away from him. Say you are going to measure his temperature or blood pressure instead.

Relationships with Patients

Many things make a difference in a patient's behavior and attitude during an illness. The patient may be frightened, angry, or sad. Some factors or influ-

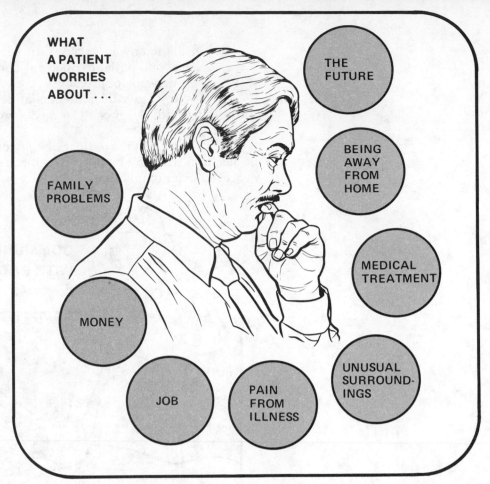

WHAT A PATIENT WORRIES ABOUT . . .

- THE FUTURE
- BEING AWAY FROM HOME
- MEDICAL TREATMENT
- UNUSUAL SURROUND-INGS
- PAIN FROM ILLNESS
- JOB
- MONEY
- FAMILY PROBLEMS

ences are the diagnosis, seriousness of the illness, age, previous illnesses and past experience in hospitals, and mental condition. Other things that can make a difference are the patient's personality and disposition and perhaps his financial condition.

Each patient is different in his reaction to pain, treatment, annoyances, and even kindness. Always treat each patient as an individual, a person who needs your help. Practice the kind of special consideration that all patients need on an individual basis.

RELATIONSHIPS WITH PATIENTS

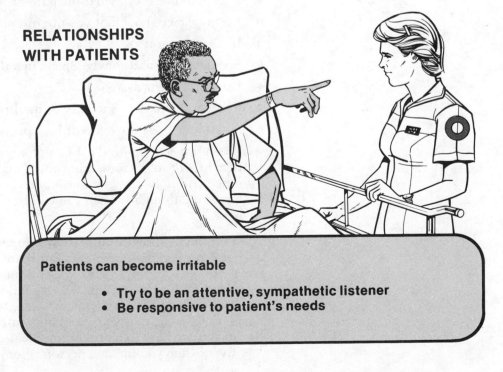

Patients can become irritable

- **Try to be an attentive, sympathetic listener**
- **Be responsive to patient's needs**

Never talk to anyone except your supervisor about a patient's condition. Never discuss one patient's medical condition with another patient. That would be an invasion of privacy.

Always try to give the patient confidence in the hospital, the doctors, and the nursing staff. Never criticize any of your fellow staff members in front of a patient.

Remember that the patient's behavior is the result of things that worry or bother him. He may be hostile or mean and nasty. You may simply be the nearest person to talk to.

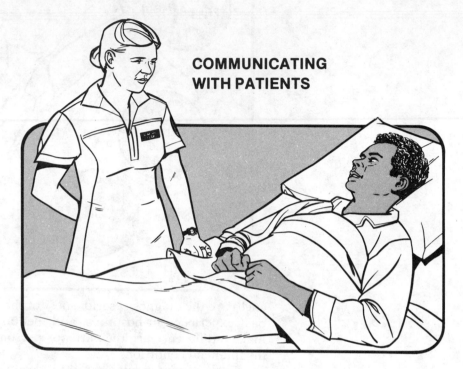

COMMUNICATING WITH PATIENTS

Communicating with Patients

- Show an interest in what the patient is saying.
- Let your face show that you are interested.
- Use good manners.
- Speak clearly and slowly. Speak in a pleasant tone.
- Use normal words.
- Respect the patient's moods. Sometimes silence can help.
- Make your body movements look pleasing and energetic.
- When someone in need asks you for assistance—whether to bathe him or turn him or to get something out of his reach—you should give your assistance willingly and graciously, no matter whose patient it is. It helps to have kind thoughts. Then you will be able to handle a situation with kindness.

Communicating through Body Language. Spoken and written words are used for most communications. But there are other ways—sometimes better ways—to get a message across. Hand movements (gestures), expressions on your face, and body movements may tell the story better than words.

As a nursing assistant, you are close to the patient during his stay in the hospital. Often he tells you about his wants, his pains, and his worries. As you listen, you are both in close communication.

Every time you touch a person's body, whether you speak any words or not, you are communicating something to him. How you assist him in any action that involves touching his body tells him something. If you are careful, firm, and gentle, it tells him something far different than if you are rough and jerk him around.

Pay attention to your posture. The way you move when you enter a patient's room or how you stand by his bed are ways of communicating through body language. Try to make these movements communicate energy, a sense of interest, and a willingness to help. A frown or an impatient body movement, a shrug, may give the patient the message, "Do not bother me." Also, a certain way of standing or walking may send the message, "I am lazy."

Look at the patient when you speak to him. This tells him that he has your attention. If you are looking away as you talk with him, he gets the impression that your attention is elsewhere. Speak clearly and distinctly. This is especially necessary when you are talking with older people. Some of them, as part of the aging process, may have a hearing loss. Talk with the patient, not just to or at him. Ask him what he likes and dislikes. Ask what he thinks or what he wants. Listen to his responses in an interested manner.

Communicating through Words. Slang or coarse or vulgar words are not appropriate or necessary. Also, do not use medical terms or abbreviations when talking to patients and their visitors. If you do use medical language, you might give the patient the wrong idea about what is happening to him.

Keep your voice pleasant, not too loud or too high pitched. Speak clearly and slowly enough to be easily understood. Never whisper or mumble, even when you think the patient is asleep or cannot hear you. This is annoying to the patient. Besides, he may hear more than you think.

Remember that although some patients seem to be unconscious, they may be fully aware of what is happening around them. Therefore, always speak and behave as if the patient can hear every word.

Be sensitive to those times when the patient does not want to talk. Respect his moods. At times saying nothing may have more meaning than any words or facial expressions on your part. Sometimes a pat on the shoulder or hand means more to a patient than anything you might say. Simply being near the stretcher or bed at the moment of trouble may be the most comforting message of all.

Relationships with Children and Their Parents

Several important things need to be considered and remembered with the pediatric patient:

- Parents need to be with their children, and children need their parents.
- Parents are normally concerned and often are worried, frightened people.
- Most children first learn about the world from their parents.
- The younger the child, the more he needs his parents.

Things You Can do to Help:

- Do the best possible job of caring for the child. This is usually reassuring to the parents.
- Show interest and concern about the parents' welfare. Ask, "Is there something we can do?"
- Do not make judgments about the parents' attitudes or behavior, even if they seem strange to you.
- Let the parents help to take part in the child's care, when possible and if permitted.
- Sometimes parents seem to be worried about something concerning their child in the hospital and are afraid to talk about it. If you suspect this, tell your team leader or head nurse.

Relationships with Visitors

Visiting hours are often the highlight of the day for patients. Knowing his family and friends are interested and concerned about him can do a lot to relax his tensions, ease his feelings of loneliness or isolation, relieve his fears, and cheer his spirit.

Visitors may be worried and upset over the illness of a member of the family. They need your kindness and patience. Pleasant comments about flowers or gifts brought by visitors for the patient may be helpful.

If it appears that visitors are upsetting the patient or making him tired, notify the head nurse or team leader. She can caution visitors or ask them to leave.

If the patient is seriously ill or is an obstetrical patient, visiting hours may be different. Your instructor will tell you about the visiting hours and any rules for visitors in your health care institution. These rules, of course, must be followed. Three main rules usually apply to visitors in all health care institutions:

- Visitors are not allowed to take institutional property away with them.

- Visitors are not allowed to give nursing or medical care to a patient.

- Visitors cannot bring food or drink to the patient unless permission has been given by the head nurse or team leader.

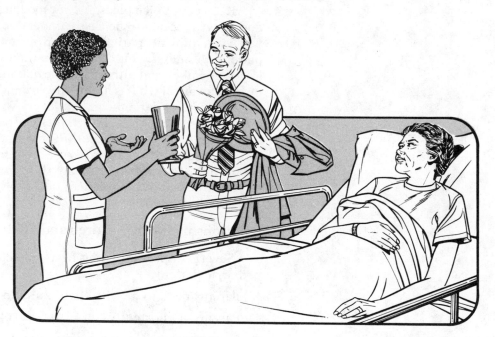

Certain Ways to Act are Helpful in Your Contacts with Visitors

- Listen to the family member. Whether it is a suggestion, a complaint, or "passing the time of day," listen to the person. Some suggestions by visitors can be very helpful. Some complaints may be valid, others not. When a complaint is first presented, you probably need to get more information. You might ask, "Where did this happen?" or "What did you do?" Say to the person, "I will tell the head nurse about this," and then report it to the head nurse or team leader.

- Do not get involved in the family's private affairs and feelings. Never take sides in family quarrels. Never give information or opinions to someone about other family members.

- Be prepared to give information to visitors. Tell them under what circumstances family members are allowed to eat in the employee cafeteria.

Mention where the coffee shop is and what hours it is open. Tell them where a public telephone is. Direct them to other places in the institution, for example, the business office or the gift shop.

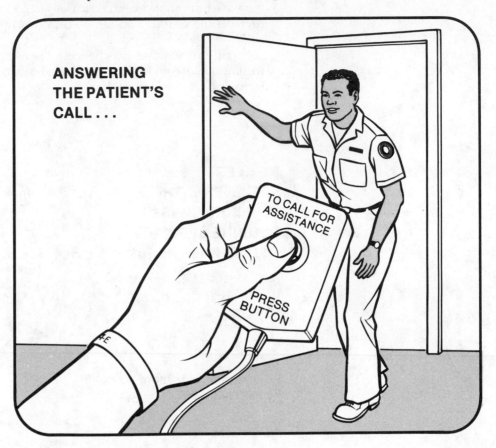

ANSWERING THE PATIENT'S CALL . . .

TO CALL FOR ASSISTANCE

PRESS BUTTON

Answering the Patient Call Signal

Every patient has a way of sending a signal to the nursing staff when he wants something. One thing you will do often in a health care institution is answer the patient's call for service or help without delay.

All patients have a signal cord. When the patient presses a button on the end of the cord, a light flashes in the head nurse's station and over the patient's door. This device may be called a signal cord or call bell. You should always keep alert for such signals. Answer the signal as soon as it flashes. Every minute seems forever to the patient who is waiting. When the patient signals:

- Go to the patient at once, quietly and in a friendly way.
- Turn off the call signal, and address the patient by name.
- Say, "Mr. Jones, what can I do for you?"
- Do whatever the patient asks, but be sure it is correct and safe for this patient. If you are in doubt, ask the head nurse or team leader. Tell her what the patient wants and then follow her directions.
- When necessary, use the emergency signal to get qualified personnel to assist you.
- Replace the signal cord where the patient can reach it easily.
- Caution: A young child or a helpless adult may not be able to use the signal cord. Listen for calls for help from these patients and go quickly to see what they need. Check these patients often to see if they need something.

When the Patient is Blind or Deaf. For patients who have serious hearing and vision losses, the signal cord is used differently. BLIND OR VISUALLY HANDICAPPED PATIENTS MUST BE SHOWN HOW TO USE THE SIGNAL.

Have them feel around for the cord and practice using it while you are there.

If the signal is the kind that you push to turn on, you can call it a "push" button. If it works like a light switch, you can compare it to that. When working with patients who have serious visual losses, you should not expect them to turn off the signal. You can do that routinely when you respond to the signal call.

Patients with serious hearing losses can easily learn how to pull or push the signal cord on if you show them how to do it. Show them, do not tell them. Remember, they cannot hear you.

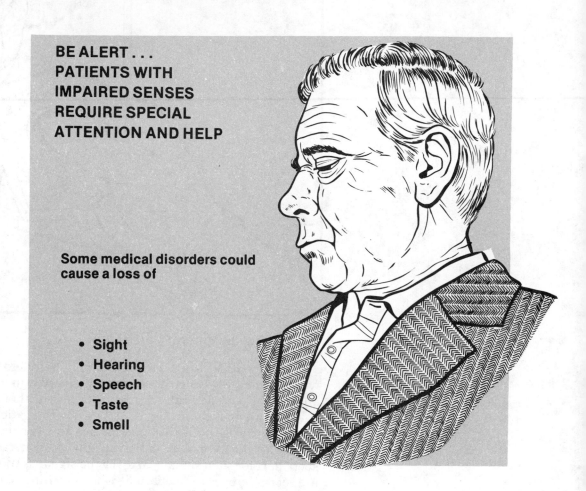

BE ALERT . . .
PATIENTS WITH
IMPAIRED SENSES
REQUIRE SPECIAL
ATTENTION AND HELP

Some medical disorders could cause a loss of

- **Sight**
- **Hearing**
- **Speech**
- **Taste**
- **Smell**

Using the Telephone

When you use the telephone or an intercommunication system (intercom), speak clearly and slowly. When you answer the telephone, for example, say, "Third floor, west. Mrs. Brown, nursing assistant, speaking." When you take a message for someone else, write it down immediately. Then, if possible, repeat it to the person calling to make sure it is correct. Ask the caller how to spell his name so you are sure you have it right. Record the following:

- The person being called
- The time the call was received
- The caller's name
- The message
- Your name and title

SECTION 3: OBSERVING THE PATIENT

OBJECTIVES: WHAT YOU WILL LEARN

When you have completed this section, you will be able to:

- Use your senses of sight, touch, hearing, and smell to observe the patients you care for.
- Notice changes in patients' appearance or behavior.
- Describe the difference between objective and subjective reporting.
- Report your observations promptly, accurately, and objectively.

KEY IDEAS: OBSERVING THE PATIENT

Get into the habit of observing the patient during all your contacts with him. These contacts include the bed bath, bed making, meal times, visiting hours, and any other time you are with him. Observation of the patient is a continuous process. Observing begins the first time you see a patient and ends when he is discharged from the hospital.

Observation means more than just careful watching. It includes listening to the patient, talking to him, and asking questions. It means being aware of a situation and interpreting it. Be extra alert to anything unusual whenever you are with a patient. Notice any changes in the patient's condition or appearance that may be important. Watch also for changes in the patient's attitude, his moods, his emotional condition. Pay attention to any complaints. For example, report to the head nurse or team leader if:

- A patient who had an abdominal operation two or three days ago says, "The calf of my leg is sore."
- A patient who is being given a blood transfusion says, "I feel itchy."

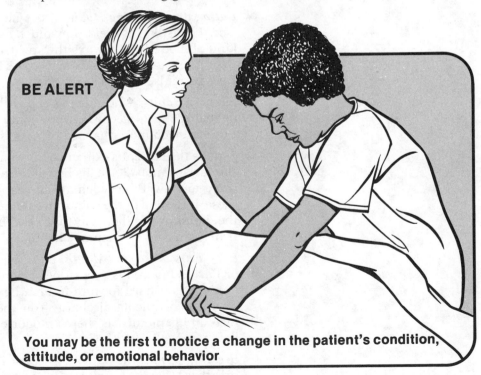

BE ALERT

You may be the first to notice a change in the patient's condition, attitude, or emotional behavior

Methods of Observation

USE ALL OF YOUR SENSES WHEN MAKING OBSERVATIONS:

- You can see some signs of change in a patient's condition. By using your eyes, you can observe a skin rash (breaking out), reddened areas, or swelling (edema).

- You can feel some signs with your finger—a change in the patient's pulse rate, puffiness in the skin, dampness (lots of perspiration).

- You can hear some signs, such as a cough or wheezing sounds, when the patient breathes.

- You can smell some signs, such as an odor on the patient's breath.

- Listen to the patient talking, for other changes in his condition. Some can be felt and described only by the patient himself. Examples are pain, nausea, dizziness, a ringing in the ears, or headache.

Making useful observations is one of the most important things you will do in your work. Learning how to make useful observations will give you satisfaction, a feeling of achievement. The process never ends. You learn by doing. Doctors and nurses never stop learning more about observing a patient. This is because observations are so important in the total medical care of the patient.

Things to Observe in a Patient

- *General Appearance.* Has this changed? If so, in what way? Is there a noticeable odor (smell)?

- *Mental Condition or Mood.* Does the patient talk a lot? Very little? Does he talk about the future or the past? Does he talk about where he hurts? Is the patient anxious and worried? Is he calm? Or is he very excited? Is he talking sensibly? Or not making sense? Is he speaking rapidly? Slowly? Is he cooperative? Uncooperative?

- *Position.* Does the patient lie still? Or does he toss around? Does he like to lie in one position better than others? Does he prefer being on his back? Or on his side? Is he able to move easily?

- *Eating and Drinking Habits.* Does he complain that he has no appetite? Does he dislike his diet? How much does he eat? Does he eat some of each kind of food? Is he always thirsty? Or does he very seldom drink water? Does he eat all of the food on his tray? Does he eat half the food on his tray? Does he refuse to eat?

- *Sleeping Habits.* Is he able to sleep? Is he restless? Does he complain about not being able to sleep? Do these complaints agree with your observations? Does he sleep more than is normal? Is he constantly asleep?

- *Skin.* Is the patient's skin unusually pale (pallor)? Is it flushed (red)? Is the skin dry or moist? Are his lips and fingernails turning blue (cyanotic)? Is there any swelling (edema) noticeable? Are there reddened areas? Are these at the end of the spine, or on the heels, or at other pressure points? Is the skin shiny? Is there any puffiness? Is there puffiness in the legs and feet? Is his skin cold or clammy? Is it hot?

- *Eyes, Ears, Nose, and Mouth.* Does the patient complain that he sees spots or flashes before his eyes? Does bright light bother him? Are his eyes inflamed? Is it hard for him to breathe through his nose? Does he seem to have a lot of mucous discharge from the nose? Does he say that he has a bad taste in his mouth? Is there an odor on his breath? Is the patient able to hear you?

- *Breathing.* Does the patient wheeze? Does he make other noises when he breathes? Does he cough? Does he cough up sputum? Lots of it? What is the color? Is it bloody? Does he have difficulty breathing (dyspnea)?

- *Abdomen, Bowels, and Bladder.* Does the patient's stomach appear to be distended (puffed up)? Does he complain of gassiness, belching, or nausea? Is he vomiting (having emesis)? What is the appearance of the vomitus? Does it contain red blood? Does it look like coffee grounds? Is the patient constipated? How often does he have a bowel movement? What is the color and consistency (hard or soft) of feces (stool)? Does the stool look like black tar or coffee grounds? Is the amount large or small? Is there any blood, or clumps of mucus, or pieces of white material in the feces? How often does the patient void (urinate)? How much does he void each time? Does he say that he has pain during urination? That it is difficult to start to urinate? Is there sediment (cloudiness) or blood in the urine? Does the urine have a peculiar odor or color? Is the patient unable to control his bowels or urine (incontinent)?

- *Pain.* Where is the pain? How long does the patient say he has had it? How does he describe the pain? Is it constant? Does it come and go? Does he say that it is sharp, dull, aching, or knifelike? Has he had medicine for the pain? Does the patient say that the medicine relieved the pain?

- *Daily Activities.* Does he dress himself? Does he walk without help? Does he walk with help? Does he avoid walking altogether?

- *Personal Care.* Without help, does the patient brush his teeth? Comb his hair? Go to the bathroom? Wash his face? Does he ask for assistance?

- *Movements.* Is he shaking (having tremors or spasms)? Is he limp? Are his movements jerky, shaky, or jumpy?

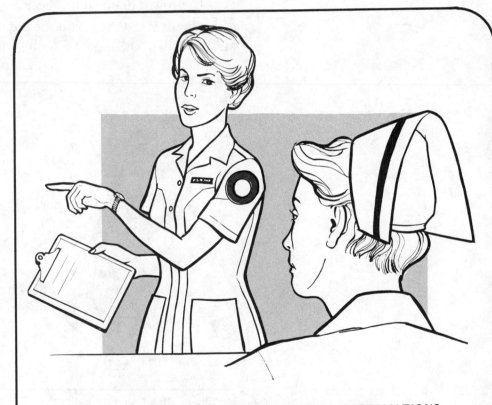

RULES TO FOLLOW WHEN REPORTING YOUR OBSERVATIONS

Write down patient's name, room number, and bed number

Write or report your observations to the head nurse or team leader as soon as possible

Report the time you made the observation

Report the location of the abnormal or unusual sign

Report exactly, but report only what you observe, that is, report objectively

Reporting

Objective and Subjective Reporting. It is very important for you to understand the difference between objective reporting and subjective reporting.

Objective reporting means reporting exactly what you observe—that is, reporting what you see, hear, feel, or smell. The nursing assistant must always use objective reporting.

Subjective reporting means giving your opinion about something, or what you think might be the case. One might report, for example, what he or she thinks is the cause of a change in a patient's condition or what might be the proper treatment. The nursing assistant should never use subjective reporting.

Objective Reports. Here are some examples of objective reporting:

a) Mrs. Smith (404-B bed) is breathing rapidly and the breaths appear to be shallow.

b) Mr. Williams's (204-B bed) urine looks as if there is blood in it.

c) Cindy Jones (107-A bed) says that she has pain in her right upper abdomen.

d) Mr. Jones (101-A bed) picked up his selective menu but could not read it. He asked me to read it for him.

e) For Mr. Brown (104-B bed) to hear me, I had to speak louder than normal.

f) Mrs. Adams (119-C bed) said she did not want to get out of bed.

g) Mr. Cass (103-D bed) cannot hold a glass without spilling its contents.

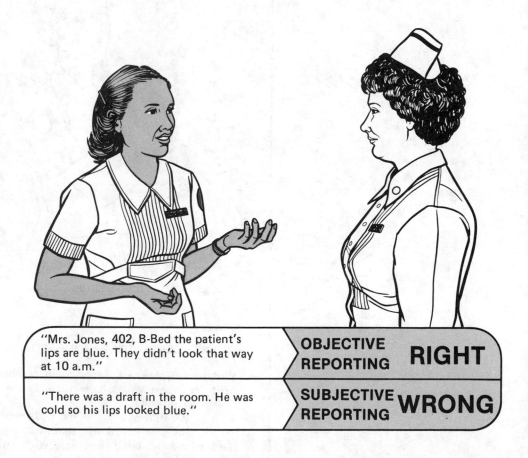

"Mrs. Jones, 402, B-Bed the patient's lips are blue. They didn't look that way at 10 a.m." — **OBJECTIVE REPORTING RIGHT**

"There was a draft in the room. He was cold so his lips looked blue." — **SUBJECTIVE REPORTING WRONG**

Observation of an Infant or Child

Observing an infant or a child means looking at his appearance and physical condition, his bodily functions and secretions, his movements, and his behavior. When you observe changes in any of these, it is very important that you report them to the head nurse or team leader right away. Report things that can be measured, such as a high temperature. Also report the things you see in a pattern of change, such as the child's behavior. Your careful observation and quick reporting could save a baby's life. The following are things to report when you observe them in infants or children:

Appearance and Physical Condition.

- The child's temperature is high or very low.
- The pulse is unusually fast, slow, or irregular.
- The child is breathing rapidly or is having trouble breathing.
- The abdomen seems to be swollen.
- The child's skin does not look right. It may be yellow, or show purplish patches, or appear unusually pale, or have a blue cast. There may be blueness (cyanosis) in the fingernails or lips.
- There are secretions, bleeding, or odor coming from the baby's navel (umbilicus).

Bodily Functions and Secretions.

- The child has not urinated during your hours of work or has voided very little.
- The child has diarrhea.
- There is a large amount of mucus being secreted in the mouth or nose.
- The child is producing a large amount of saliva.
- The child is having trouble swallowing.
- The child is coughing or choking.
- The child is vomiting.

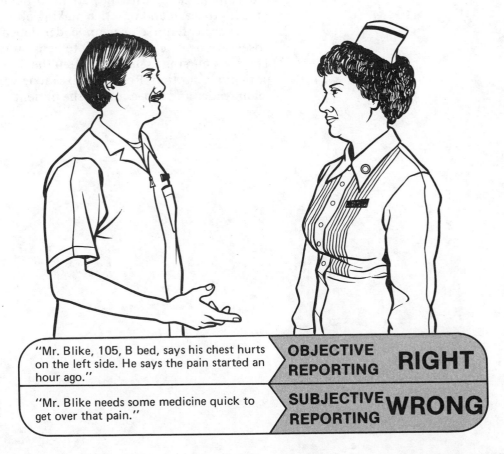

"Mr. Blike, 105, B bed, says his chest hurts on the left side. He says the pain started an hour ago."

OBJECTIVE REPORTING **RIGHT**

"Mr. Blike needs some medicine quick to get over that pain."

SUBJECTIVE REPORTING **WRONG**

Movement and Behavior.

- The child is lying in an abnormal position.
- The muscles are twitching.
- There is no movement in the legs or arms.
- The child is lying very quietly or seems unusually still.
- The child is crying or is very irritable.

WHAT YOU HAVE LEARNED

Patients who have the same illness or medical condition often show the same behavior and have similar needs. Knowing what certain patients look like, how they act, and what their problems are likely to be will help you in your work. You will be better able to meet each patient's needs. You will be a more effective nursing assistant and will give better care.

Your attitude is very important in your relationships with patients and visitors. A good attitude by everyone makes good relationships. The result is a pleasant working environment. The work in the unit goes more smoothly. In this pleasant atmosphere, patients and visitors have more confidence. Everyone feels better and the patients get the benefit.

Your attitude toward visitors should be just as courteous and friendly as it is toward patients and other staff members. Try always to be sympathetic and a good listener.

Be sure every patient knows how to use the signal cord. Always leave the cord where the patient can reach it easily.

Keep improving your skills in communication. The better you can communicate with everyone—patients, visitors, other staff members—the better you will feel about your work and the more self-confidence you will have.

You are in the best position to note changes in the patient's condition and report them. Being with the patient so much of the time gives you many opportunities to learn and practice making observations.

Your head nurse or team leader depends on you to make good objective observations. She expects you to be prompt and accurate in reporting them. The alert nursing assistant is often the first person to see a major change in a patient's condition. Reporting it can be very important to the head nurse or team leader and especially to the patient.

3 HUMAN ANATOMY AND PHYSIOLOGY

OBJECTIVES: WHAT YOU WILL LEARN
    When you have completed this chapter, you will be able to:

- Describe the structure and function of cells, tissues, organs and systems.
- Explain how the body systems work together.
- Carry out instructions accurately which specify particular parts of the anatomy.
- Apply your understanding of how the body works to clinical procedures.

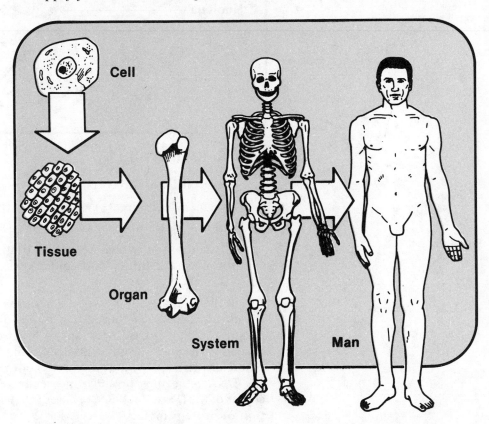

Cell

Tissue

Organ

System   Man

**KEY IDEAS:
THE CELL**

Anatomy is the study of the structure of the body. **Physiology** is the study of the bodily functions. Knowledge of these subjects will help you give better care to your patients. The vocabulary of these subjects will help you understand the instructions your head nurse or team leader gives you. The study of anatomy and physiology is the basis for understanding all the clinical procedures you will be doing as a nursing assistant.

The Cell

The cell is the fundamental building block of all living matter. Cells are microscopic in size. They are the living parts of organisms. The human body is made up of millions of cells. There are many kinds of cells. Each one has a special task within the body. Living cells have many things in common:

- They come from pre-existing cells.
- They use food for energy.
- They use oxygen to break down the food.
- They use water to transport various substances such as sodium.
- They grow and repair themselves.
- They reproduce themselves.

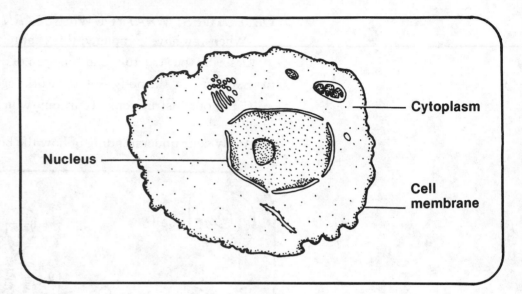

Structure of the Cell

Cells consist of three main parts:

- Nucleus, which directs cellular activities.
- Cytoplasm, where the activities of the cell take place.
- Cell membrane, which keeps the living substance of the cell, called the protoplasm, within bounds and allows certain materials to pass in and out of the cell.

Cells are made up of two main compartments: a **nucleus** which contains the chromosomes (the hereditary material) and a surrounding mass of cytoplasm. The nucleus is important to the process of heredity, growth, and cell division. The **chromosomes** are threadlike structures which contain deoxyribonucleic acid (**DNA**) and therefore control inheritance.

DNA molecules produce messenger **RNA** molecules which are partial copies of the DNA. Each RNA passes into the cytoplasm and directs the formation of protein molecules necessary to maintain life. Through the RNA the nucleus controls the kinds of chemical reactions carried out by the cell.

Cells reproduce by **division**. In any cell preparing for division, the nucleus exactly duplicates its chromosomes. As the cell divides, the pairs of chromosomes pull apart and move to opposite sides of the nucleus. When division is complete the new cells are identical.

Most current research to discover what is causing diseases involves studying the cell and its immediate environment. We are living in a time when there is an explosion of scientific knowledge about the cell. It is hoped from this kind of study scientists will someday find out how to cure or prevent cancer or the common cold.

Tissues

Cells usually do not work alone. They are organized together in tissues. Groups of cells of the same type that do a particular kind of work are called **tissues**.

Some of the primary kinds of tissues in the human body are:

- **Epithelial Tissue**—The duty of this tissue is to protect (skin), secrete (hormones), absorb (intestines), and receive sensations.

- **Connective Tissue**—The duty of this tissue is to connect (tendons), to support (bones), and to cover, ensheath, or line (the thin and sometimes fatty layer of connective tissue under the skin, the tough sheet of fibrous tissue over the limbs) and to pad or protect (bursal sacs).

- **Muscle Tissue**—The duty of this tissue is movement. Striated tissue is found in voluntary muscles, those you can move consciously. Smooth tissue is found in the involuntary muscles such as those that push food and water through the gastrointestinal tract. Smooth muscle allows such action as a dilation and contracting of the pupil of your eye and of blood vessels.

- **Cardiac Muscle Tissue**—is found only in the heart and is involuntary.

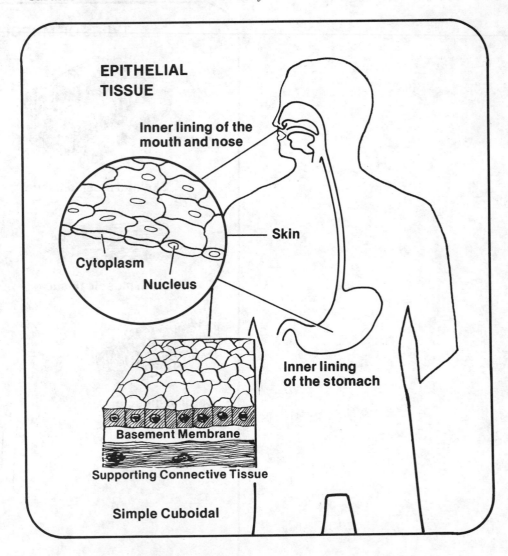

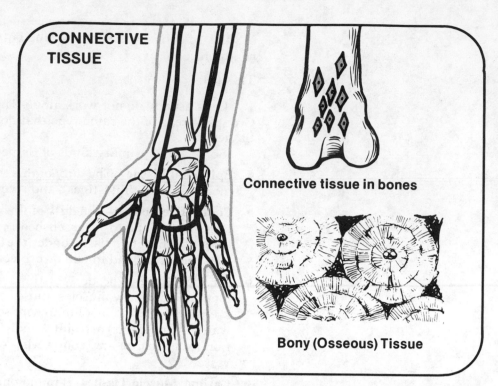

CONNECTIVE TISSUE

Connective tissue in bones

Bony (Osseous) Tissue

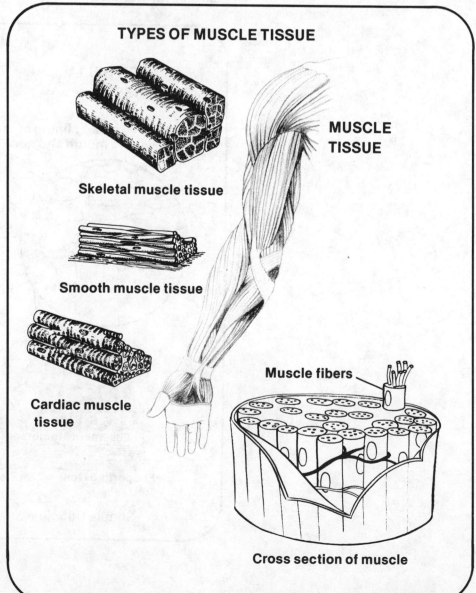

TYPES OF MUSCLE TISSUE

Skeletal muscle tissue

Smooth muscle tissue

Cardiac muscle tissue

MUSCLE TISSUE

Muscle fibers

Cross section of muscle

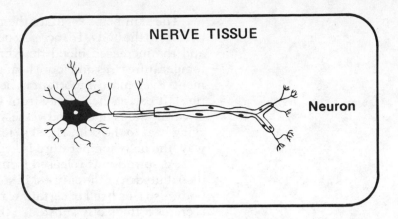

NERVE TISSUE

Neuron

- **Nerve Tissue**—The duty of this tissue is to carry nervous impulses from a portion of the brain or spinal cord to all parts of the body. The body cannot renew nervous tissue. A healthy baby is born with a specific amount and this is all he will ever have.

- **Blood and Lymph Tissue**—In this type of tissue the cells are singular and move within a fluid to every part of the body.

Cells to Systems

Tissues are grouped together to form **organs**, such as the heart, lungs, and liver. Each organ has specific jobs. Organs that work together to perform similar tasks make up **systems**. It is easier to study anatomy and physiology by systems. Always remember that a system cannot work by itself. Systems are dependent, one upon the other.

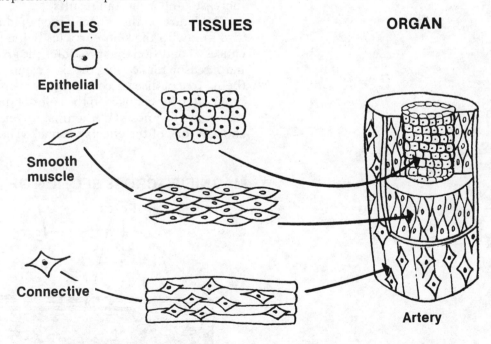

CELLS   TISSUES   ORGAN

Epithelial

Smooth muscle

Connective

Artery

Cells combine to form tissues, and tissues combine to form organs

The skin covers and protects underlying structures from injury or bacterial invasion. Skin also contains nerve endings from the nervous system, which aid the body in awareness of its environment.

**KEY IDEAS:
THE INTEGUMENTARY
SYSTEM (THE SKIN)**

The skin helps regulate the body temperature by controlling the loss of heat from the body. To increase heat loss, the blood vessels near the skin dilate, and the increased blood flow brings more heat to the skin. Then the skin temperature rises and more heat is lost from the hot skin to the cooler environment. Even more important in heat loss is the evaporation of sweat (perspiration). It carries heat away from the skin. When the body is conserving heat, sweating stops and blood vessels contract. This prevents the blood from carrying heat to the skin. The skin temperature falls, decreasing heat loss. In this way, the body temperature is kept almost constant.

Perspiration is released from the body through sweat glands, which are distributed over the entire skin surface. The glands open by ducts or pores. The body also rids itself of certain waste products through perspiration. Skin also secretes a thick oily substance through ducts that lead to oil glands. In this way, the skin is lubricated and kept soft and pliable. The oil also provides a protective film for the skin, which limits the absorption and evaporation of water from the surface. In elderly persons, these oil glands sometimes fail to function properly and the skin becomes quite dry, scaly, and delicate.

Appendages of the skin, in addition to the sweat and oil glands, include the hair and the nails. Each hair has a root embedded in the skin, into which the oil glands of the skin open. Fingernails and toenails grow from the nail bed at the base underneath. If the nail bed is destroyed, the nail stops growing.

The skin covers the entire body. The outer layer of the skin (the layer you can see) is called the **epidermis**. Cells are constantly flaking off or being rubbed off this outer layer of skin. Beneath the epidermis is the **dermis**. In this layer of skin are the new cells that will replace the cells that are lost from the epidermis. Pigment is found in the epidermis. This is responsible for the color of the skin. In sunlight, through a chemical reaction, the amount of pigment increases and a sun tan results.

Moisture on the skin can pick up dust and dirt from the air. Moisture can also mix with the skin particles being flaked off the epidermis. This process causes a condition that promotes the growth and spread of bacteria. This is the main reason for keeping the skin clean. The skin is where the battle for asepsis (being free of disease causing organisms) begins.

Watch for changes in the color of the patient's skin. Watch for blueness or darkening (cyanosis) of the lips, fingernails, or eyelids. **Cyanosis** is a sign of shock or one of the effects of shock. The primary functions of the skin are:

MAGNIFIED CROSS SECTION OF THE SKIN

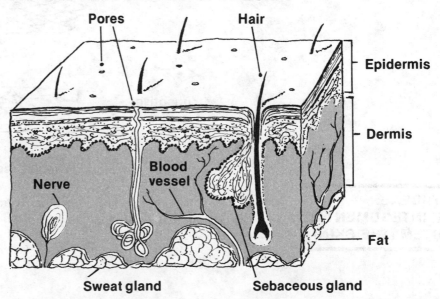

Pores · Hair · Epidermis · Dermis · Nerve · Blood vessel · Fat · Sweat gland · Sebaceous gland

- To cover and protect underlying body structures from injury and bacterial invasion.
- To help regulate body temperature by controlling loss of heat from the body.
- Storage of energy in the form of fat and vitamins.
- Elimination of wastes by perspiration.
- Sensory perception—the sense of touch (the skin can sense heat, cold, pain, and pressure).

KEY IDEAS: THE SKELETAL SYSTEM

The skeletal system is made up of 206 bones. The bones act as a framework for the body, giving it structure and support. They are also the passive organs of motion. They do not move by themselves. They must be moved by muscles, which shorten or contract. A muscle is stimulated to contract by a nerve impulse. This is an example of how systems interact. It is necessary to learn the names of the bones because they are like landmarks.

There are four types of bones:

- Long bones, such as the big bone in your thigh, the femur.
- Short bones, like the bones in your fingers, the phalanges.
- Irregular bones, such as the vertebrae that make up the spinal column.
- Flat bones, like the bones of the rib cage.

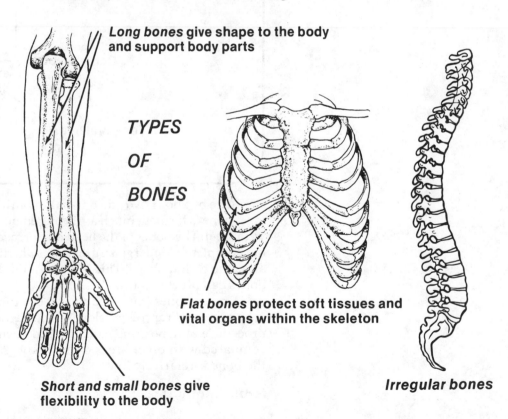

Long bones give shape to the body and support body parts

TYPES OF BONES

Flat bones protect soft tissues and vital organs within the skeleton

Short and small bones give flexibility to the body

Irregular bones

Bones are not inactive. They are dynamic and usually busy parts of the body. They store vital minerals that are necessary for many other body activities. The bones of the head are designed to protect the very delicate tissue of the brain. They are joined by sutures, similar to a zigzag embroidery pattern, and totally surround the brain and cranial nerves. Some other bones that protect vital organs include the vertebrae of the spinal column, which protects the spinal nerve cord and the rib cage, which guards the heart and lungs.

When the fetus is developing in the uterus, the entire skeleton is formed in

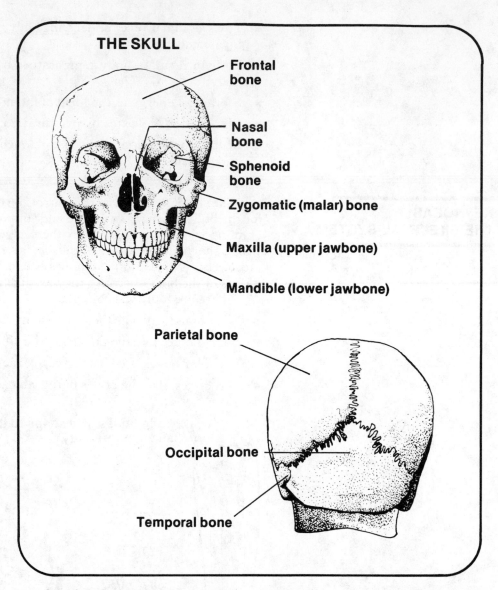

THE SKULL

Frontal bone

Nasal bone

Sphenoid bone

Zygomatic (malar) bone

Maxilla (upper jawbone)

Mandible (lower jawbone)

Parietal bone

Occipital bone

Temporal bone

cartilage by about two and one-half months after conception. From this cartilage, bone is formed, much as if you replaced a wooden bridge, piece by piece, with steel. The bones of the head are formed from strong membranes. They do not completely undergo **ossification** (which means development of bone) until after the child is born. This is a great aid during childbirth, when the baby's bones can overlap a little.

Broken bones can mend solidly but the process is slow and gradual. Bone cells grow and reproduce slowly. The hardening of the new bone is a gradual procedure of depositing calcium. Blood supply to bone tissue is poor, when compared with other areas of the body. Therefore, resistance to infection in the bone is relatively low.

Joints (Motion)

The systems of the body must all work together. No one system can stand alone. All the systems operate simultaneously in a healthy human body. The skeletal system, muscular system, nervous system, and circulatory system are all interacting during each body movement. Movement of the body occurs at the joints. This is a perfect example of how several systems must work together.

Joints are areas in which one bone connects with one or more bones. They are necessary levers in all motion. Joints are made up of many structures. The tough white fibrous cord, the **ligament** , connects bone to bone. The **tendons**

SKELETON AND SURFACE MUSCLES

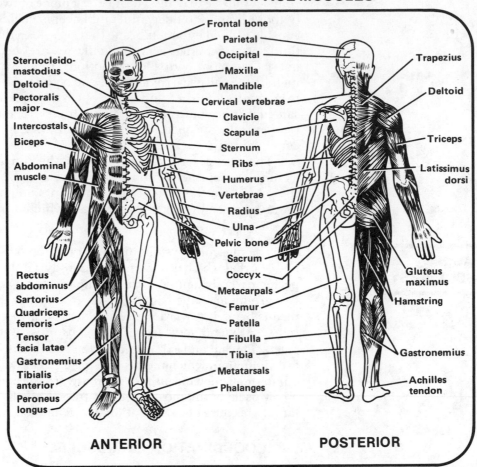

Frontal bone
Parietal
Occipital
Maxilla
Mandible
Cervical vertebrae
Clavicle
Scapula
Sternum
Ribs
Humerus
Vertebrae
Radius
Ulna
Pelvic bone
Sacrum
Coccyx
Metacarpals
Femur
Patella
Fibulla
Tibia
Metatarsals
Phalanges

Sternocleido-mastodius
Deltoid
Pectoralis major
Intercostals
Biceps
Abdominal muscle

Rectus abdominus
Sartorius
Quadriceps femoris
Tensor facia latae
Gastronemius
Tibialis anterior
Peroneus longus

Trapezius
Deltoid
Triceps
Latissimus dorsi
Gluteus maximus
Hamstring
Gastronemius
Achilles tendon

ANTERIOR

POSTERIOR

SYNOVIAL (MOVABLE) JOINTS

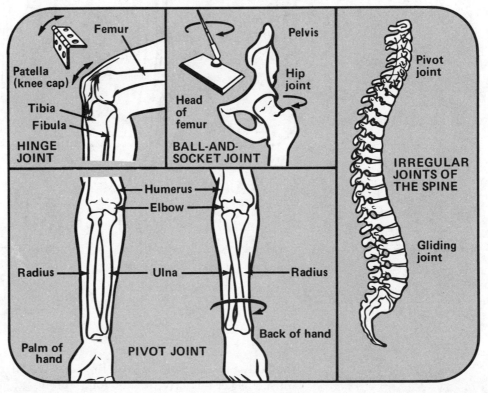

Femur
Patella (knee cap)
Tibia
Fibula
HINGE JOINT

Pelvis
Hip joint
Head of femur
BALL-AND-SOCKET JOINT

Pivot joint
IRREGULAR JOINTS OF THE SPINE
Gliding joint

Humerus
Elbow
Radius
Ulna
Radius
Palm of hand
Back of hand
PIVOT JOINT

connect muscle to bone. The meeting place of two bones—the joint—especially those in the shoulder, hip, and knee, is enclosed in a strong capsule. This capsule is lined by a membrane that secretes a fluid called **synovial fluid**. This fluid acts as a buffer, very much like a water bed, so the ends of the bones do not get worn out with a lot of motion. Other structures that protect the bone include the pad of cartilage at the end of the bone, a sac of synovial fluid (which is known as a **bursa**), and a disc of cartilage called the **meniscus**. Many such safeguards are built into the body. Injury to joints may cause a ligament or tendon to be strained in what we call a sprain. Inflammation of the bursa causes bursitis.

There are several kinds of joints in the human body. The hinge joint, such as in the knee, is freely movable. There are also less movable joints, such as those between the vertebrae. Some joints do not move at all. An example is joints between the bones of the head, which protect the brain.

KEY IDEAS: THE MUSCULAR SYSTEM

The muscular system makes all motion possible, either that of the whole body or that which occurs inside the body. Groups of muscles work together to perform a body motion. Other groups perform just the opposite motion. These two groups are called antagonistic groups. For example, flex your arm, which means bring it toward your shoulder. Your biceps contracts, and the triceps relaxes. Extend your arm. The biceps muscle relaxes while the triceps contracts. **Flexion** and **extension** are the two terms you should know. Two others are **abduction**, which means moving a part away from the body midline, and **adduction** which means moving it toward the body.

Muscle is the most infection free of all the body's basic tissues. This is largely because of its exceptionally rich blood supply. Muscles not only move

COORDINATION OF MUSCLES

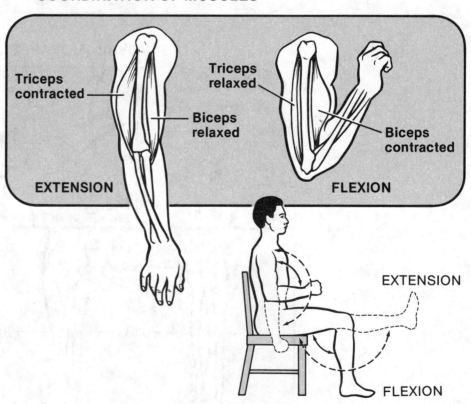

Triceps contracted

Biceps relaxed

Triceps relaxed

Biceps contracted

EXTENSION

FLEXION

EXTENSION

FLEXION

the body but also help to keep the body warm, especially during activity. If a muscle is kept inactive for too long, it tends to shrink and waste away. This is called **atrophy**. **Contracture** is a permanent muscle shortening. This is the reason that regular exercise is so important to good health. Range of motion exercises are often given to inactive patients to prevent these problems.

When you are helping to lift a patient or when you are making a bed, remember to use the strong muscles of your legs rather than those of your back. This will prevent you from seriously hurting yourself. Use the large thigh muscles, the quadriceps femoris, on the ventral portion of the thigh, and the hamstrings on the dorsal portion. This will also save you from straining your muscles.

ADDUCTION　　　　　　　**ABDUCTION**

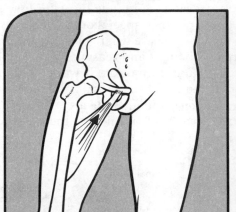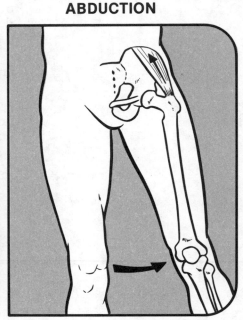

KEY IDEAS: THE NERVOUS SYSTEM

The nervous system controls and organizes all body activity, both voluntary and involuntary. The nervous system is made up of the brain, the spinal cord, and the nerves. The nerves are spread throughout all areas of the body in an orderly way.

Nervous tissue is made up of cells called **neurons** and other supporting cells called **neuroglia**. A typical neuron is made up of a cell body with one long column called the **axon** and many small outbranchings called **dendrites**. Nerve impulses move from the dendrites through the cell body along the axon. Inside and outside our bodies, we have structures called **receptor-end organs**. Any change in our external or internal environment that is strong enough will set up a nervous impulse in these receptor-end organs. This impulse is carried by a sensory neuron to some part of the brain or spinal cord where it connects with an interneuron. The connection is called a **synapse**. This interneuron often makes hundreds of synapses (particularly in the cerebrum, the part of the brain in which we think) before a decision is made. Once that happens, the proper impulses are sent down a motor neuron to the **effector-end organs**, those organs that are going to respond to the nerve impulse.

Most nerve cells outside the brain and spinal cord have a protective covering known as the **myelin sheath**. The task of the myelin sheath is to insulate the nerve cell. The nerve cell can be compared to an electrical wire that requires insulation to keep the current in the correct pathway. This sheath helps prevent damage to the cells and often helps the nerve return to healthy function, or regenerate, if it has been injured. Nerve cells with a myelin sheath also carry an impulse faster than those without myelin. The neurons in the brain do not have this kind of protection. When they are injured, as they are by a stroke or **cerebral vascular accident** (C.V.A.), it is necessary for another part of the brain to take over the function of the part that has been damaged. The rehabilitation department in your health care institution helps patients learn to do things again after such damage has been done.

The brain is well protected by bones, membranes, the meninges, and a cushion of fluid called **cerebral spinal fluid**. This fluid circulates outside of and within the brain as well as around the spinal cord. The brain is a very complicated organ. It is made up of five portions. The **cerebrum** is divided into two halves, called hemispheres. They are connected to one another by white material known as **corpus callosum**. The right hemisphere controls most of the activity on the left side of the body. And the left hemisphere of the cerebrum controls the activity on the right side of the body. The cerebrum has many indentations, which are known as **convolutions**. It is here that all learning, memory, and associations are stored so that thought is possible. Also, it is here that decisions are made for voluntary action. Certain areas of the cerebrum seem to perform special organizing activities. For example, the **occipital lobe** is the place where what you see is interpreted. The **frontal lobe** is the primary area of thought and reason. The **cerebellum** is the part of the brain that controls voluntary motion. It works with part of the inner ear, the semicircular canals, to enable us to walk and move smoothly through our world. The **midbrain, pons,** and **medulla** are primarily pathways through which nervous impulses reach the brain from the spinal cord.

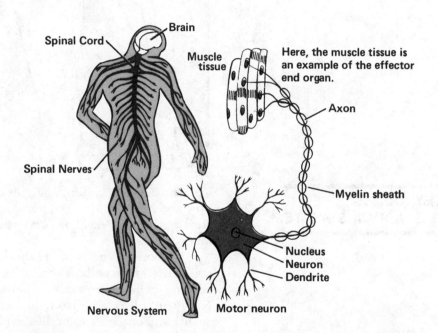

Spinal Cord
Brain
Muscle tissue
Here, the muscle tissue is an example of the effector end organ.
Axon
Spinal Nerves
Myelin sheath
Nucleus
Neuron
Dendrite
Nervous System
Motor neuron

Nerves throughout the body send messages into the tracts of white matter in the spinal cord, from which they rise to higher centers in the brain. There are 12 pairs of cranial nerves and 32 pairs of spinal nerves. These have many branches that go to all parts of the body.

One of the most important areas of the brain is an area called the **diencephelon**. It is here that small structures surround one of the ventricles of the brain. These structures help circulate cerebral spinal fluid and exercise an almost dictatorial control over the body's activities. They screen all nervous impulses going to the brain, either getting them there faster or slowing them down. One of these tiny structures is the **hypothalamus**, which in times of stress, emergency, excitement, or danger actually takes control of the body by controlling the **pituitary gland**, the body's master gland. Although it can be mapped, like the subways of a great city, we still know very little about the actual activity of the pituitary gland. We do know that it has tremendous control over most body activities. It seems to be the link between the mind and the body. It receives messages from the cerebrum, from the cerebellum, and from impulses coming up the spinal cord, and it has direct control over all the endocrine glands.

Much of the activity of the organs of the body is involuntary. In other words, we do not think about it. Or, for the most part, we have no conscious control over this activity. The part of the nervous system that controls such things as digestion and the functions of other **visceral** (abdominal) organs is the autonomic nervous system. This is really not separate from the brain and the spinal cord. The neurons that make up the autonomic nervous system use the same pathways as those neurons that control our voluntary actions. However, the two divisions of this part of the nervous system direct and control the activity of our internal organs. Each organ is supplied with neurons from each division of the autonomic nervous system.

SENSORY AND MOTOR PROCESSES IN OPERATION

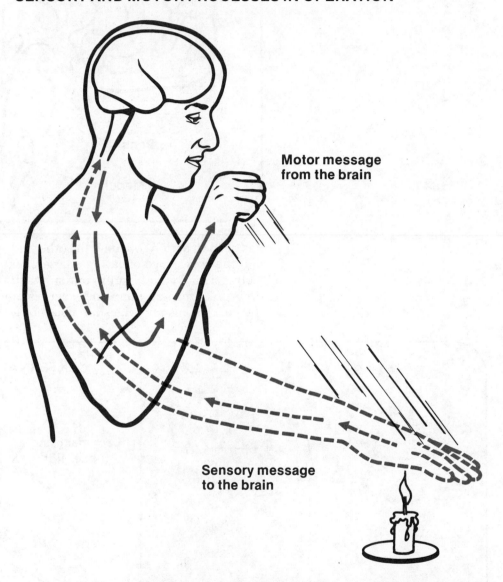

Motor message from the brain

Sensory message to the brain

One division is called the **sympathetic division**. The neurons that make up this division become active during stress, danger, excitement, or illness. These neurons cause the pupils of our eyes to become larger, so we can see more clearly and can see better at a distance. These neurons also cause the heart to beat more strongly and to send more oxygen to the large muscles of the body in case it is necessary to fight or run. In today's fast paced world, we are all subject to stress and sometimes we cannot run away from it or fight it. The action of the neurons from the sympathetic system then causes changes in the shape or activity of some of our organs. This action may also cause illness.

The **parasympathetic division** of the autonomic nervous system is in control when we are relaxed. It is known to conserve our energy. Fortunately, there is a checks-and-balances system between the two divisions. When one

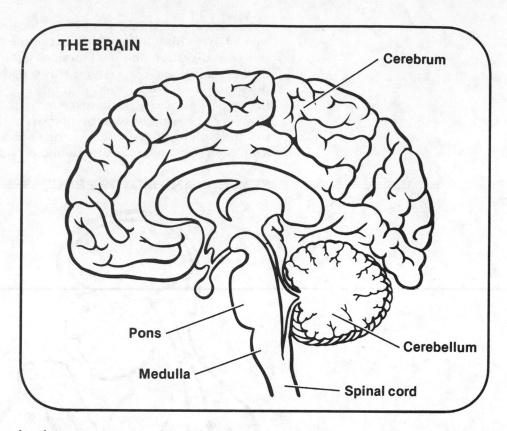

THE BRAIN

Cerebrum

Pons

Cerebellum

Medulla

Spinal cord

has been in action too long, the other automatically switches on. We have all had the experience of eating a large meal after being emotionally upset and feeling as if we had lead in our stomach. This is because of the sympathetic division of the autonomic nervous system. **Peristalsis** (which is movement of the gut) lessens and digestion does not go on.

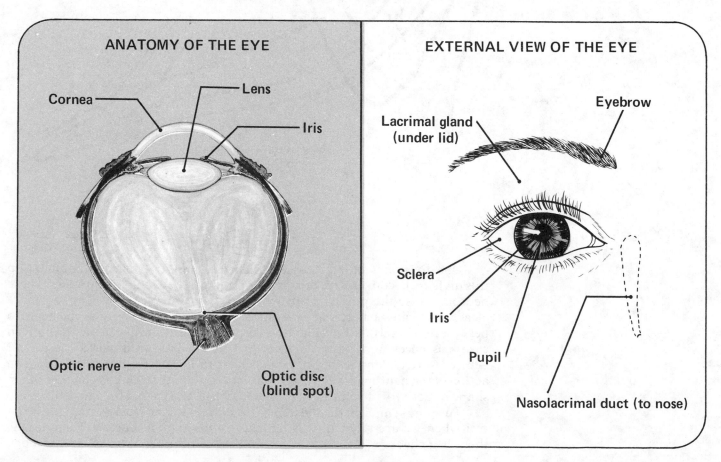

ANATOMY OF THE EYE

Cornea

Lens

Iris

Optic nerve

Optic disc (blind spot)

EXTERNAL VIEW OF THE EYE

Lacrimal gland (under lid)

Eyebrow

Sclera

Iris

Pupil

Nasolacrimal duct (to nose)

The Sense Organs. The sense organs contain specialized endings of the sensory neurons. These are excited by sudden changes in the outside environment, called **stimuli**.

- Eyes respond to visual stimuli.
- Ears respond mainly to sound stimuli.
- Membranes of the nose respond to smells.
- Taste buds, located chiefly on the tongue, respond to sweet and sour and other sensations.
- Skin responds to touch, pressure, heat, cold, and pain.

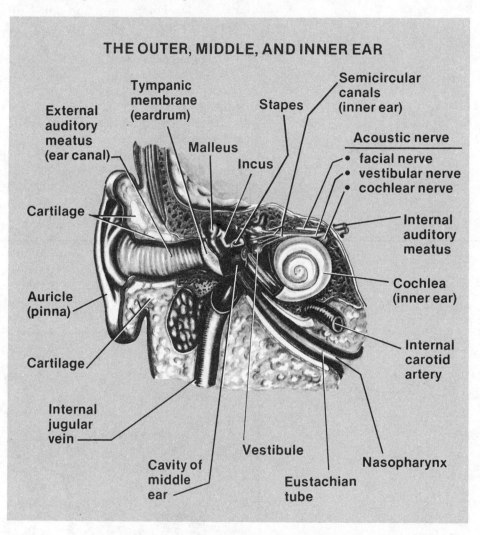

THE OUTER, MIDDLE, AND INNER EAR

KEY IDEAS: HORMONES AND THE ENDOCRINE SYSTEM

The endocrine glands secrete liquid called **hormones**. These help the nervous system organize and direct the activities of the body. The hormones are secreted (flow) directly into the bloodstream. Exocrine glands, such as the salivary glands, deliver their products through ducts into a body cavity.

The hormones from the pituitary gland, both the anterior and posterior portions, regulate all metabolism of our billions of cells. The anterior portion manufactures and releases seven hormones.

The **pituitary gland** is the master gland. Its hormones directly affect the other endocrine glands, stimulating them to produce their hormones. Its hormones are especially important in reproduction and in all functions leading to puberty. This is the time at which a child takes on the physical characteristics of an adult man or woman. Hormones from the pituitary gland regulate the menstrual cycle in the female and sperm production in the male. Without these hormones, it would not be possible for us to reproduce.

The pituitary gland and all of these important hormones are under the direct control of the **hypothalamus**, a tiny fragment of tissue lying near the base of the brain. This structure seems to be the real link between our thinking, our emotions, and our body functions.

The **thyroid** gland produces a hormone that regulates growth and general metabolism. The **thymus** gets smaller after puberty, but it plays an important part in the body's immunity system. It is this immunity system that prevents us from getting many diseases.

The **parathyroids** are located within the capsule of the thyroid. They produce a hormone that regulates, along with one of the hormones in the thyroid gland, the level of calcium and potassium in the blood. Calcium is important for many functions of the body, such as muscle contraction and conduction of nerve impulses.

The **pancreas** is both an endocrine gland and an exocrine gland, or a gland that has a duct. Its endocrine portion produces the hormone **insulin**. Insulin regulates the sugar content of the blood. If the body does not have enough insulin, the person becomes diabetic. He must be treated by reducing the carbohydrate or sugar intake and by regulating the balance between insulin and blood sugar.

The **adrenal glands** lie on top of the kidneys. They are very important in helping the body adapt to stress conditions, giving a lot of help to the autonomic nervous system.

The **ovaries** in the female are responsible for secreting the hormones estrogen and progesterone. The rise and fall of the levels of these hormones in the blood determine the menstrual cycle. The hormones are also important in causing an ovum, or egg, to develop and in maintaining a pregnancy.

The **testes** in the male produce testosterone, the primary sex hormone of the male, which also causes the production of sperm.

ENDOCRINE GLANDS

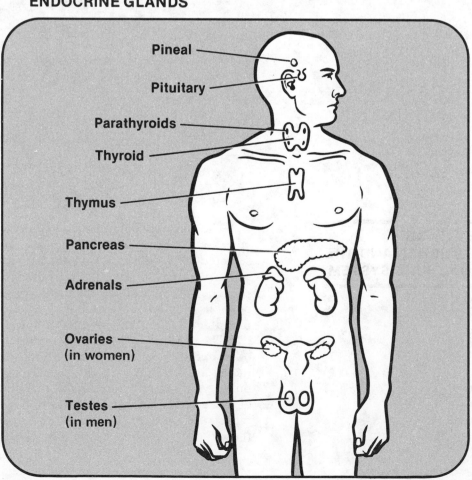

Pineal
Pituitary
Parathyroids
Thyroid
Thymus
Pancreas
Adrenals
Ovaries
(in women)
Testes
(in men)

The circulatory system is made up of the blood, the heart, and the blood vessels—**arteries, veins,** and **capillaries.** The heart actually acts as a pump for the blood, which carries the nutrients, oxygen, and other elements needed by the cells. Important facts to know about blood include:

- The blood carries oxygen from the lungs to the cells.
- Carbon dioxide is carried by the blood from the cells to the lungs.
- Nutrients (food) are picked up (absorbed) by the blood from the duodenum (small intestine) and brought to the cells.
- Waste products from the cells are carried by the blood to the kidneys to be eliminated in urine.
- The hormones from the endocrine glands are transported by the blood.
- Dilation (enlargement) and contraction (narrowing) of the blood vessels help regulate body temperature.
- The blood helps maintain the fluid balance of the body.
- The white cells of the blood defend the body against disease.

THE HEART

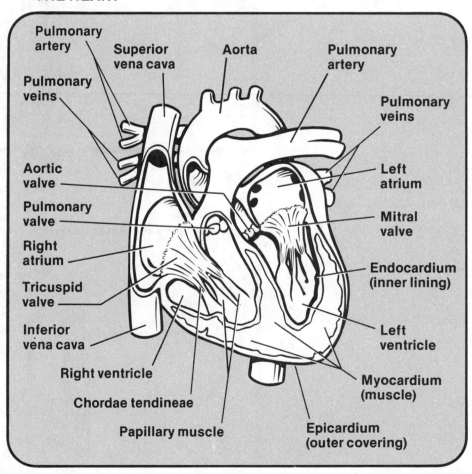

The heart is made up of four chambers—two **auricles** (the atria) and two **ventricles.** The atria are the two smaller chambers. The right ventricle sends the blood only as far as the lungs. Here, in the **pulmonary** circulation, the blood picks up oxygen and gets rid of carbon dioxide. This blood then returns to the heart, carrying its load of oxygen, which is pushed into **systemic** circulation by the left ventricle.

The ventricles have thick walls of muscle. When they contract, the left ventricle pushes the blood through the largest blood vessel, the **aorta,** to all

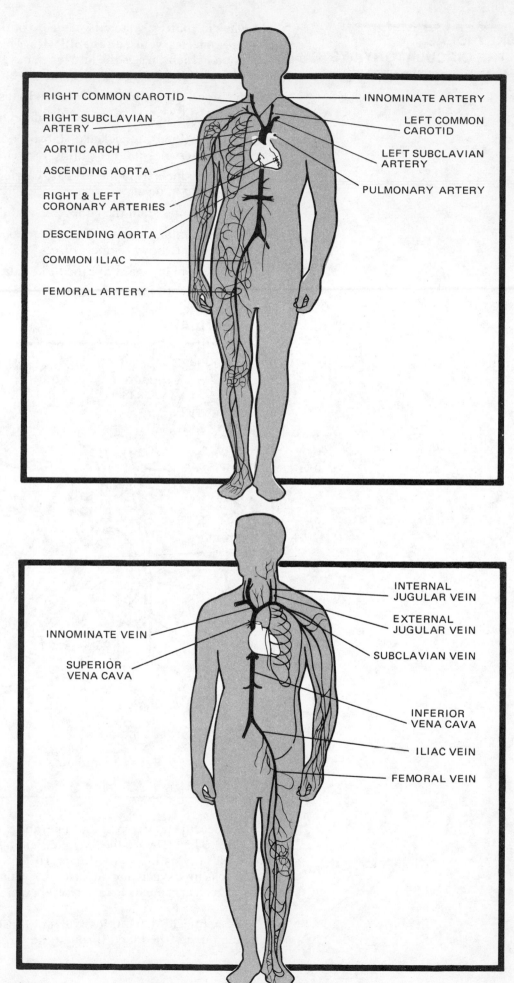

RIGHT COMMON CAROTID — INNOMINATE ARTERY

RIGHT SUBCLAVIAN ARTERY — LEFT COMMON CAROTID

AORTIC ARCH — LEFT SUBCLAVIAN ARTERY

ASCENDING AORTA — PULMONARY ARTERY

RIGHT & LEFT CORONARY ARTERIES

DESCENDING AORTA

COMMON ILIAC

FEMORAL ARTERY

INNOMINATE VEIN — INTERNAL JUGULAR VEIN

SUPERIOR VENA CAVA — EXTERNAL JUGULAR VEIN

SUBCLAVIAN VEIN

INFERIOR VENA CAVA

ILIAC VEIN

FEMORAL VEIN

parts of the body. The blood vessels that carry blood having a lot of oxygen are called **arteries**. The only exception is the pulmonary artery, which carries the blood to the lungs. Arteries branch into a vast network throughout the body. As they branch, the blood vessels become smaller and smaller until finally they are so thin they become **capillaries**. The walls of the capillaries are only one cell-layer thick. Through these walls, gases, nutrients, waste products, and other substances are exchanged among the blood in the capillaries, the tissue fluid, and the individual cell. After the blood has given up its oxygen, which is carried on the surface of the red blood cells, it is returned to the heart through the **veins**. Other important points are:

- All arteries carry blood away from the heart.
- All veins carry blood back to the heart.
- All arteries carry oxygenated blood except the pulmonary artery.
- All veins carry deoxygenated blood except the four pulmonary veins.

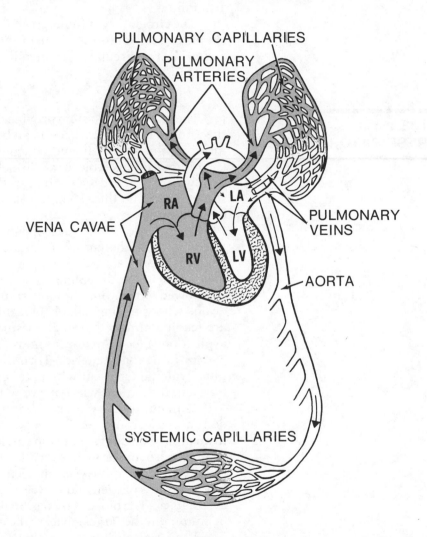

It is necessary that the heart muscle be supplied with blood carrying oxygen. The first branches of the aorta, which come from the heart's left ventricle, are the coronary arteries, which surround the heart. These carry needed oxygen to cardiac (heart) muscle tissue. If one of these branches of the coronary arteries is blocked by a blood clot (embolism), the patient has a heart attack (coronary thrombosis). This can result in the death of some heart tissue. The event is called a myocardial infarction (MI).

The liquid portion of the blood is called **plasma**. The cells are **red blood cells**, which carry oxygen, and **white blood cells**, which fight infection. If a patient has an inflammation in some area of the body, a physician often prescribes warm, moist compresses. These are applied to dilate (widen) the blood vessels in the area and to bring more of those important white blood cells to the place of infection to help fight it. People who have too few red blood cells have some type of anemia. People with too few white blood cells have a lowered resistance to disease. An increase in white blood cells in the blood means that an infection is present somewhere in the body.

A patient's circulation of blood tends to slow down when he is in bed. Sometimes this can cause clotting of the blood. A blood clot is dangerous.

If you have orders to help a patient out of bed for the first time after an illness or after surgery, remember that his circulation is slower. Therefore make sure he moves carefully and slowly. Allow the patient to sit at the edge of the bed until his circulation stabilizes, that is, comes back to normal. Then assist him carefully to a standing position. Sometimes this procedure will cause the blood to leave the brain suddenly. Then the patient may be dizzy or feel faint.

The circulatory system is responsible for getting all of the necessary ingredients to a cell for its metabolism and for carrying away its products and waste material. The circulatory system works in close harmony with the respiratory system.

The respiratory system provides a route or pathway for oxygen to get from the air into the lungs, where it can be picked up by the blood. The organs that make up this system include the **nose** and **mouth**, **pharynx** (throat), **trachea** (windpipe), **larynx** (voicebox), **bronchi**, and **lungs**. Because we must have oxygen to live, it is necessary to keep this pathway open. The structures themselves help to do this. The trachea and bronchi are kept open by incomplete cartilage rings.

On the top of the trachea, opening from the pharynx (the throat), is a structure known as the larynx. It is not only the opening to the trachea, it also contains the vocal cords, which make it possible for us to talk. An important piece of cartilage, the **epiglottis**, covers the opening to the trachea when food is swallowed, preventing the food from going into the lungs. A very weak patient or one who is having trouble breathing must be watched carefully when you are feeding him so that food does not get into the trachea. This is known as aspiration of food. An unconscious patient who vomits may also be in danger of aspirating that material. Turn the patient's head to one side at once. You must watch the patient with great care, because if the pathway for oxygen is blocked, the patient will not live without immediate treatment.

As in our other systems, the important work of the respiratory system is done at the level of the cell. The exchange of oxygen and carbon dioxide occurs in an area of the lungs that is so small you must use a microscope to see it. The last branch of the bronchus is called the **alveolar duct**. At its end is a small sac, the **alveolus**. Many oxygen molecules fill this sac after you breathe in. The blood has less oxygen and therefore is able to pick up a lot of oxygen from the alveolar sac. The blood is then returned to the heart to be sent around the body beginning in the largest artery, the aorta.

The respiratory system, then, is responsible for getting oxygen to the blood. **Internal respiration** occurs when those cells that need the oxygen receive it in exchange for carbon dioxide, which is the cells' gas waste product. Both functions are equally important.

Breathing is regulated by a center in the **medulla**, a part of the brain. Often, especially after surgery, a patient must be encouraged to breathe deeply in order to keep all the air sacs open and inflated. Sometimes you will be asked to help the patient cough, especially if there is inflammation of the lung tissue. Placing one of your hands gently under the diaphragm and the other on the patient's back will assist the muscles of respiration. In many of the larger health care institutions the Pulmonary Medicine Department (Respiratory Therapy) will, by a doctor's order, institute a treatment that will force the patient to breathe deeply and cough.

THE RESPIRATORY SYSTEM

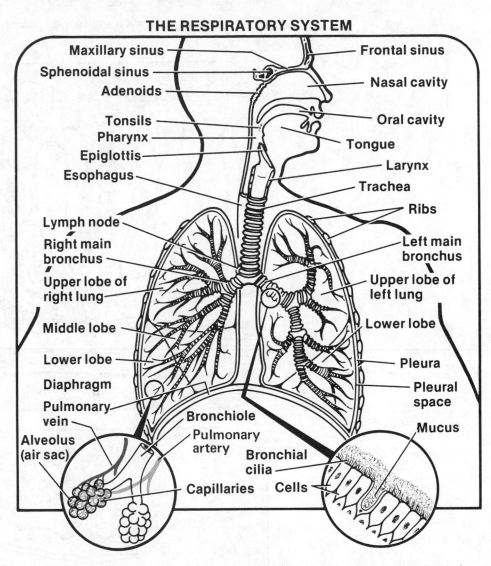

- Maxillary sinus
- Sphenoidal sinus
- Adenoids
- Tonsils
- Pharynx
- Epiglottis
- Esophagus
- Lymph node
- Right main bronchus
- Upper lobe of right lung
- Middle lobe
- Lower lobe
- Diaphragm
- Pulmonary vein
- Alveolus (air sac)
- Frontal sinus
- Nasal cavity
- Oral cavity
- Tongue
- Larynx
- Trachea
- Ribs
- Left main bronchus
- Upper lobe of left lung
- Lower lobe
- Pleura
- Pleural space
- Mucus
- Bronchiole
- Pulmonary artery
- Bronchial cilia
- Capillaries
- Cells

**KEY IDEAS:
THE DIGESTIVE SYSTEM
(GASTROINTESTINAL
SYSTEM)**

The digestive system is responsible for breaking down the food that is eaten into a form that can be used by the body cells. This action is both chemical and mechanical. The digestive tract is about 30 feet long. All of it is important in reducing food to simple compounds.

Digestion begins in the mouth, where food is chewed and mixed with the substance called **saliva**. During swallowing, the food moves in a moistened ball down the esophagus to the stomach. The stomach churns and mixes the food at the same time it is being broken down chemically. The most important area of digestion is the **duodenum**. This is the first loop of the **small intestine**. It is here that the digestive juices, not only from the duodenum itself but also from the pancreas, finish the job of breaking down food into usable parts. In addition, bile, which has been stored in the gallbladder after being manufactured in the liver, also enters the duodenum and helps the reduction process.

A lot of water is necessary for the chemical reduction of food into its end products. It is moved by the rhythmic contraction, called peristalsis, of the muscle walls of the organs of digestion.

Some of the final products of digestion are also absorbed in the area of the duodenum. These end products are:

- Amino acids, the building blocks for all growth and repair of body tissue, which come from dietary proteins.
- Fatty acids and glycerols, from fat.
- Simple sugars, such as glucose, from carbohydrates.
- Water and vitamins.

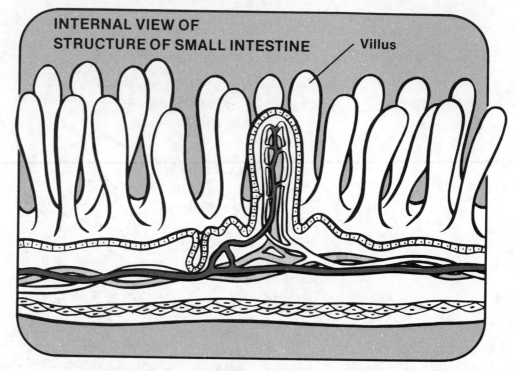

INTERNAL VIEW OF STRUCTURE OF SMALL INTESTINE

Villus

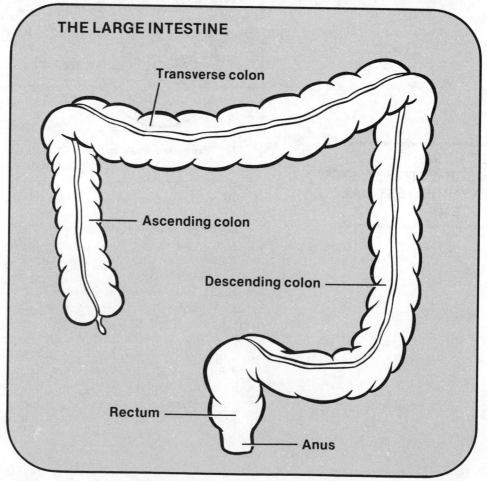

THE LARGE INTESTINE

Transverse colon

Ascending colon

Descending colon

Rectum

Anus

THE DIGESTIVE SYSTEM

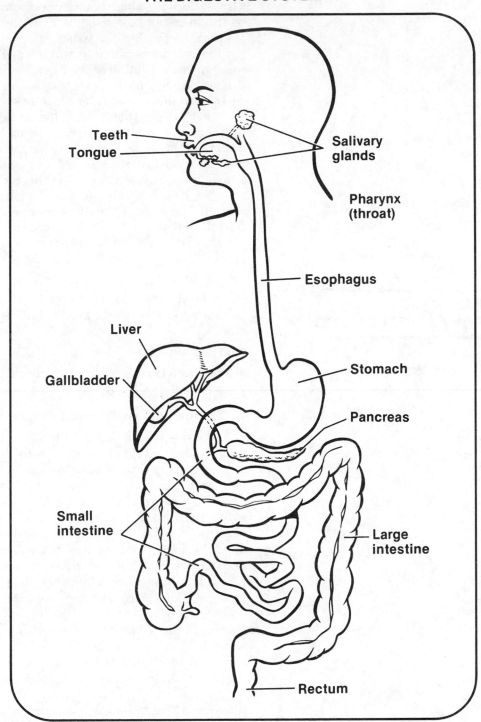

Teeth

Tongue

Salivary glands

Pharynx (throat)

Esophagus

Liver

Stomach

Gallbladder

Pancreas

Small intestine

Large intestine

Rectum

The lining of the duodenum is composed of thousands of tiny fingerlike projections called **villi**. Each villus is capable of absorbing these end products of digestion. The products are then moved into the bloodstream, where they are carried to individual cells.

Some digestion continues to take place in other parts of the small intestine. What is left of the food moves through the large intestine, where water is reabsorbed into the body. The material that cannot be used by the body is excreted from the rectum through the anus as feces.

The **liver** has important responsibilities aside from manufacturing bile. The liver is a storage area for glucose. This form of sugar is released in large amounts when the cells need it for energy to carry on their activities. The liver also is the place where toxins, or poisons, are removed from the blood. Damage to the liver can be caused by drinking alcoholic substances or taking drugs that are harmful to its tissues, such as alcoholic beverages. The liver is also responsible for production and storage of some proteins which are necessary for proper circulation of the blood and for blood clotting. Blood clots are not all bad. When a blood vessel has been injured, a clot may form that holds the blood within a closed tube (the blood vessel) until healing occurs.

On the right side of the colon, at the junction between the small intestine and the large intestine, there is a pouch with a projection of tissue called the **appendix**. Because there is very little peristalsis in this area, the appendix has a tendency to become infected, in a condition known as appendicitis. Surgery is usually performed to correct this condition.

The lowest portion of the large intestine curves in an S-shape into the **rectum**. The rectum is made of very delicate tissue. It has an internal sphincter muscle and an external sphincter muscle. Sometimes blood vessels that supply this area become enlarged and filled with blood clots, causing hemmorrhoids.

KEY IDEAS: THE EXCRETORY SYSTEM

A vital body system in maintaining homeostasis is the excretory system (which gets rid of waste products). The organs that make up this system include:

- The **kidneys**.
- The **ureters** (tubes leading from the kidneys).
- The **urinary bladder**.
- The **urethra** (which leads from the bladder to the outside of the body).

The other organs that help rid the body of waste material include the lungs, which get rid of carbon dioxide by exhalation (breathing out); the skin, which not only is protective but contains glands that secrete moisture and so help maintain body temperature; and, of course, the large intestine.

The functional unit of the kidneys is called a **nephron**. An exchange of substances takes place between the blood capillaries and a part of the nephron. A network of capillaries, called the **glomerulus**, lies within a cupping of a tube, known as Bowman's Capsule. Materials from the blood that are not needed by the body are filtered into Bowman's Capsule. They are then carried through a series of tubules, which help make up the nephron. As the filtered material flows through these tubules, the blood vessels surrounding them reabsorb those materials still needed by the body, particularly the water. Near the end of the winding tubules, substances from the blood, such as toxins and some drugs, pass into the urine. The filtrate that is left is collected in a larger tube. This tube joins those of all the other nephrons in a basin-like portion of the kidney. From here it drips steadily through the ureter, helped by a peristaltic motion very similar to that of the gastrointestinal tract, to the urinary bladder. There are stretch receptor-end organs in the muscular wall of the bladder. The bladder is capable of expanding greatly. When these receptors are stimulated by a full bladder, messages are sent to the brain that cause the person to urinate.

Because the urethra is open to the outside of the body, it may also provide a passageway for disease-causing organisms. These organisms may go up to the bladder, infecting it and causing a disease known as cystitis. The infection may also spread through the ureters to the kidney, causing kidney damage.

The urinary system is perhaps the most important system for maintaining homeostasis. This is because the system determines the content of the blood. The blood content, in turn, determines the content of the tissue fluid, which is the immediate environment of the cells. Many changes in kidney function, some normal, can be found in urine samples. Such changes are also revealed in accurate measurement of intake and output. Sometimes in illness, especially after surgery, the patient is unable to void (urinate).

THE URINARY SYSTEM

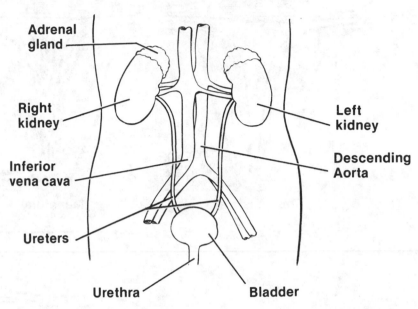

**KEY IDEAS:
THE REPRODUCTIVE
SYSTEM**

In the female the primary reproductive organs are the two **ovaries**. The main task of the ovary is the production of **ova** (eggs). These are specialized cells that are able to unite with a sperm cell released from the male during intercourse and then grow over a period of forty weeks into a new human being. Developing ova lie in a lake of estrogen, a hormone that enters the blood stream during ovulation. **Ovulation** is the process whereby an ovum is re-

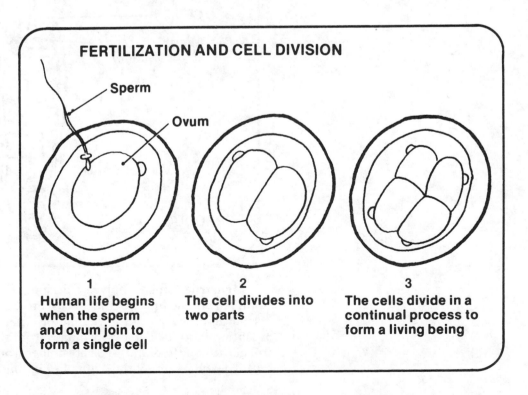

FERTILIZATION AND CELL DIVISION

1
Human life begins when the sperm and ovum join to form a single cell

2
The cell divides into two parts

3
The cells divide in a continual process to form a living being

leased from one ovary into the opening of the oviduct (Fallopean tube) and moves to the **uterus** (womb). This occurs once each month, usually fourteen days before the onset of the next menstrual period. During this time a woman is fertile (able to become pregnant). During ovulation, release of estrogen causes a buildup of the lining of the uterus (endometrium), preparing it for a possible pregnancy.

THE MENSTRUAL CYCLE

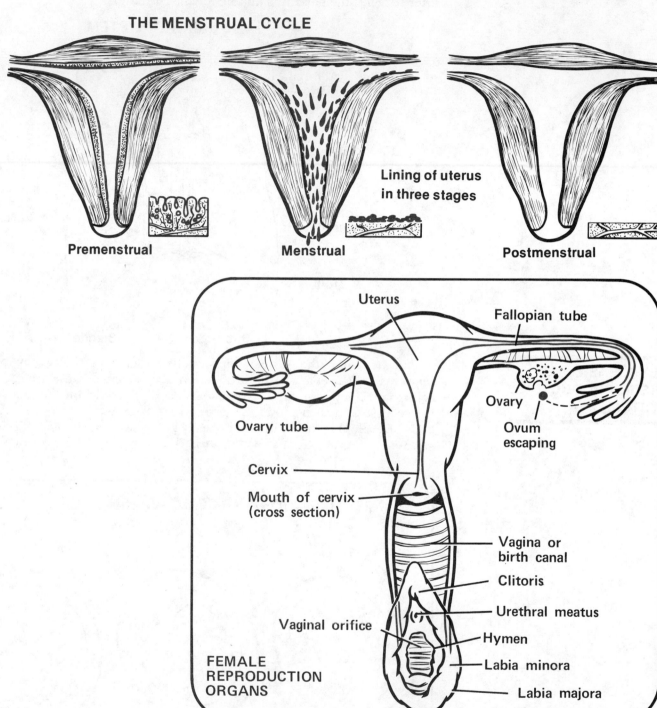

Lining of uterus in three stages

Premenstrual   Menstrual   Postmenstrual

Uterus

Fallopian tube

Ovary tube

Ovary

Ovum escaping

Cervix

Mouth of cervix (cross section)

Vagina or birth canal

Clitoris

Urethral meatus

Vaginal orifice

Hymen

FEMALE REPRODUCTION ORGANS

Labia minora

Labia majora

Menstruation is simply the periodic (monthly) loss of some blood and a small part of the lining of the uterus, an organ that is full of blood vessels. The discharge flows out of the vagina for a period of 4 to 7 days. The process of ovulation is controlled by hormones from the pituitary gland, under the control of the hypothalamus. The hormones from the pituitary gland are involved in the development of the ovum and in maintaining pregnancy.

In the human female there are three openings in the perineal area. 1) The external urinary **meatus**, the end of the urethra. 2) The **vagina**, which is not only the organ for intercourse but also the birth canal. 3) The **anus**, the last portion of the gastro-intestinal tract.

Many women who find it necessary to have a hysterectomy, or surgical removal of the uterus, are afraid of what will happen to their bodies after surgery. Although such women will not be able to become pregnant, they usually are not affected in any other way.

In the male the primary reproductive organs are the testes, which produce sperm. **Testicles**, or **testes**, are paired glands that lie in a sac called the **scrotum** outside the body, posterior to the **penis**, which is the primary male sex organ. During intercourse, sperm travel up the **vas deferens**, or sperm duct, to a point where they enter the urethra. The entrance is made along with secretions from other glands in the male reproductive system. These glands—the **seminal vesicles**, the **prostate gland**, and **Cowper's glands**—contribute water, nutrients, and vitamins, which, added to the sperm, make up the **semen**, a fluid that is ejaculated (expelled) at the same time the male has an orgasm. There is only one duct in the penis. It is used for the flow of urine and for the ejaculation of sperm in its carrying medium, the semen. During intercourse the internal sphincter of the male's urinary bladder closes tightly, so there is no chance for the urine to become mixed with the semen. The penis has three columns of spongy or cavernous tissue. During sexual excitement, blood rushes in through the penile artery and the veins constrict, trapping the blood so it fills these spaces. Then the penis becomes erect and turgid. All of this activity occurs under the influence of **testosterone**, the primary male sex hormone, which is also manufactured in the testes. It is secreted into the blood through the influence of the hormones from the anterior pituitary, which is under the control of the hypothalamus.

Sometimes during the aging process the **prostate gland**, which encircles the urethra like a doughnut, becomes enlarged. When the prostate expands, it squeezes the urethra, causing painful urination. Many men fear surgery on their prostate glands, because they believe it will end their sex life. The amount of semen ejaculated will be less but otherwise, men who have had a prostatectomy are almost always capable of having normal sexual relations.

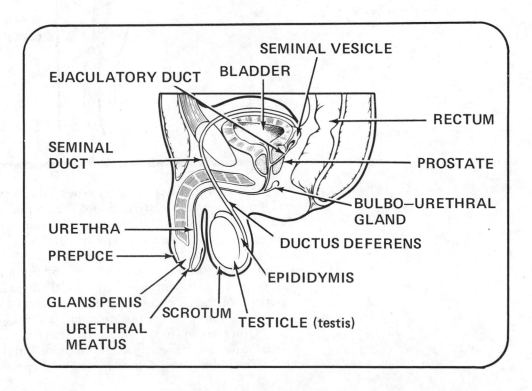

As part of the study of each system, it would be wise to take an overall look at the body and to become familiar with the names given to body areas and cavities. In any demonstration or diagram, the body or body part shown is in the **anatomical position**. The person is standing up straight, facing you, palms out and feet together. When you look at a person in the anatomical position, remember that the left side is always on your right, as in a mirror. This is especially important in studying diagrams. The front of a person is referred to as the **anterior** side. The back, containing the backbone, is called the **posterior** side. The areas of the body closer to the head are called **superior**. Those closer to the feet are called **inferior**. These terms may also be used to describe the position of an organ in the body. For example, the liver is inferior to the diaphragm. The shoulder is superior to the elbow.

WORDS THAT SHOW WHERE BODY PARTS ARE LOCATED

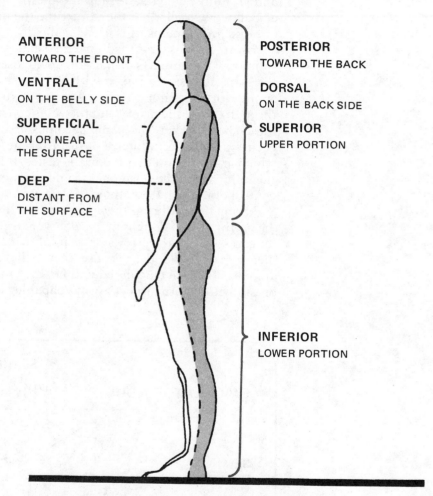

ANTERIOR
TOWARD THE FRONT

VENTRAL
ON THE BELLY SIDE

SUPERFICIAL
ON OR NEAR
THE SURFACE

DEEP
DISTANT FROM
THE SURFACE

POSTERIOR
TOWARD THE BACK

DORSAL
ON THE BACK SIDE

SUPERIOR
UPPER PORTION

INFERIOR
LOWER PORTION

The body has two major cavities—the **dorsal** cavity and the **ventral** cavity. The dorsal cavity is divided into the cranial and spinal cavities. The cranial cavity is in the head. It contains the brain, its protecting membranes, large blood vessels, and nerves. The spinal cavity contains the spinal cord.

The ventral cavity is divided by a large, dome-shaped muscle—called the **diaphragm**—into the thoracic and abdominal cavities. The **thoracic** cavity is in your chest. It contains the lungs, the heart, the major blood vessels, and a portion of the esophagus. The esophagus is the food tube. It penetrates the diaphragm and enters the stomach, which is in the **abdominal** cavity.

Other organs in the abdominal cavity include the liver, spleen, pancreas, small and large intestines, and in the female, the ovaries and uterus.

The kidneys are located in the dorsal portion of the abdominal cavity. The kidneys are outside the large membrane that envelops all of the other organs. This membrane is known as the **peritoneum**. When this membrane becomes infected, the disease is known as peritonitis. The peritoneum, like all membranes in the body, is made up of both epithelial and connective tissue. It protects organs and prevents friction when they move.

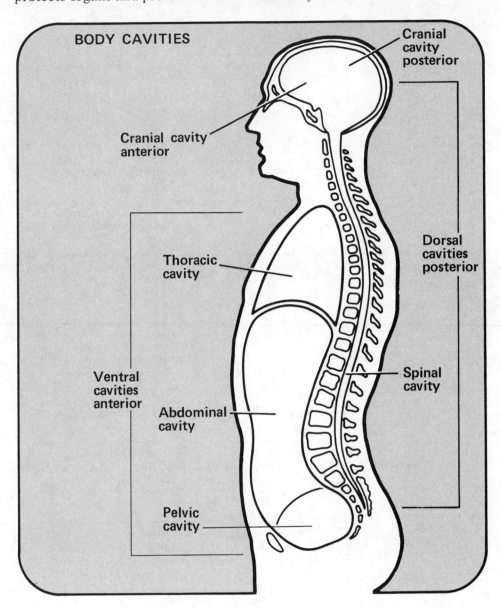

BODY CAVITIES

Cranial cavity posterior

Cranial cavity anterior

Dorsal cavities posterior

Thoracic cavity

Ventral cavities anterior

Spinal cavity

Abdominal cavity

Pelvic cavity

The Body Systems

System	Function	Organs
Skeletal	Supports and protects the body	Bones; joints
Muscular	Gives movement to the body	Muscles; tendons; ligaments
Gastrointestinal (digestive, GI)	Takes and absorbs nutrition and eliminates wastes	Mouth; teeth; tongue, esophagus; salivary glands; stomach; duodenum; intestines; liver; gallbladder; ascending, transverse, and descending colon; rectum; anus; appendix
Nervous	Controls activities of the body	Brain; spinal cord; nerves
Excretory	Removes wastes from the blood, produces urine, and eliminates urine	Kidneys; ureters; bladder; urethra
Reproductive	To reproduce, allows a new human being to be born	Male; testes, scrotum, penis Female; ovaries, uterus, breasts, fallopian tubes, vagina
Respiratory	Eliminates carbon dioxide and gives the body air to supply oxygen to the cells through the blood	Nose; pharynx; larynx; trachea; bronchi; lungs
Circulatory	Carries food, oxygen, and water to the body cells and removes wastes	Heart; blood; arteries; veins; capillaries; spleen; lymph nodes; lymph vessels
Endocrine	Secretes hormones directly into the blood and regulates body function.	Thyroid and parathyroid glands; pineal gland; adrenal glands; testes; ovaries; thymus; pancreatic islands of Langerhans; pituitary gland
Integumentary	Provides first line of defense against infection, maintains body temperature, provides fluids and gets rid of wastes.	Skin; hair; nails; sweat and oil glands

WHAT YOU HAVE LEARNED

The cell is the basic unit of all living matter. The human body is made up of millions of cells. Cells reproduce by a process called cell division, which eventually produces groups of similar cells. When the cells that are similar in form and function become specialized, they are called tissues. When two or more tissues work together to perform a certain function, they form an organ, such as the heart. A system, such as the circulatory system, is formed when a group of organs act together to perform complex body functions. All cells, tissues, organs, and systems operate together to form a human being.

Good reasons for studying human anatomy are: to deliver more effective health care to the patient, to better understand the instructions your head nurse or team leader gives you, and to have the knowledge necessary to act as a teacher to your patients.

The best reason of all is that an appreciation of the design of the healthy human body and how it works will help you deliver a good quality of patient care.

4 INFECTION CONTROL

SECTION 1: MEDICAL ASEPSIS

OBJECTIVES: WHAT YOU WILL LEARN

When you have completed this section, you will be able to:

* Define medical asepsis.
* Explain how microorganisms are destroyed.
* Demonstrate the procedure for handwashing.

**KEY IDEAS:
MICROORGANISMS**

People who work in health care institutions must learn the importance of cleanliness. Everyone tries constantly in many ways to achieve ideal sanitary conditions. You, too, take part in this team effort to keep everything absolutely clean. Why? Because cleanliness is a part of every health care institution's effort to control disease and keep communicable diseases from spreading.

You will understand the importance of cleanliness in the health care institution if you know something about germs—the microorganisms that cause diseases. It may help to know what they are, how they spread, and how they can be destroyed.

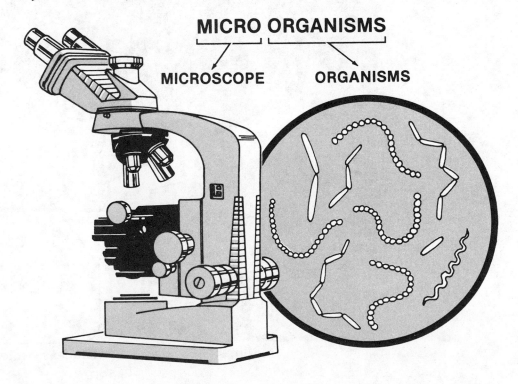

MICRO ORGANISMS

MICROSCOPE   **ORGANISMS**

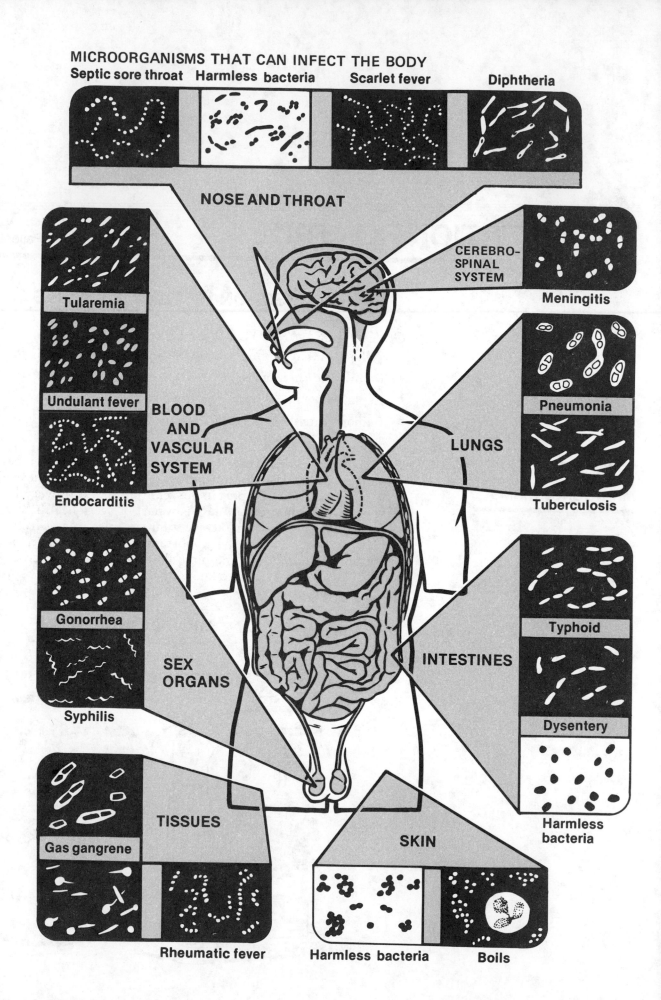

MICROORGANISMS THAT CAN INFECT THE BODY

Septic sore throat   Harmless bacteria   Scarlet fever   Diphtheria

NOSE AND THROAT

CEREBRO-SPINAL SYSTEM

Meningitis

Tularemia

Undulant fever

BLOOD AND VASCULAR SYSTEM

LUNGS

Pneumonia

Endocarditis

Tuberculosis

Gonorrhea

SEX ORGANS

INTESTINES

Typhoid

Syphilis

Dysentery

Gas gangrene

TISSUES

SKIN

Harmless bacteria

Rheumatic fever

Harmless bacteria

Boils

The Causes of Disease

People once believed that sickness was caused by evil spirits. About 500 years ago scientists began to suspect that some diseases were caused by very small living things they called germs.

A germ is a **microorganism**. Micro means very small. Germs can be seen only under a microscope. Organism means a living thing. Different kinds of microorganisms (also called microbes) are:

- Viruses
- Bacteria (microscopic plants)
- Rickettsiae
- Fungi, including molds and yeasts
- Protozoa (microscopic animals)

The Nature of Microorganisms

Some microorganisms are helpful to people. For example, certain microbes cause a chemical change in food called **fermentation**. Fermentation is the change that produces cottage cheese from milk, beer from grains, cider from apples, and sauerkraut from cabbage. Other microorganisms in the human digestive system break down the foods not used by the body and turn them into waste products (feces).

There are other kinds of microorganisms, however, that are harmful to man. These are the microbes that cause disease and infection. Disease-producing microorganisms are called **pathogens**. They grow best at body temperature, 98.6°F (37°C). Pathogens destroy human tissue by using it as food. They also give off waste products called **toxins**. These are absorbed into and poison the body.

Organisms each have their own normal environment or home called their natural habitat. When organisms gain access to areas of the body in which they do not belong, that is, they move out of their normal habitat and into a foreign area, they become pathogens. For example, E. Coli belongs in the colon where it helps to digest our food. When it gets into the bladder or into the blood stream it can cause a urinary infection or a blood infection called bacteremia.

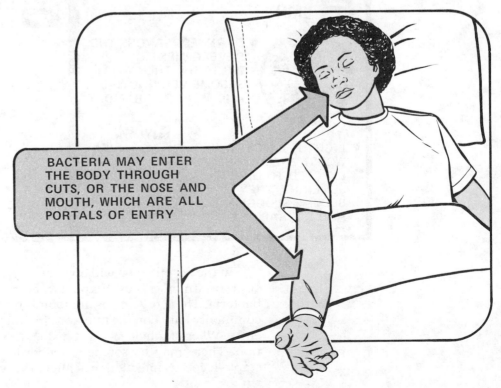

BACTERIA MAY ENTER THE BODY THROUGH CUTS, OR THE NOSE AND MOUTH, WHICH ARE ALL PORTALS OF ENTRY

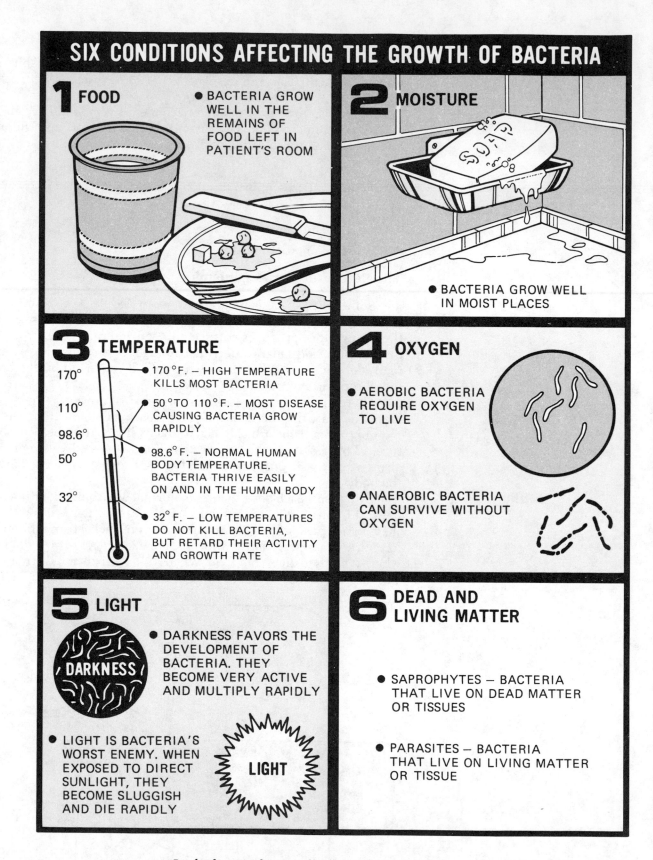

SIX CONDITIONS AFFECTING THE GROWTH OF BACTERIA

1 FOOD

- BACTERIA GROW WELL IN THE REMAINS OF FOOD LEFT IN PATIENT'S ROOM

2 MOISTURE

- BACTERIA GROW WELL IN MOIST PLACES

3 TEMPERATURE

170°
110°
98.6°
50°
32°

- 170°F. – HIGH TEMPERATURE KILLS MOST BACTERIA
- 50° TO 110°F. – MOST DISEASE CAUSING BACTERIA GROW RAPIDLY
- 98.6°F. – NORMAL HUMAN BODY TEMPERATURE. BACTERIA THRIVE EASILY ON AND IN THE HUMAN BODY
- 32°F. – LOW TEMPERATURES DO NOT KILL BACTERIA, BUT RETARD THEIR ACTIVITY AND GROWTH RATE

4 OXYGEN

- AEROBIC BACTERIA REQUIRE OXYGEN TO LIVE
- ANAEROBIC BACTERIA CAN SURVIVE WITHOUT OXYGEN

5 LIGHT

- DARKNESS FAVORS THE DEVELOPMENT OF BACTERIA. THEY BECOME VERY ACTIVE AND MULTIPLY RAPIDLY
- LIGHT IS BACTERIA'S WORST ENEMY. WHEN EXPOSED TO DIRECT SUNLIGHT, THEY BECOME SLUGGISH AND DIE RAPIDLY

6 DEAD AND LIVING MATTER

- SAPROPHYTES – BACTERIA THAT LIVE ON DEAD MATTER OR TISSUES
- PARASITES – BACTERIA THAT LIVE ON LIVING MATTER OR TISSUE

In the hospital you will often hear the words staph or staphylococcus and strep or streptococcus. **Staphylococcus** and **streptococcus** are two types of bacteria. These organisms are found in all health care institutions. They are commonly found on the human skin. They enter the body through a portal of entry. When staphylococci get inside the skin, they may produce a local infection. There may be soreness, tenderness, redness, and/or pus. Sometimes staphylococcus infections can affect the whole body. When streptococci enter the body, they may cause a septic sore throat, a local infection, or rheumatic fever, a general infection.

A **virus** is another type of microorganism. Viruses are much smaller than bacteria, and they cause many of man's diseases. Examples are measles, smallpox, and influenza. Viruses can survive only in living cells.

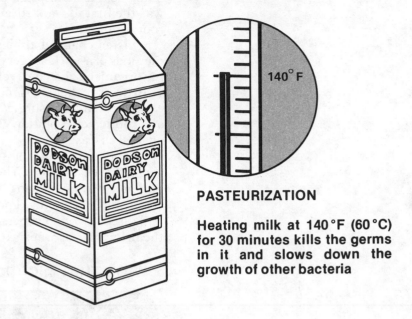

PASTEURIZATION

Heating milk at 140 °F (60 °C) for 30 minutes kills the germs in it and slows down the growth of other bacteria

History of Infection Control

The germ theory of disease was not actually proved until about 100 years ago. A French scientist named Louis Pasteur made two important discoveries about bacteria. First, he discovered that many diseases are caused by bacteria. Second, he discovered that bacteria could be killed by heat.

Pasteur's name has been used to refer to this method of killing germs. For

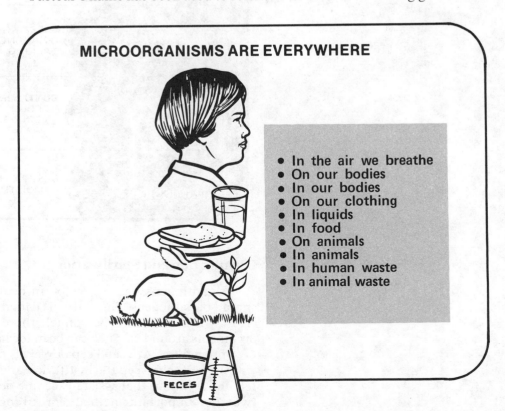

MICROORGANISMS ARE EVERYWHERE

- In the air we breathe
- On our bodies
- In our bodies
- On our clothing
- In liquids
- In food
- On animals
- In animals
- In human waste
- In animal waste

FECES

example, **pasteurization** is the process of heating milk to about 140°F (60°C) and keeping it at that temperature for one-half hour. Pasteurization kills harmful bacteria and makes milk safe for us to drink.

A few years after Pasteur's discoveries, a British surgeon, Joseph Lister, found that germs could also be killed by carbolic acid. Lister recognized that many deaths in hospitals seemed to be connected with unclean conditions. He was the first to want surgical wounds kept clean and the air in the operating room kept pure.

Lister changed things in hospitals by introducing the principles and methods of aseptic surgery. **Aseptic** means germ-free, without disease-producing organisms. Lister developed a technique to keep germs out of open wounds or to destroy them. His method was to spray the skin around the wound with carbolic acid. Also, surgical instruments were made aseptic by being dipped in a carbolic acid solution. This technique was a major advance in the battle against disease.

People working in hospitals began to realize that some disease-producing germs are everywhere. They are in the air, on the furniture, on and inside the patients' bodies, and on all the equipment. Doctors knew that germs multiply very rapidly. They also knew that if germs are not killed, they spread infection and disease from one person to another. Therefore, it was necessary to apply the principles of asepsis to the entire health care institution.

WAYS THAT MICROORGANISMS ARE SPREAD

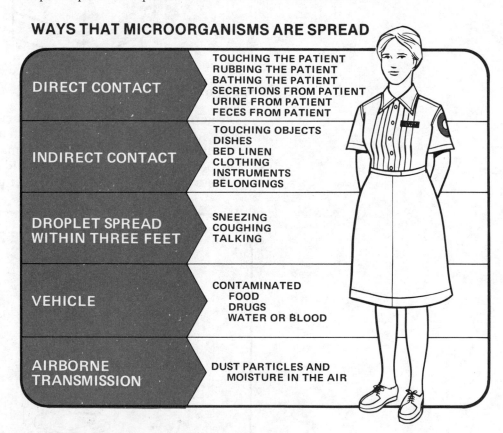

DIRECT CONTACT	TOUCHING THE PATIENT RUBBING THE PATIENT BATHING THE PATIENT SECRETIONS FROM PATIENT URINE FROM PATIENT FECES FROM PATIENT
INDIRECT CONTACT	TOUCHING OBJECTS DISHES BED LINEN CLOTHING INSTRUMENTS BELONGINGS
DROPLET SPREAD WITHIN THREE FEET	SNEEZING COUGHING TALKING
VEHICLE	CONTAMINATED FOOD DRUGS WATER OR BLOOD
AIRBORNE TRANSMISSION	DUST PARTICLES AND MOISTURE IN THE AIR

Disinfection and Sterilization

A continuous battle goes on in health care institutions to prevent the spread of pathogens. This battle is called **medical asepsis**. In spite of the best efforts of health care personnel, there are always some harmful microorganisms around us. They can be made harmless, however, by simple cleanliness procedures. We can keep ourselves clean by bathing and frequent handwashing. We can keep the institution and its equipment clean with soap, water, and solutions that assist in keeping down bacterial growth. Also, there are two very important methods for killing microorganisms or keeping them under control. These methods are:

- Disinfection—the process of destroying as many harmful organisms as possible. It also means slowing down the growth and activity of the organisms that cannot be destroyed.

- Sterilization—the process of killing all microorganisms, including spores, in a certain area.

Spores are bacteria that have formed hard shells around themselves as a defense. These shells are like a protective suit of armor. Spores are very difficult to kill. Some can even live in boiling water. Spores can be destroyed, however, by being exposed to pressurized steam at a high temperature. Machines called **autoclaves** can produce this high-temperature, pressurized steam. Autoclaves are used to kill spores and other disease-producing bacteria. Another method of sterilization uses a chemical gas instead of heat to destroy microorganisms. This method can be used to sterilize equipment made of plastics without melting them. When an object is free of all microorganisms, it is called **sterile**. These are both effective ways of sterilizing objects used in a health care institution.

Sterilization is necessary if the article comes in direct contact with a wound, as in the case of surgical instruments. Most supplies and equipment used in the care of patients can be disinfected to prevent them from spreading disease or infection.

AUTOCLAVE

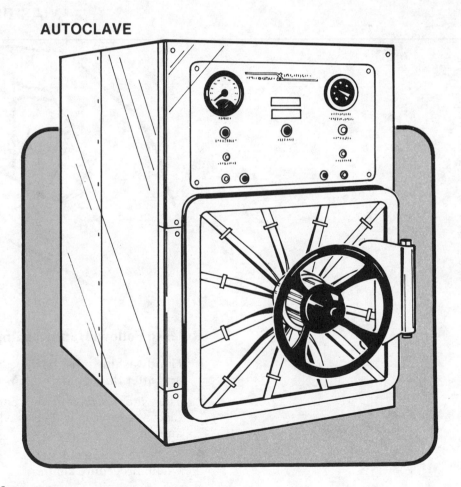

Medical Asepsis

Medical asepsis means preventing the conditions that allow pathogens to live, multiply, and spread. As a nursing assistant, you will share the responsibility for preventing the spread of disease and infection by using aseptic techniques. The main purposes for medical asepsis in caring for patients are:

- Protecting the patient against becoming infected a second time by the same microorganism. This is called **reinfection.**

- Protecting the patient against becoming infected by a new or different type of microorganism from another patient or a member of the hospital staff. This is called **cross infection.**

- Protecting all other patients and hospital staff against becoming infected by microorganisms passing from patient to patient, staff to patient, or patient to staff.

- Protecting the patient from becoming infected with his own organisms. This is called **self-inoculation.**

Handwashing

In your work you will be using your hands constantly. You will often be touching sick patients. You will handle supplies and equipment used in the treatment and care of patients. Germs will get on your hands.

They will come from the patient or from the things he or she has touched. Your hands could carry these germs to other persons and places. The germs could also be moved to your own face and mouth. Washing your hands frequently will help to prevent this transfer of germs.

WASHING YOUR HANDS

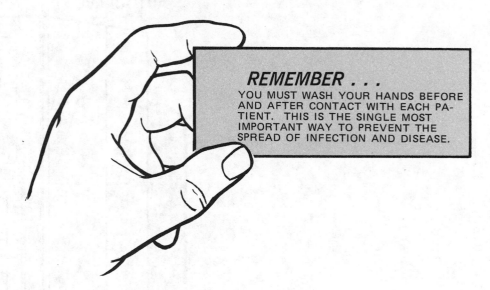

REMEMBER . . .
YOU MUST WASH YOUR HANDS BEFORE AND AFTER CONTACT WITH EACH PATIENT. THIS IS THE SINGLE MOST IMPORTANT WAY TO PREVENT THE SPREAD OF INFECTION AND DISEASE.

Rules to Follow: Handwashing

- Handwashing must be done before and after each nursing task and before and after direct patient contact.

- The water faucet is always considered contaminated. This means there are disease germs on it. This is why you use paper towels to turn the faucet on and off.

- If your hands accidentally touch the inside of the sink, start over. Do the whole procedure again.

- Take soap from a dispenser, if possible, rather than using bar soap. Bar soap accumulates pools of soapy water in the soap dish, which is then considered contaminated.

- Handwashing is effective only when:
  a) You use enough soap to produce lots of lather.

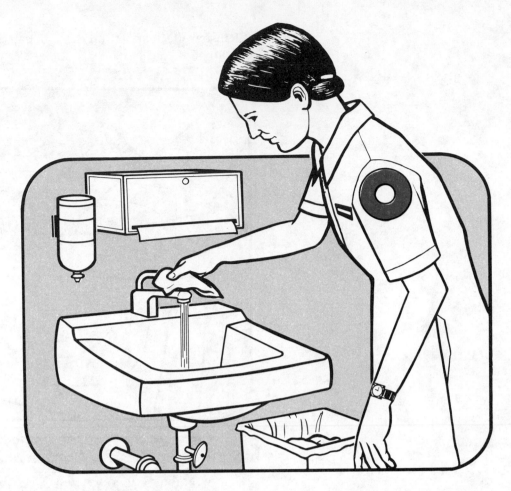

b) You rub skin against skin to create friction, which helps to eliminate microorganisms.
c) You rinse from the clean to the dirty parts of your hands. Rinse with running water from 2 inches above the wrists to hands and then to the fingertips.

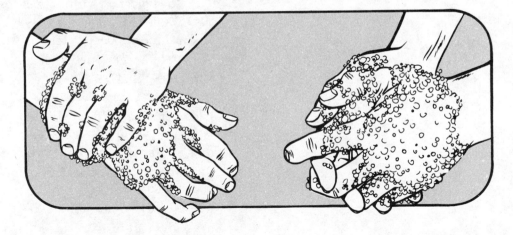

- Hold your hands lower than your elbows while washing. This is to prevent germs from contaminating your arms. Holding your hands down prevents backflow over unwashed skin.
- Have the temperature of the water comfortable for you.
- Add water to the soap while washing. This keeps the soap from becoming too dry.
- Never use the patient's soap for yourself.

- Rinse well. Soap left on the skin causes drying and can cause skin irritation.

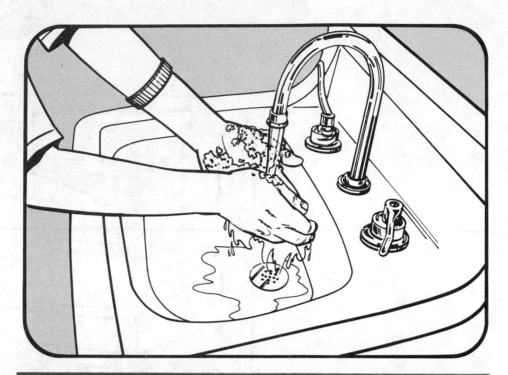

Procedure: Handwashing

1. Assemble your equipment. The equipment used for handwashing is found at all times at every sink in all health care institutions.
   a) Soap or detergent
   b) Paper towels
   c) Warm running water
   d) Wastepaper basket

2. Turn the faucet on with a paper towel held between your hands and the faucet. Adjust the water to a temperature comfortable for you.

3. Discard the paper towel in the wastepaper basket.

4. Completely wet your hands and wrists under the running water. Keep your fingertips pointed downward.

5. Apply soap or detergent.

6. Hold your hands lower than your elbows while washing.

7. Work up a good lather. Spread it over the entire area of your hands and wrists. Get soap under your nails and between your fingers.

8. Clean under your nails by rubbing your nails across the palms of your hand.

9. Use a rotating and rubbing (frictional) motion for one full minute:
   a) Rub vigorously.
   b) Rub one hand against the other hand and wrist.
   c) Rub between your fingers by interlacing them.
   d) Rub up and down to reach all skin surfaces on your hands and between your fingers.
   e) Rub the tips of your fingers against your palms to clean with friction around the nail beds.

10. Wash two inches above your wrists.

(continued next page)

11. Rinse well. Rinse from two inches above your wrists to hands. Hold your hands and fingertips down, under running water.

12. Dry thoroughly with paper towels.

13. Turn off the faucet. Use a paper towel between your hands and the faucet. Never touch the faucet with your hands, after washing.

14. Throw the paper towel into the wastepaper basket. Do not touch the basket.

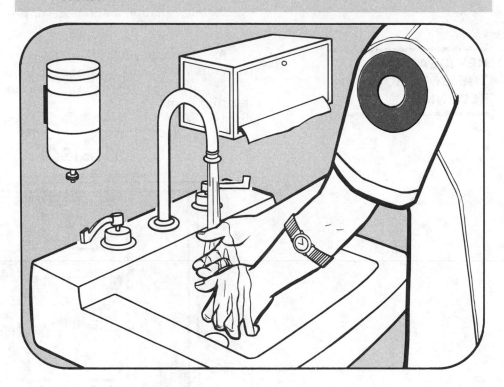

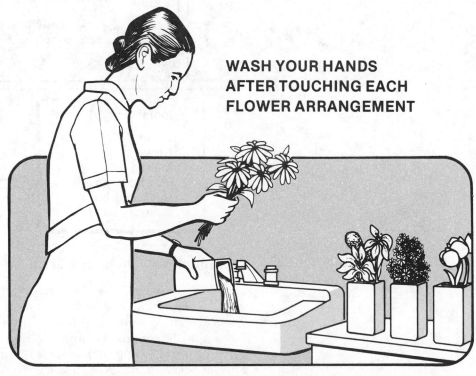

**WASH YOUR HANDS
AFTER TOUCHING EACH
FLOWER ARRANGEMENT**

SECTION 2: THE PATIENT IN ISOLATION

OBJECTIVES: WHAT YOU WILL LEARN

When you have completed this section, you will be able to:

- Demonstrate double bagging.

- Demonstrate mask and gown technique.

- Define clean and dirty.

- Explain isolation and reverse or protective isolation.

**KEY IDEAS:
THE ISOLATION
TECHNIQUE**

Aside from handwashing, special methods are used to prevent communicable diseases from spreading. Isolation technique, including use of masks and gowns, keeps disease germs away from equipment and personnel. Certain health care areas need extra precautions to prevent the spread of infection and disease.

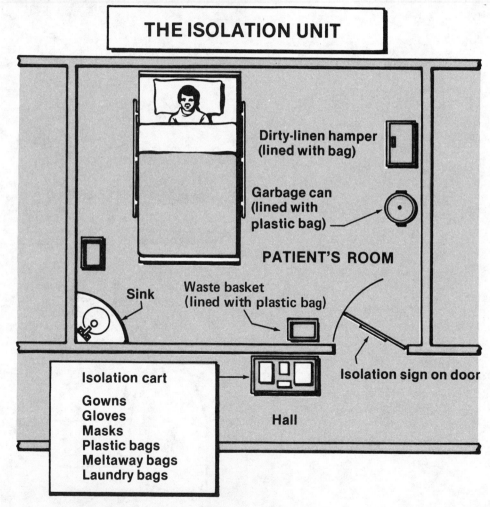

THE ISOLATION UNIT

Dirty-linen hamper (lined with bag)

Garbage can (lined with plastic bag)

PATIENT'S ROOM

Sink

Waste basket (lined with plastic bag)

Isolation cart

Gowns
Gloves
Masks
Plastic bags
Meltaway bags
Laundry bags

Isolation sign on door

Hall

Communicable Diseases and Infections

Communicable diseases spread very quickly and easily from one person to another. Examples are hepatitis and the common cold. Sometimes the more general term, communicable conditions, is used because it includes both diseases and infections. Ordinary cleanliness alone will not protect you and others from catching such diseases. When a patient has one of these diseases, special precautions are necessary. These safety measures are called isolation technique. The patient is separated (in **isolation**) from other patients and personnel.

The purpose of isolation technique is to keep the germs that cause the disease inside the isolated patient's unit. As you know, these disease germs are everywhere in the sick room. They are on the floor, furniture, bedding, articles brought to the bedside and on the patient himself. The area, the articles, and the patient are said to be contaminated. When you touch or brush your clothes against any of these, disease germs are almost sure to contaminate your hands or clothing. Isolation technique is used to prevent the germs from leaving the unit on your hands, arms, or on clothing or articles used in the unit.

The following special precautions and procedures tell you how to protect yourself from catching the patient's disease and how to avoid carrying it outside his unit to other persons.

Clean and Dirty

The words clean and dirty have a special meaning when we are talking about health care isolation technique. **Clean** means uncontaminated. It refers to those articles and places from which disease has not spread. **Dirty** means contaminated. Articles or places near the patient who has a communicable condition are dirty. These are things and areas from which disease can spread. For example, before a patient receives his meal tray, the tray is clean. After the tray has been in his room, no matter what he has or has not touched or eaten, it is dirty and can spread disease. *Clean* refers to all articles and places that have not been contaminated with or come in contact with pathogens. *Dirty* refers to those articles and places that a patient has been near or touched. They may be "dirty" or contaminated with pathogens. Consider the floor heavily contaminated (dirty). Discard or put in a hamper any item if it falls to the floor. One good way to control the spread of disease is to have two areas:

- A *clean utility room.* Things are stored or prepared here that have *never* been near or had contact with a patient or any articles belonging to the patient.

- A *dirty utility room.* Things or articles are brought here after having been in contact with the patient or with the patient's belongings.

Equipment kept in these utility rooms varies greatly from one institution to another. In most facilities there is a special area in the dirty utility room for items to be put that have to be returned to the central supply room (CSR) after having been used for a patient. Dirty linen hampers should be stored in the dirty utility room.

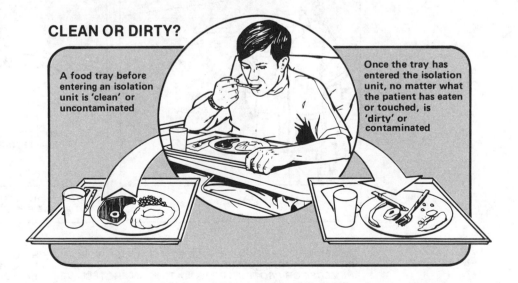

CLEAN OR DIRTY?

A food tray before entering an isolation unit is 'clean' or uncontaminated

Once the tray has entered the isolation unit, no matter what the patient has eaten or touched, is 'dirty' or contaminated

ISOLATION

PURPOSE OF ISOLATION

A HOSPITAL ISOLATES A PATIENT WITH A DISEASE THAT IS EASILY SPREAD TO REDUCE THE POSSIBILITY OF SPREADING THE DISEASE. THIS IS DONE TO PROTECT PATIENTS AND STAFF.

REGULAR ISOLATION

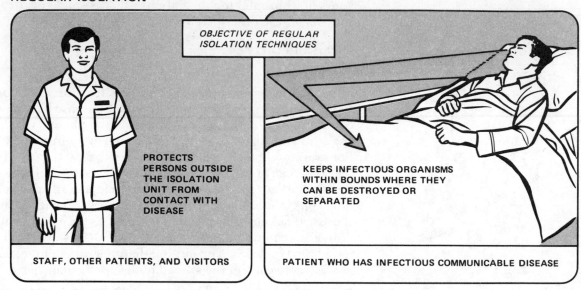

OBJECTIVE OF REGULAR ISOLATION TECHNIQUES

PROTECTS PERSONS OUTSIDE THE ISOLATION UNIT FROM CONTACT WITH DISEASE

KEEPS INFECTIOUS ORGANISMS WITHIN BOUNDS WHERE THEY CAN BE DESTROYED OR SEPARATED

STAFF, OTHER PATIENTS, AND VISITORS

PATIENT WHO HAS INFECTIOUS COMMUNICABLE DISEASE

IN REGULAR ISOLATION, CONTAMINATION IS PREVENTED FROM SPREADING FROM THE ROOM.

REVERSE OR PROTECTIVE ISOLATION

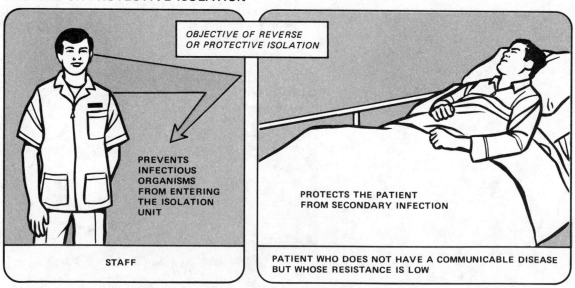

OBJECTIVE OF REVERSE OR PROTECTIVE ISOLATION

PREVENTS INFECTIOUS ORGANISMS FROM ENTERING THE ISOLATION UNIT

PROTECTS THE PATIENT FROM SECONDARY INFECTION

STAFF

PATIENT WHO DOES NOT HAVE A COMMUNICABLE DISEASE BUT WHOSE RESISTANCE IS LOW

SOMETIMES A PATIENT WHOSE RESISTANCE IS LOW AND WHO COULD EASILY CATCH A DISEASE IS ISOLATED FROM POSSIBLE INFECTIONS' THIS IS COMMONLY DONE FOR BURN PATIENTS. IT IS CALLED *REVERSE* OR *PROTECTIVE* ISOLATION. IN PROTECTIVE ISOLATION, CONTAMINATION MUST BE PREVENTED FROM ENTERING THE ROOM.

Special Areas for Preventive Measures

Certain patient care areas in the health care institution need special attention to ensure cleanliness. Precautions to prevent communicable conditions from spreading are more strict than in other areas. This is because the patients in these areas may have a low resistance to disease. However, they do not have any communicable conditions. These areas include:

- Newborn nursery
- Premature care nursery
- Postpartum patient care unit
- Surgical patient care unit (operating room)
- Delivery room
- Cardiac care unit
- Intensive care unit
- Dialysis unit

Protective Isolation Card: Color-coded Blue*

Protective Isolation

Visitors - Report to Nurses' Station Before Entering Room.

1. **Private Room**–*necessary;* door must be kept closed.
2. **Gowns**–must be worn by all persons entering room.
3. **Masks**–must be worn by all persons entering room.
4. **Hands**–must be washed on entering and leaving room.
5. **Gloves**–must be worn by all persons having direct contact with patient.
6. **Articles**–see manual text.

ONE OF THE FOLLOWING CARDS IS ALWAYS HUNG ON THE DOOR OF THE ISOLATED UNIT TO IDENTIFY THE TYPE OF ISOLATION AND TO GIVE INSTRUCTIONS TO EVERYONE ENTERING THE ISOLATED UNIT.

*Public Health Service Publication no. 2054: Isolation technique for use in hospitals. Washington, DC, U.S. Government Printing Office.

Wound & Skin Precautions
Visitors - Report to Nurses' Station
Before Entering Room

1. **Private Room**–desirable.
2. **Gowns**–must be worn by all persons having direct contact with patient.
3. **Mask**–not necessary except during dressing changes.
4. **Hands**–must be washed on entering and leaving room.
5. **Gloves**–must be worn by all persons having direct contact with infected area.
6. **Articles**–special precautions necessary for instruments, dressing, and linen.
7. **NOTE:** See manual for Special Dressing Techniques to be used when changing dressings.

*Public Health Service Publication no. 2054: Isolation technique for use in hospitals. Washington, DC, U.S. Government Printing Office

Respiratory Isolation
Visitors - Report to Nurses' Station
Before Entering Room

1. **Private Room**– *necessary;* door must be kept closed.
2. **Gowns**–not necessary.
3. **Masks**–must be worn by all persons entering room if susceptible to disease.
4. **Hands**–must be washed on entering and leaving room.
5. **Gloves**–not necessary.
6. **Articles**–those contaminated with secretions must be disinfected.
7. **Caution**–all persons susceptible to the specific disease should be excluded from patient area: if contact is necessary susceptibles must wear masks.

*Public Health Service Publication no. 2054: Isolation technique for use in hospitals. Washington, DC, U.S. Government Printing Office

Strict Isolation Card: Color-Coded Yellow*

Strict Isolation

Visitors - Report to Nurses' Station Before Entering Room

1. **Private Room**—*necessary;* door must be kept closed.
2. **Gowns**—must be worn by all persons entering room.
3. **Masks**—must be worn by all persons entering room.
4. **Hands**—must be washed on entering and leaving room.
5. **Gloves**—must be worn by all persons entering room.
6. **Articles**—must be discarded, or wrapped before being sent to Central Supply for disinfection or sterilization.

*Public Health Service Publication no. 2054: Isolation technique for use in hospitals. Washington, DC, U.S. Government Printing Office

Enteric Precautions Card: Color-Coded Brown*

Enteric Precautions

Visitors - Report to Nurses' Station Before Entering Room

1. **Private Room**—*necessary for children only.*
2. **Gowns**—must be worn by all persons having direct contact with patient.
3. **Mask**—not necessary.
4. **Hands**—must be washed on entering and leaving room.
5. **Gloves**—must be worn by all persons having direct contact with patient.
6. **Articles**—special precautions necessary for articles contaminated with urine and feces. Articles must be disinfected or discarded.

*Public Health Service Publication no. 2054: Isolation technique for use in hospitals. Washington, DC, U.S. Government Printing Office

Face Masks

When a patient's communicable condition can be spread by breathing, face masks are very important. Before you put on or take off a face mask, be sure your hands are thoroughly clean. Face masks are effective for 30 minutes only. If you stay in an isolated area longer, you must wash your hands and remove the old mask. Then wash your hands again and put on a clean mask. Masks are used only once and then thrown away. If the mask gets wet, it must be changed. Never let the face mask hang around your neck.

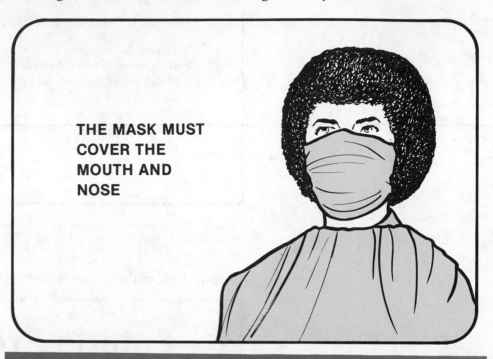

THE MASK MUST COVER THE MOUTH AND NOSE

Procedure: Mask Technique

1. Assemble your equipment: A disposable paper mask.
2. Wash your hands.
3. Remove a clean mask from its container.
4. Hold the mask firmly, avoiding unnecessary handling. Do not touch the part of the mask that will cover your face. Hold the mask by the strings only.
5. Place the mask over your nose and mouth. Tie the top strings over your ears first. Then tie the lower strings.
6. Be sure the mask covers your nose and mouth during your task or procedure with the patient.
7. When you are ready to take off the mask, wash your hands.
8. Untie the bottom ties first, to avoid contamination. Hold the mask by the strings or loops only.
9. Untie the top strings. Remove the mask from your face. Discard it in the proper container inside the patient's room.
10. Wash your hands.

KEY IDEAS: ISOLATION GOWNS

You will wear an isolation gown when you are caring for a patient in isolation. You will wear the gown if there is any possibility that your clothes could touch the patient or brush against any articles in the unit. Remember, all of this is considered contaminated. There are three types of isolation gowns:

- Cotton twill, which is reusable after proper washing.

- A paper disposable gown, which is thrown away after one use.
- A plastic disposable apron, which is worn once and thrown away.

Individual Gown Technique

This means that a gown should be used only once. It is then discarded in the proper dirty linen hamper or trash can. This is done before you leave the isolated room.

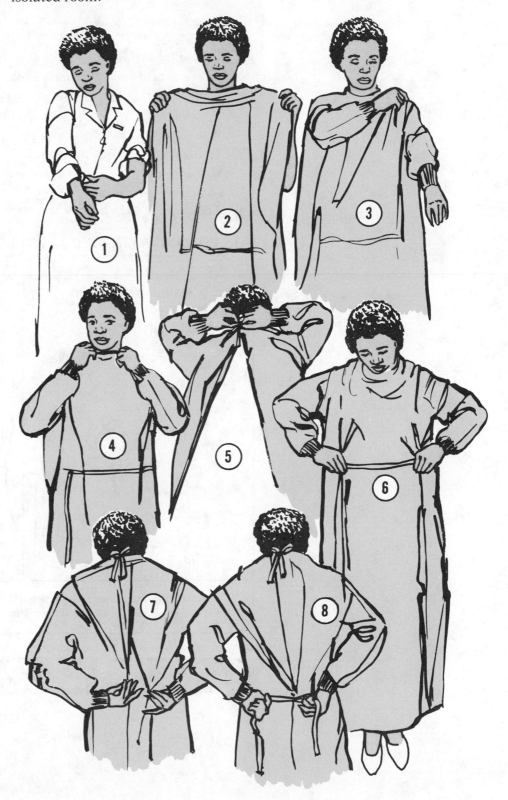

To be effective, the isolation gown must cover your uniform completely. Therefore, it is made wide enough to lap over in the back.

Put on a clean gown in the hall before you enter the patient's room. Take off the dirty gown in the patient's room before leaving the unit.

Procedure: Putting on an Isolation Gown in the Hall Before Entering the Patient's Room

1. If you are wearing a long sleeve uniform, roll your sleeves above your elbows. Wash your hands.
2. Unfold the isolation gown so the opening is at the back.
3. Put your arms into the sleeves of the isolation gown.
4. Fit the gown at the neck, making sure your uniform is covered.
5. Reach behind and tie the neck band with a simple shoelace bow or fasten adhesive strip.
6. Grasp edges of gown and pull to back.
7. Overlap edges of gown; roll gown edges together in back, completely closing the opening and covering your uniform completely.
8. Tie waist tapes in a bow, or fasten adhesive strip.

SOILED, CONTAMINATED LINEN DOUBLE-BAGGING TECHNIQUE

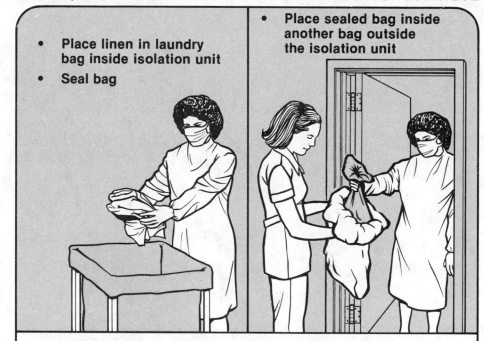

- Place linen in laundry bag inside isolation unit
- Seal bag

- Place sealed bag inside another bag outside the isolation unit

The double bag technique should be applied when removing specimens, linen, trash and other contaminated articles from the isolation room.

Procedure: Removing an Isolation Gown Inside the Patient's Room Before Leaving the Unit

1. Untie the waist tapes and loosen the gown.
2. If you are not wearing gloves:
   a) Use a paper towel to turn on the faucet. Do not touch the faucet with your hands.

(continued next page)

Procedure continued

b) Throw the paper towel into the wastepaper basket.
c) Wash your hands and dry them with a paper towel.
d) With a dry paper towel, turn off the faucet.

3. If you are wearing disposable gloves, remove them and discard.

4. Open the neck band of the isolation gown.

5. Remove gown by rolling it away from yourself into a ball.

6. Roll the gown with the contaminated portion inside.

7. If the gown is washable, put it in the dirty linen hamper inside the patient's room. If the gown is disposable, place it in the trash container inside the patient's room.

8. Wash your hands, using paper towels to turn on the faucet and to turn off the faucet.

9. Remove face mask.

10. Wash your hands.

11. Use a paper towel to open the door to leave the room. Put the towel into the wastepaper basket inside the patient's room as you leave.

KEY IDEAS: PERSONAL CARE OF THE PATIENT IN ISOLATION

The patient in isolation needs the same personal care as any other patient. It is very important to combine normal patient care with good isolation technique. These tasks should be performed in your usual pleasant and supportive style. Make it clear that it is the disease-causing microorganisms that are unwanted and not the patient. You will make continuous observations to note any pattern of change in the patient's appearance or behavior.

The Nursing Assistant's Watch

When a gown and gloves are to be worn, the nursing assistant must be prepared to use a watch without contaminating it or oneself. Before entering the patient's room the nursing assistant places the wrist watch on a clean piece of paper towel. On entering the patient's room the paper towel with the watch must be placed so that the assistant can read it easily without touching it. The nursing assistant must wash her hands before picking up the watch when leaving the isolated unit. Some hospitals have a policy that central ser-

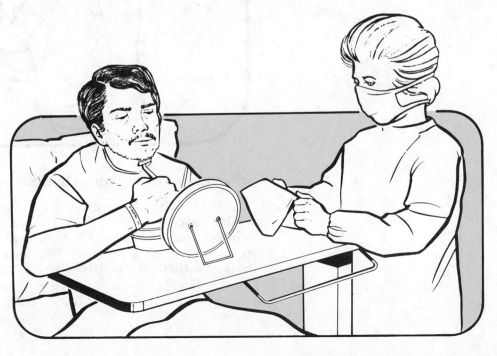

vice provides a watch in a plastic covering, which stays inside the patient's room for the entire isolation period. Follow your institution's policy regarding a watch in an isolation unit.

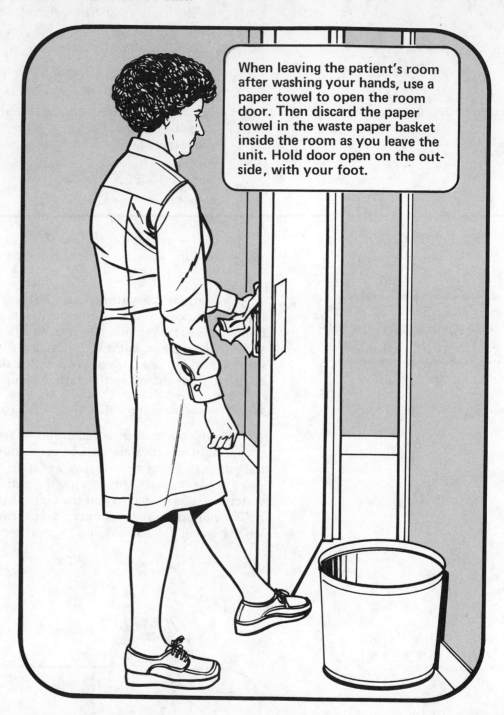

When leaving the patient's room after washing your hands, use a paper towel to open the room door. Then discard the paper towel in the waste paper basket inside the room as you leave the unit. Hold door open on the outside, with your foot.

Serving Food to the Patient in Isolation

Many health care institutions do not require you to wear a gown when serving meals to patients in isolation. If you are serving a patient, be careful that your uniform does not become contaminated. You must wear a gown if you feed a patient or stay with him during his meal to help him eat. Food for the isolated patient should be served in disposable dishes on a disposable tray. Uneaten food is considered to be contaminated. Scraps are disposed of in a trash container inside the patient's room.

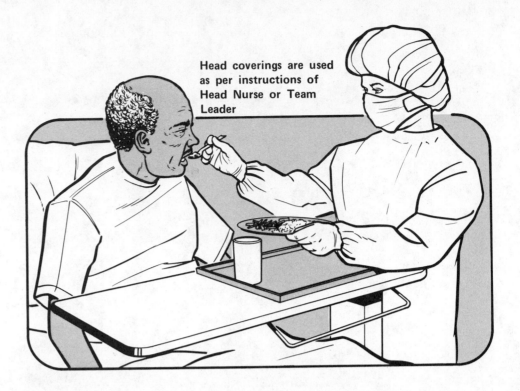

Head coverings are used as per instructions of Head Nurse or Team Leader

Handling the Contaminated Articles of the Patient in Isolation

For some patients in isolation it is necessary to take special precautions with articles contaminated by urine or feces. For example, it may be necessary to disinfect (or discard) a bedpan and excreta. Follow your health care institution's procedure and the instructions of your head nurse or team leader.

WHAT YOU HAVE LEARNED

Diseases are caused by microorganisms. The spread of pathogens is reduced by keeping everything clean. Being extra careful to avoid contamination is a way of keeping the environment safe.

Isolation technique is especially important. Each step in every isolation procedure must be done carefully.

Washing your hands before and after contact with patients is the best example of protection for health care personnel as well as for patients.

5 YOUR WORKING ENVIRONMENT

1. The Patient's Unit and Equipment
2. Bedmaking
3. Safety and Fire Prevention

SECTION 1: THE PATIENT'S UNIT AND EQUIPMENT

OBJECTIVES: WHAT YOU WILL LEARN

When you have completed this section you will be able to:

- Describe the patient's unit.
- Check the unit.
- Define disposable equipment.
- List the equipment contained in the unit.
- Identify and describe the purpose of each piece of equipment.

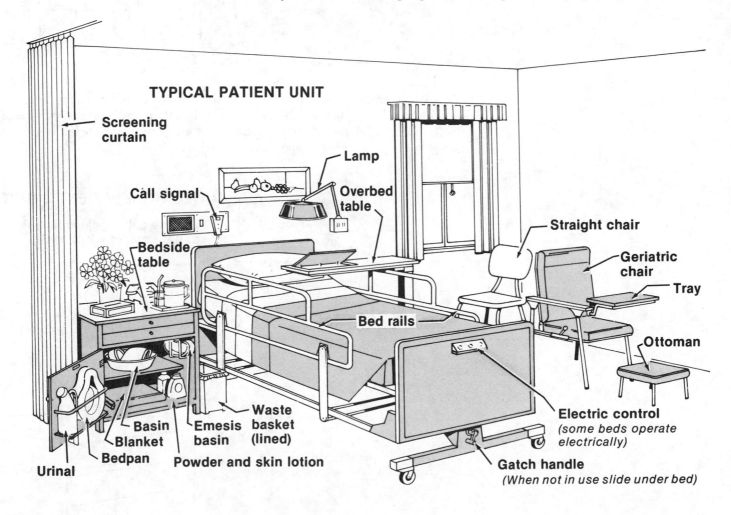

TYPICAL PATIENT UNIT

Screening curtain

Call signal

Lamp

Overbed table

Bedside table

Straight chair

Geriatric chair

Tray

Bed rails

Ottoman

Basin
Blanket
Bedpan

Emesis basin

Waste basket (lined)

Powder and skin lotion

Electric control *(some beds operate electrically)*

Urinal

Gatch handle *(When not in use slide under bed)*

A patient's unit consists of all of the room space, furniture, and equipment provided by the hospital for one patient. Each unit can be screened off for privacy by movable screens or draw curtains.

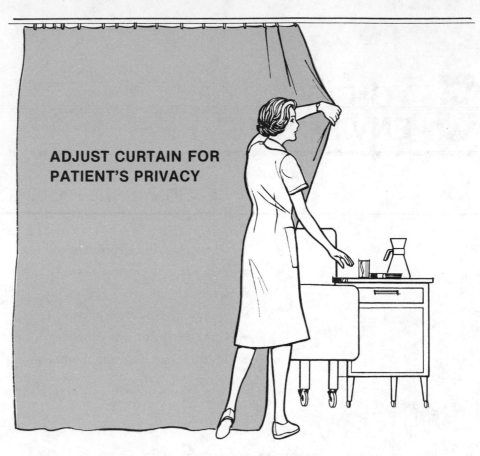

**ADJUST CURTAIN FOR
PATIENT'S PRIVACY**

After a patient has been assigned to the unit for which you are responsible, make sure everything that belongs in the unit is there and in its proper place. If the patient is left handed, put the table and signal cord near the left hand; if the patient is right handed, place them near the right hand.

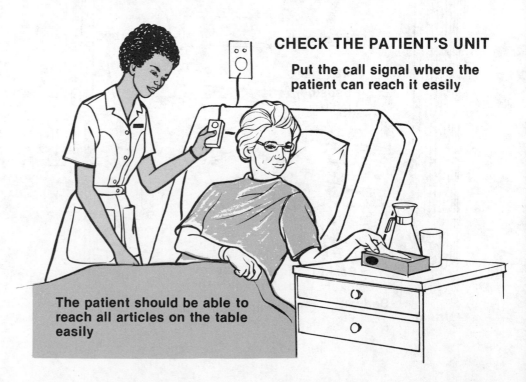

CHECK THE PATIENT'S UNIT

Put the call signal where the patient can reach it easily

The patient should be able to reach all articles on the table easily

A hospital unit designed for children may be different from an adult unit. A child's age and the reason he is in the hospital will determine how his unit is arranged and the equipment that will be needed.

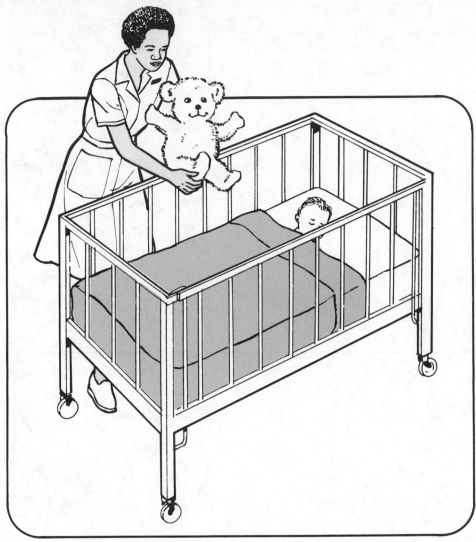

Today in most health care institutions, standard equipment has been replaced by disposable equipment. Standard equipment requires washing, disinfecting, and sterilizing. Disposable equipment needs almost no care and is usually prepackaged. It may be made of plastic, styrofoam, or paper. Some of this equipment is used only one time and then thrown away. Other disposable equipment may be used several times for one patient only, being cleaned between uses, and thrown away when the patient is discharged.

Nursing assistants usually get disposable equipment from the Central Supply Room (CSR) as needed. Central supply may also be called Special Purchasing Department (SPD) or Central Supply Department (CSD). This is a central place for storing supplies and equipment. You will need a requisition slip to get equipment from CSR.

Equipment

The modern health care institution has many pieces of large equipment needed for patient care and treatment. This equipment might include:

● *Intravenous poles*. These are often called IV poles, IV standards, or a stan-

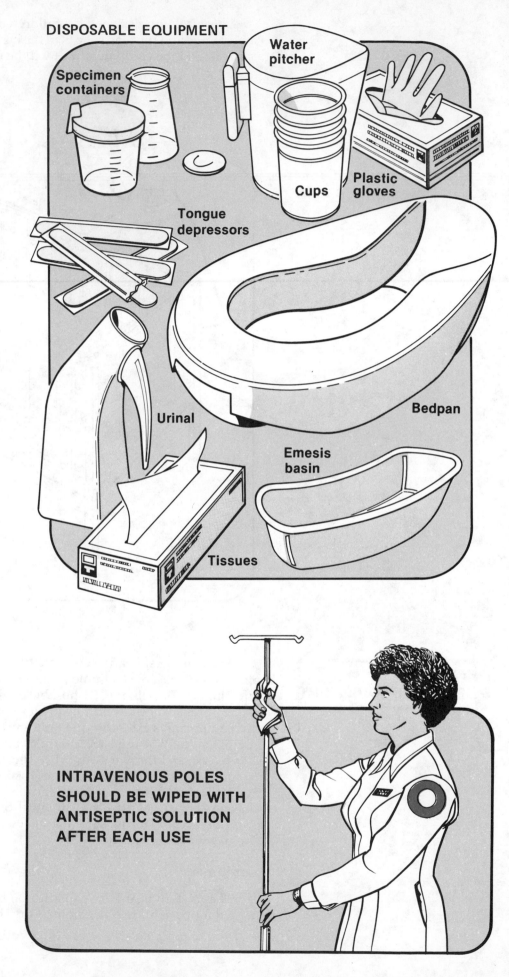

DISPOSABLE EQUIPMENT

Specimen containers

Water pitcher

Cups

Plastic gloves

Tongue depressors

Urinal

Bedpan

Emesis basin

Tissues

INTRAVENOUS POLES SHOULD BE WIPED WITH ANTISEPTIC SOLUTION AFTER EACH USE

dard. These support the containers or tubes used in various treatments. Some IV poles are on casters or rollers for easy movement. Other IV poles fit right into the bed frame.

- *Portable patient lift.* A mechanical device used to move the patient from bed to chair and back again. It is used when the patient needs full assistance.
- *Bed cradle.* This cradle looks like a half barrel cut the long way. It is used to cover a part of the patient's body where he is having great pain, so as to support the weight of the bedspread and top sheet, to eliminate additional pain in the area, or when you do not want anything to touch that area.

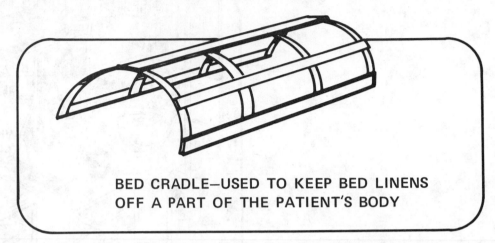

BED CRADLE—USED TO KEEP BED LINENS OFF A PART OF THE PATIENT'S BODY

- *Heat cradle.* The heat cradle is the same as a regular bed cradle, but it has an electric light in it. It acts as a heat lamp. The heat cradle is sometimes ordered alone (dry). Sometimes it is ordered when the patient is having continuous warm compresses applied to an arm or leg. Here the purpose would be to keep the compress warm.
- *Wheelchair.* This is a chair with wheels used to transport patients.
- *Stretcher.* This is a narrow table on wheels used to transport patients. Also called a litter or gurney.
- *Walker.* The walker is an aluminum frame used by the patient to help himself to walk.
- *Air or rubber rings.* These look like small inner tubes. They are used to relieve pressure on the lower back or buttocks. The rings are used in the treatment or prevention of pressure areas.
- *Alternating-pressure (A-P) mattress.* A device like an air mattress placed beneath the bedridden or elderly patient. It reduces pressure on the shoulders, back, heels, and elbows.
- *Roto-Rest Bed.* Used to eliminate pressure points and prevent bedsores.
- *Bed-board.* A large board placed beneath the mattress to provide additional support for patients with back muscle or bone problems.
- *Binders.* These are strips of heavy cotton cloth. Binders are wrapped securely around the patient's body over the abdomen to give support and comfort after abdominal surgery. Binders are also used to give support to female patients' breasts or abdomen after childbirth.
- *Foot-board.* This is a small board placed upright at the foot of the bed and used to keep the patient's feet aligned properly to prevent foot drop.
- *Lamb's wool.* Wide strips of lamb's wool cloth (or soft synthetic materials) used to relieve pressure in treatment or prevention of bedsores.
- *Protective devices.* Devices, usually of cotton, used to restrain a patient's arms, legs, or body to prevent him from injuring himself.

EQUIPMENT

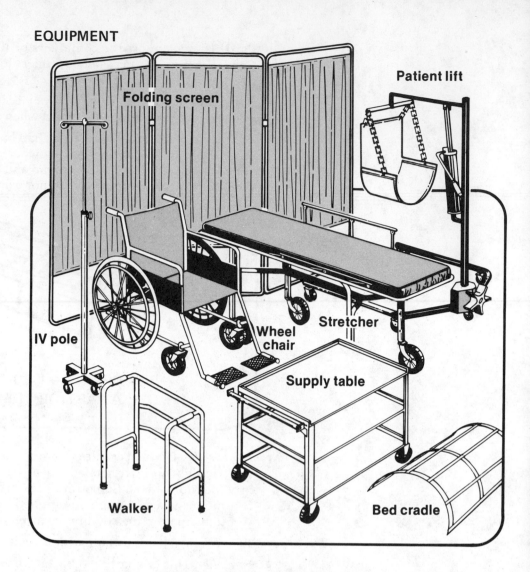

Folding screen

Patient lift

IV pole

Wheel chair

Stretcher

Walker

Supply table

Bed cradle

SECTION 2: BEDMAKING

OBJECTIVES: WHAT YOU WILL LEARN

   When you have completed this section, you will be able to:

- Make the closed bed.
- Make the open fan-folded or empty bed.
- Make the operating room bed (OR, stretcher, post-operative bed, surgical bed, recovery room bed).
- Make the occupied bed.

**KEY IDEAS:
BEDMAKING**

   Patients spend most of their time in bed. Some patients are unable or not permitted to get out of bed. As a result of this, many patients are fed, bathed, and use a bedpan in bed. Therefore, it is important to make the patient's bed with great care.

   Nursing assistants should make beds without any wrinkles in the sheets. Wrinkles are not only uncomfortable but restrict the patient's circulation and can cause painful bedsores **(decubitus ulcers)**. Making the bed carefully is very important to the patient's comfort and well being.

Four Basic Beds

- *The Closed Bed:*
  This bed is made after environmental service personnel have cleaned the unit following a patient's discharge. The bed is made up CLOSED so it will stay clean until a new patient is assigned to it.

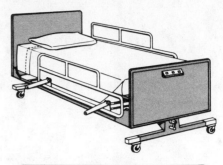

- *The Open Bed:*
  When a patient is assigned to a unit, the closed bed is made into an open bed by fan-folding the top sheets down.

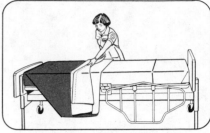

- *The Occupied Bed:*
  Sometimes a patient is completely bedridden. Complete bed rest (CBR) is the way it appears on the record of activities of daily living. The bed must be made with the patient in the bed.

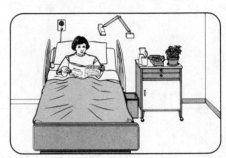

- *The Postoperative Bed:*
  This also may be called the OR, surgical, recovery, or stretcher bed. A special method is used to make this bed for a patient who is returning to the unit after surgery.

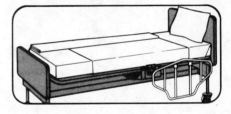

Rules to Follow: Bedmaking

- Return torn linen to a "repair box" in the linen closet for repair. Never use a torn piece of linen. It will probably tear even more and could be dangerous.
- Never use a pin on any item of linen.
- Never use bed linen for any purpose other than that for which it was intended.
- Report to the head nurse or team leader if you see patients or visitors trying to remove articles of linen from the unit for any reason.
- Most health care institutions that use wool blankets have special rules for their use. Be sure to learn and follow these rules at all times.
- Many health care institutions make the bed without the blanket or bedspread. However, the nursing assistant making the bed may leave a folded blanket at the foot of the bed to be used later, if needed.
- Do not shake the bed linen. Shaking would spread germs to everything and everyone in the room, including you.
- Never bring extra linen into a patient unit. It is considered contaminated (or dirty) and cannot be used elsewhere.

- Never allow any linen to touch your uniform.
- Dirty used linen should never be put on the floor.
- In most health care institutions the linen hamper is in the dirty utility room.
- Some health care institutions use melt-away plastic bags for laundry bags. These bags dissolve during the washing process. The dirty linen is put into these bags at the patient's bedside. Then it is carried to the dirty laundry hamper.
- Some health care institutions today use fitted bottom sheets. Others still use flat sheets where the nursing assistant makes the mitered corners. A mitered corner is also called a hospital corner. The mitered corner keeps the sheets firm and smooth and makes the bed neat and attractive.
- The bottom sheet must be firm and smooth under the patient. This is very important for the patient's comfort. Always make sure that the bottom sheet is tight and unwrinkled.
- By fan-folding the top of the bed you make it easy for the patient to get back into his bed.
- The cotton draw sheet is about half the size of a regular sheet. When cotton draw sheets are not available, a large sheet can be folded in half widthwise (with small and large hems together) and used to cover plastic draw sheets. The fold must always be placed toward the head of the bed and the hems toward the foot of the bed.
- Plastic should never touch a patient's skin. When using a plastic draw sheet, be sure to cover it entirely with a cotton draw sheet.
- The plastic draw sheet and disposable bed protectors protect the mattress.
- Some health care institutions do not use a draw sheet at all. Instead, small disposable bed protectors are placed on the bed under the patient as necessary.
- Bottom of the bed refers to the mattress pad, if used, the bottom sheet, and the draw sheets.
- Top of the bed refers to the top sheet, blanket, if used, and bedspread.
- Remember that you save time and energy by first making as much of the bed as possible on one side before going to the other side.

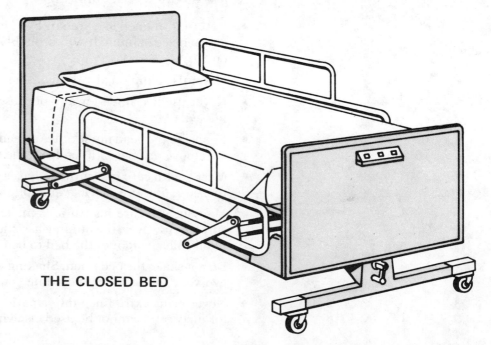

THE CLOSED BED

Procedure: Making the Closed Bed

1. Assemble your equipment: Mattress cover, if used in your institution, bottom sheet, cotton and plastic draw-sheet (or disposable bed protector), top sheet, blanket, bedspread, pillowcase, pillow, and pillow protector, if used in your institution.

2. Wash your hands.

3. Place a chair near the bed.

4. Put the pillow on the chair.

5. Stack the bedmaking linen items on the chair in the order that you will use them. First things to be used on top, last things to be used on the bottom.

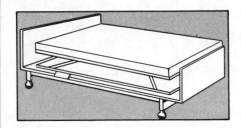

6. Adjust the bed to its highest horizontal position. Lock the bed in place.

7. Pull the mattress to the head of the bed, until it touches the headboard.

8. Place the mattress pad on the mattress even with the head edge of the mattress, if used by your health care institution.

9. Fold the bottom sheet lengthwise and place it on the bed:

   a) Place the center fold of the sheet at the center of the mattress from head to foot.

   b) Put the small hem at the foot of the bed, even with the edge of the mattress.

   c) Place the large hem to the head of the bed.

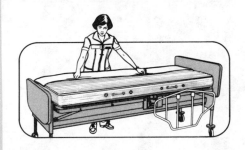

10. Open the sheet. It should now hang evenly the same distance over each side of the bed. The rough edges of the hem are now facing down toward the mattress, and away from the patient.

11. There should be 18 inches of the sheet to tuck smoothly under the head of the mattress. Tuck it in tightly.

    (continued next page)

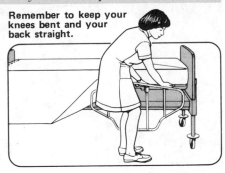

Remember to keep your knees bent and your back straight.

Procedure continued

12. To make a mitered corner:

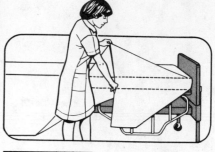

a) Pick up the edge of the sheet at the side of the bed 12 inches from the head of the mattress.

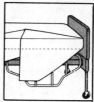

b) Place the triangle (the folded corner) on top of the mattress.

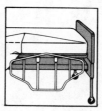

c) Tuck the hanging portion of the sheet under the mattress.

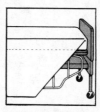

d) While you hold the fold at the edge of the mattress, bring the triangle down over the side of the mattress.

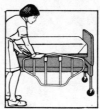

e) Tuck the sheet under the mattress from head to foot.

13. Stand and work entirely on one side of the bed until that side is finished.

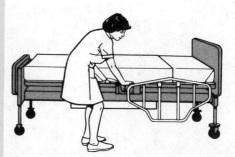

14. Place the plastic draw sheet 14 inches (two open hand spans) down from the head of the bed. Tuck it in.

(continued next page)

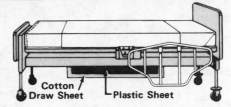

15. Cover the plastic draw sheet with the cotton draw sheet, and tuck it in.

16. Fold the top sheet lengthwise and place it on the bed:
    a) Place the center fold on the center of the bed from the head to foot.
    b) Put the large hem at the head of the bed, even with the top edge of the mattress.
    c) Open the sheet, with the rough edge of the hem up.
    d) Tightly tuck the sheet under at the foot of the bed.
    e) Make a mitered corner at the foot of the bed.
    f) Do not tuck in at the side of the bed.

17. Fold the blanket lengthwise and place on the bed.
    a) Place the center fold of the blanket on the center of the bed from head to foot.
    b) Place the upper hem 6 inches from the top edge of the mattress.
    c) Open the blanket.
    d) Tuck it under the foot tightly.
    e) Make a mitered corner at the foot of the bed.
    f) Do not tuck in at the sides of the bed.

18. Fold the bedspread lengthwise and place it on the bed.
    a) Place the center fold on the center of the bed from head to foot.
    b) Place the upper hem even with the head edge of the mattress.
    c) Have the rough edge down.
    d) Open the spread.
    e) Tuck it under at the foot of the bed tightly.
    f) Make a mitered corner at the foot of the bed.
    g) Do not tuck in at the sides of the bed.

19. Now go to the other side of the bed. Start with the bottom sheet.

    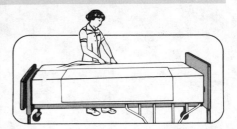

    a) Pull the sheet tight to get rid of all wrinkles.
    b) Miter the top corner.
    c) Pull the plastic draw sheet tight and tuck it in.

    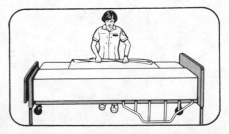

    d) Pull the cotton draw sheet tight and tuck it in.

(continued next page)

Procedure continued

e) Straighten out the top sheet, making the mitered corner at the foot of the bed.

f) Miter the corner of the blanket.

g) Miter the corner of the bedspread.

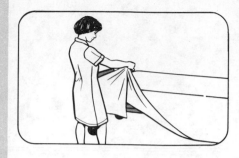

20. To make the cuff:

a) Fold the top hem of the spread under the top hem of the blanket.

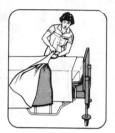

b) Fold the top hem of the sheet back over the edge of the spread and the blanket to form a cuff. The hemmed side of the sheet must be on the underside, so it does not come in contact with the patient.

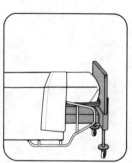

21. To put the pillowcase on a pillow:

a) Hold the pillowcase at the center of the end seam.

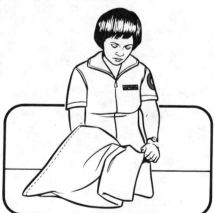

b) With your hand outside of the case, turn the case back over your hand.

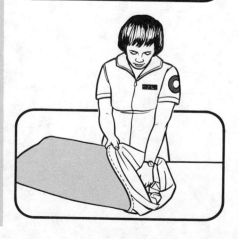

(continued next page)

Procedure continued

c) Grasp the pillow through the case at the center of one end of the pillow.

d) Bring the case down over the pillow.

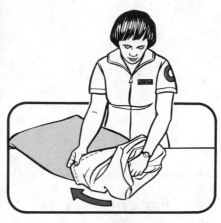

e) Fit the corner of the pillow into the seamless corner of the case.

f) Fold the extra material from the side seam under the pillow.

g) Place the pillow on the bed with the open end away from the door.

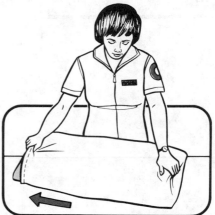

22. Adjust bed to its lowest horizontal position.

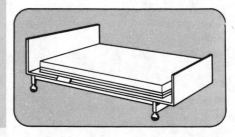

**KEY IDEAS:
THE OPEN BED,
FAN-FOLDED BED,
EMPTY BED**

The procedures for making the open bed, the fan-folded bed, and the empty bed are all the same. You will open the bed when a new patient has been assigned to a unit. You will be making an open bed when a unit is already occupied but the patient is able to get out of bed and move around while you are arranging the unit.

The open bed is made exactly like the closed bed except for one thing: The top bedding is opened so that the patient can easily get into bed.

This is done after you finish making the cuff at the head of the bed.

Procedure: Making the Open, Fan-Folded Empty Bed

1. Assemble your equipment:
   A closed bed.
2. Wash your hands.
3. Grasp the cuff of the bedding in both hands.
4. Pull it to the foot of the bed.
   (continued next page)

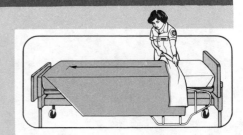

Procedure continued

5. Fold the bedding back on itself toward the head of the bed. The edge of the cuff must meet the fold.

6. Smooth the hanging sheets on each side neatly into folds you have made.

7. Wash your hands.

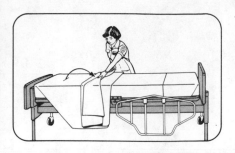

KEY IDEAS: THE OPERATING ROOM BED

The operating room bed is also known as the postoperative bed, or the stretcher bed, or sometimes the recovery bed.

The operating room bed is used by patients returning from the postoperative recovery room or the post delivery recovery room. The patient is brought in on a stretcher. The stretcher will be lined up alongside of the bed to allow the transfer of the patient from the stretcher to the bed. Some institutions make this bed with blankets, others do not. Be sure you follow the policy of the institution that employs you.

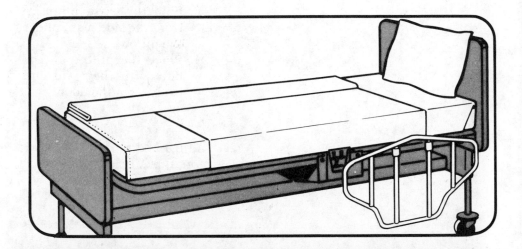

Procedure: Making the Operating Room Bed or Stretcher Bed

1. Assemble your equipment on a chair in the unit:

   a) Mattress cover, if used in your institution.
   b) Bottom sheet.
   c) Plastic draw sheet, if used in your facility.
   d) Cotton draw sheet, if used in your facility.
   e) Top sheet.
   f) Blanket.
   g) Pillowcase.
   h) Pillow.
   i) Bedspread.
   j) Two cotton bath blankets.
   k) Plastic laundry bag.
   l) Pillow protector, if used in your institution.

2. Wash your hands.

3. Strip all used linen from the bed and place in the plastic laundry bag.

4. Make the bottom part of the bed. Follow the instructions for making a closed bed.

(continued next page)

5. Spread one bath blanket across the bed, on top of the draw sheet and bottom sheet. The bottom end of the bath blanket should be even with the foot of the mattress. Tuck the edge under the mattress on your side of the bed. Blankets are not used by every health care institution. Use only if applicable to your facility.

6. Go to the other side of the bed. Tuck the bath blanket under the mattress.

7. Spread the second bath blanket across the bed. The upper edge should be about 6 inches from the head of the bed. This blanket gives the patient extra warmth.

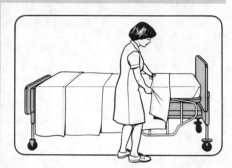

8. Put the top sheet, the regular blanket, and the spread on the bed. Do this the same way as when making the closed bed. But do not tuck them in at the foot of the bed. Instead, all the bedding at the foot end should be folded back on the bed so the folded edge is even with the foot of the mattress.

9. Make the cuff the same as the open bed, except you fold the blanket over the cuff.

10. Go to the side of the bed where the stretcher will be in place.

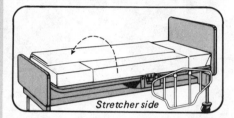

11. Grasp the top bedding at the side with both hands. Fold the bedding across the bed so the folded edge is even with the far side of the mattress.

Again, fold the bedding to the edge so it is twice folded onto itself.

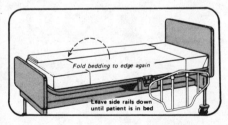

12. Put the pillow into the pillow case. Put the pillow upright against the headboard. Place it so as to protect the patient from hitting his head on the headboard during the transfer procedure. When appropriate you will place this pillow under the patient's head.

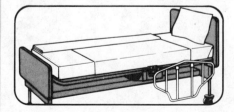

13. Move the bedside table, the chair, and any other furniture out of the way to make room for the stretcher.

14. Remove everything from the bedside table except a box of tissues and an emesis basin.

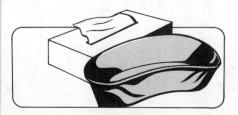

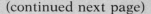

(continued next page)

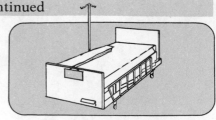

.15. Bring an IV standard into the
room and place near the head
of the bed, out of the way.

16. Wash your hands.

KEY IDEAS: THE OCCUPIED BED

The occupied bed is made when the patient is not able or not permitted to get out of bed. The most important part of making an occupied bed is to get the sheets smooth and tight under the patient, so there will be no wrinkles to rub against the patient's skin. When making the bottom of this bed, your job will be easier if you divide the bed in two parts—the side the patient is lying on and the side you are making, so the weight of the patient is never on the side where you are working. Always keep the side rail up on the patient's side. Usually the occupied bed is made after giving the patient a bed bath. The patient should be covered with the bath blanket while you are making the bed. The sheets must be placed on the bed so the rough seam edges are kept facing the mattress and away from the patient's skin.

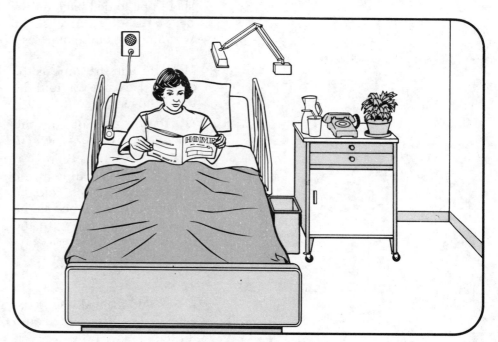

Some institutions do not use plastic draw sheets covered by cotton sheets. Instead they use disposable bed protectors, to protect the linen from getting dirty or wet. When the health care institution uses a plastic sheet covered with a draw sheet, the nursing assistant decides if the plastic sheet needs to be changed or if it can be used again according to institution policy. Usually the plastic sheet is removed and replaced with a clean one, if it is dirty or wet. If the plastic sheet does not need to be changed, follow steps # 17, 18, 23, 24, 29, and 30. If you are removing the dirty sheets from the bed of an incontinent patient, simply protect the mattress by rolling the dirty wet sheets up toward the patient's back, and place a disposable bed protector around them to keep the wetness from coming through while you are making the bed. For institutions that do not use draw sheets, omit steps # 17, 18, 23, 24, 29, and 30.

Some patients prefer the pillow to be moved with them from side to side as the bed is being made and some patients ask you to remove the pillow while making the bed. Either way is acceptable for the average patient. However, there may be instances when your head nurse or team leader instructs you to keep the patient flat in bed, elevated with a pillow, or in Fowler's position at all times. The nursing assistant must follow the instructions given by the head nurse or team leader.

Procedure: Making the Occupied Bed

1. Assemble your equipment on a chair in the unit:
   a) Two large sheets
   b) One plastic draw sheet, if used
   c) One cotton draw sheet, if used
   d) Disposable bed protectors, if used
   e) One bath blanket
   f) Pillowcase
   g) One warm blanket
   h) One bedspread
   i) One plastic laundry bag (or whatever container is used in your institution for the dirty linen in the patient's room)

2. Wash your hands.

3. Identify the patient by checking the identification bracelet.

4. Ask all visitors to step out of the room.

5. Tell the patient you are going to make the bed.

6. Pull the curtain around the bed for privacy.

7. Place a chair near the bed.

8. Place the clean linens on the chair in the order in which you will use them. That is, the last item to be put on the bed should be on the bottom of the stack.

9. Lower the backrest and kneerest until the bed is flat, if that is allowed. Raise the bed to its highest horizontal position and lock in place.

10. Loosen all the sheets around the entire bed.

11. Take the bedspread and warm blanket off the bed and fold them over the back of the chair, leaving the patient covered only with the top sheet.

12. Cover the patient with the bath blanket, by placing it over the top sheet. Ask the patient to hold the bath blanket. If the patient is unable to do this, tuck the top edges of the bath blanket under the patient's shoulders. Without exposing the patient, remove the top sheet from under the bath blanket. Fold the top sheet and place over the back of the chair.

13. If the mattress has slipped out of place, move it to its proper position touching the headboard. Ask another nursing assistant to help, if necessary.

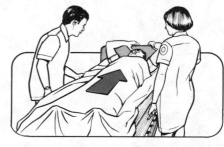

14. Raise the bedside rail on the opposite side from where you will be working and lock in place.

15. Ask the patient to turn onto his side toward the side rail. Help the patient to turn, if necessary. The patient is now on the far side of the bed.

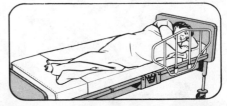

(continued next page)

16. Adjust the pillow for the patient according to instructions. (If the patient cannot sit up, lock arms with him and raise him, to remove the pillow. If you are leaving the pillow under the patient's head, then move it over to the side of the bed, adjusting it so that it is comfortable).

17. Fold the cotton draw sheet toward the patient and tuck it against his back.

18. Raise the plastic draw sheet (if it is clean) over the bath blanket and the patient.

19. Fold the bottom sheet toward the patient and tuck it against his back. This strips your side of the bed down to the mattress.

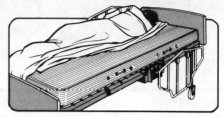

20. Take the large clean sheet and fold it in half lengthwise. Do not permit the sheet to touch the floor or your uniform.

21. Place it on the bed, still folded, with the fold running along the middle of the mattress. The small hem end of the sheet should be even with the foot edge of the mattress. Fold the top half of the sheet toward the patient. Tuck the folds against his back, below the plastic draw sheet.

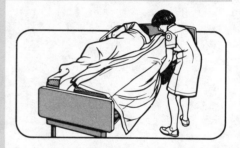

22. Miter the corner at the head of the mattress. Tuck in the clean bottom sheet on your side from head to foot of the mattress.

23. Pull the plastic draw sheet toward you, over the clean bottom sheet, and tuck in.

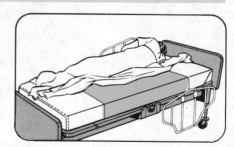

24. Place the clean cotton draw sheet over the plastic sheet, folded in half. Fold the top half toward the patient, tucking the folds under his back, as you did with the bottom sheet. Tuck the draw sheet under the mattress.

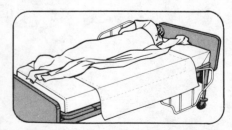

(continued next page)

25. Raise the bedside rail on your side of the bed, and lock in place.

26. Go to the opposite side of the bed.

27. Lower the bedside rail. Ask the patient, or help him, to roll over the "hump" onto the clean sheets toward you.

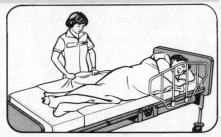

28. Remove the old bottom sheet and cotton draw sheet from the bed. Pull the fresh bottom sheet toward the edge of the bed. Tuck it under the mattress at the head of the bed and make a mitered corner. Then tuck the bottom sheet under the mattress from the head to the foot.

29. Pull the plastic draw sheet and clean cotton draw sheet toward you.

30. Then, one at a time, tuck the draw sheets under the mattress along the side.

31. Be sure to pull all the sheets tight as you tuck them in.

32. Have the patient turn on his back, or turn him yourself.

33. Change the pillowcase and place the pillow under the patient's head. If necessary, lock arms with the patient and raise him to place the pillow under his head.

34. Spread the clean top sheet over the bath blanket with the wide hem to the top. The middle of the sheet should run along the middle of the bed. The wide hem should be even with the head edge of the mattress. Ask the patient to hold the hem of the clean sheet, if he can, while you remove the bath blanket, moving toward the foot of the bed, without exposing the patient.

35. Tuck the clean top sheet under the mattress at the foot of the bed. Make sure you leave enough room for the patient to move his feet freely. Miter the corner of the sheet.

36. Spread the blanket over the top sheet. Be sure the middle of the blanket runs along the middle of the bed. The blanket should be high enough to cover the patient's shoulders.

37. Tuck the blanket in at the foot of the bed. Make a mitered corner with the blanket.

38. Place the spread on the bed in the same way. Make a mitered corner with the spread.

39. Go to the other side of the bed, turn the top covers back and miter the top sheet, then miter the blanket, then miter the spread. Be sure the top covers are loose enough for the patient to move his feet.

40. To make the cuff:
    a) Fold the top hem edge of the spread over and under the top hem of the blanket.
    b) Fold the top hem of the top sheet back over the edge of the spread and blanket to form a cuff. The rough edge of the hem of the sheet must be turned down so the patient does not come in contact with it.

(continued next page)

41. Raise the backrest and kneerest to suit the patient, if this is allowed.
42. Lower the entire bed to its lowest horizontal position.
43. Place the signal cord where the patient can easily reach it.
44. Put used linen in the plastic laundry bag and place in hamper.
45. Make the patient comfortable.
46. Wash your hands.
47. Report to your head nurse or team leader:
    - That you have made the occupied bed.
    - Report your observations of anything unusual.

SECTION 3: SAFETY AND FIRE PREVENTION

OBJECTIVES: WHAT YOU WILL LEARN

When you have completed this section, you will be able to:

- List the general rules of institutional safety.
- Describe the special safety precautions necessary when oxygen is being used.
- Explain what you can do to prevent fires.
- Explain what to do in case of fire.

**KEY IDEAS:
SAFETY AND FIRE
PREVENTION**

Patients are handicapped by illness, disabilities, worries, and medications. Many of them cannot take care of themselves in an emergency. Patients must be looked after and protected in an emergency. Therefore, health care personnel must be especially careful to guard against accidents, to prevent fires and other kinds of emergencies, and to know what to do if an emergency arises.

Rules to Follow: Safety Measures

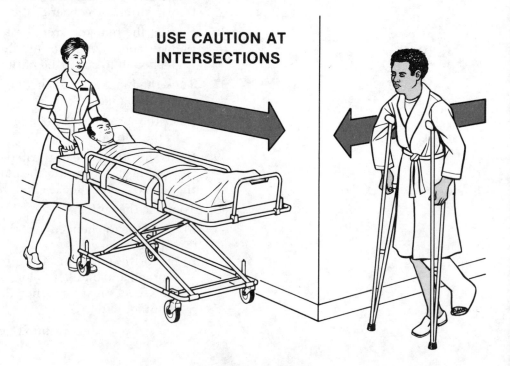

USE CAUTION AT INTERSECTIONS

- During an emergency such as a fire or tornado, move the helpless (non-ambulatory) patient on his bed to an area of safety.
- Report immediately any unsafe conditions you may notice.

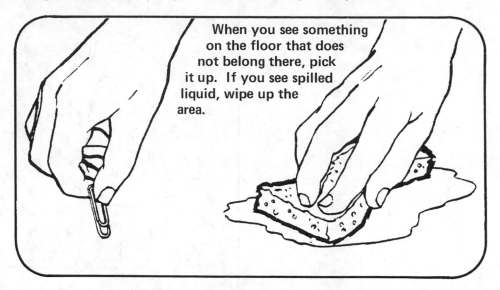

When you see something on the floor that does not belong there, pick it up. If you see spilled liquid, wipe up the area.

WATCH OUT FOR SWINGING DOORS

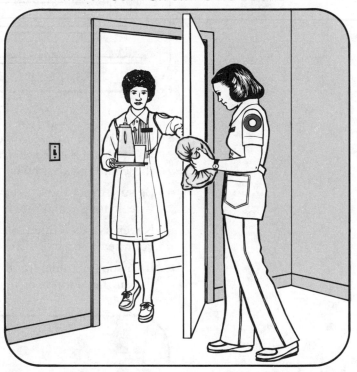

- If you are injured, even slightly, report this and get first aid immediately.
- Walk, never run, especially in halls or on stairs. Keep to the right. Use the handrails on stairways and avoid collisions. Take special care at intersections.

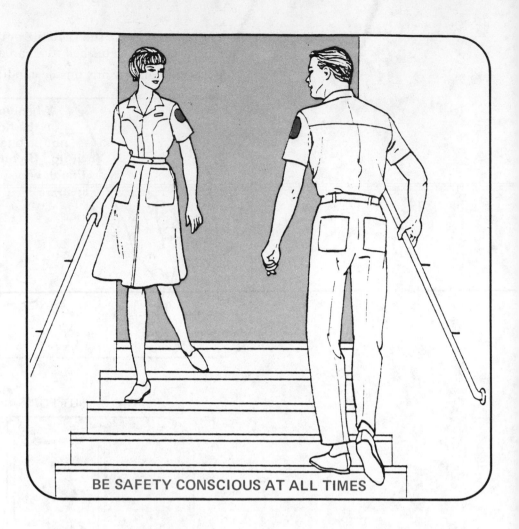

BE SAFETY CONSCIOUS AT ALL TIMES

- Check soiled linen for overlooked items before you send it to the laundry. Look for misplaced instruments, pins, needles, or other articles. Remove these and put them where they belong or dispose of them as instructed.

- Be sure to set the brakes on the wheels of stretchers, examining tables, or wheelchairs when moving patients on or off such equipment.

- Never use the contents of an unlabeled container. Take the container to your head nurse or team leader.

- If you do not understand what is written on the label of a container, take it to your head nurse or team leader and ask for an explanation.

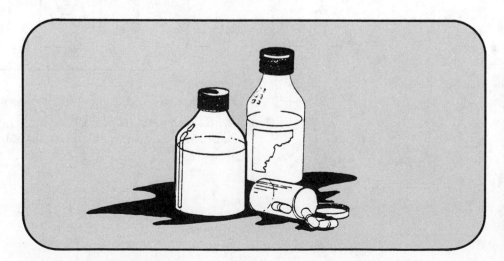

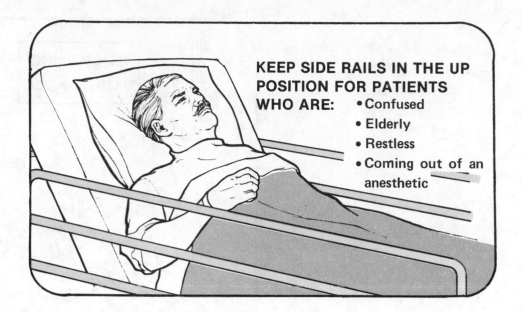

KEEP SIDE RAILS IN THE UP POSITION FOR PATIENTS WHO ARE:
- Confused
- Elderly
- Restless
- Coming out of an anesthetic

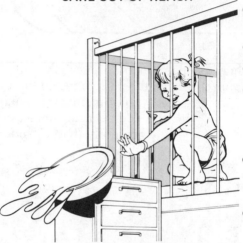

KEEP ITEMS FOR CHILD'S CARE OUT OF REACH

REMEMBER... A CHILD CAN REACH FAR AND IS QUICK

Safety for Children

- People who work with children must always be alert to things that may cause accidents.

- Small children should never be left unattended when they are awake.

- Every child in a protective device should be checked frequently.

- Articles used in the child's care should be kept out of reach of a toddler when they are not being used. Watch especially for needles, water, safety pins, medications, matches, electrical equipment, syringes, or thermometers.

- Toys should never be left carelessly on the floor. Be especially alert to pick them up, as they could cause someone to fall. Also, remember to clean up spills and messes, such as food, urine, and feces, right away.

- The sides of a child's crib should be up at all times except when someone is giving direct care to the child.

- Doors to stairways, utility rooms, and the kitchen should always be closed immediately after use. They should be locked whenever possible.

- Linen chutes should be kept locked except when they are being used by hospital personnel.

- Venetian blind cords should be kept out of the reach of children.

- Be sure there are no small toys or objects in the crib/bed that can be swallowed.

- Remove large objects that the child could stand on. The child might fall out of bed as a result. Also remove toys or objects with which the child could injure himself.

- Be sure the bedside rails are pulled up and locked in place.

Oxygen Safety

A special device is necessary when oxygen is used. This device is called a "Regulator" or "Flowmeter." It controls, or regulates the flow of oxygen. Special procedures are to be followed in the care and use of portable oxygen tanks and regulators. Follow the instructions used in your facility. Pulmonary medicine or respiratory therapy departments usually take care of this equipment in most health care institutions.

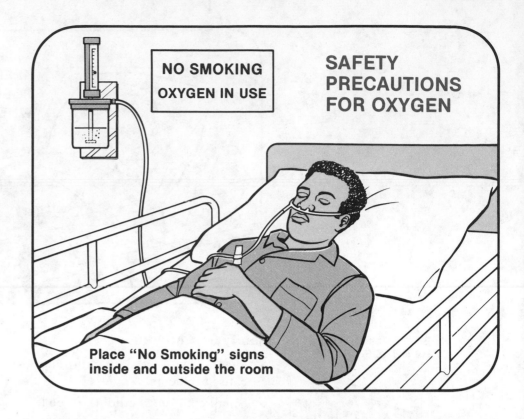

NO SMOKING
OXYGEN IN USE

SAFETY
PRECAUTIONS
FOR OXYGEN

Place "No Smoking" signs
inside and outside the room

Inhalation therapy or respiratory therapy departments are responsible in most hospitals for the inhalation therapy treatments the patient might be receiving. Such departments take care of the oxygen equipment and make adjustments in the treatments by checking with the doctor, head nurse, or team leader. Special precautions must be observed when more than the nor-

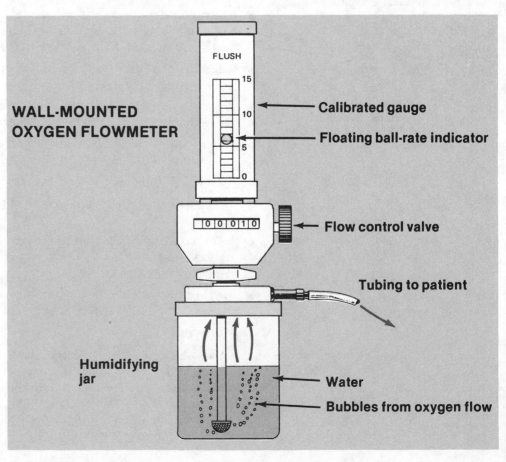

FLUSH

WALL-MOUNTED
OXYGEN FLOWMETER

Calibrated gauge

Floating ball-rate indicator

Flow control valve

Tubing to patient

Humidifying
jar

Water

Bubbles from oxygen flow

mal amount of oxygen is present in a particular area, such as the patient's unit.

Extra oxygen can make things catch fire and burn much more rapidly than they would in normal air. To prevent fires when a patient is being given oxygen, the following rules of safety must be strictly observed.

Rules to Follow: Oxygen Safety

- Check the flowmeter, a piece of equipment that shows the rate at which oxygen is being given to the patient.

- The tubing connected to the source of oxygen should be taped to the patient's gown or bedclothes. This helps to keep it in place and will prevent injury to the patient's nostrils if the tubing is accidentally pulled.

- Make sure the tubing is not kinked. Also, it should not be under any part of the patient's body. This might slow down or stop the flow of oxygen.

- A humidifying jar should be used with both the nasal oxygen cannula and the nasal oxygen catheter. The water level in the humidifying jar should be kept high enough so that it bubbles as the oxygen goes through it.

- Whenever possible, electrical appliances such as heating pads and electric shavers should be taken out of the room.

- The signal cord is replaced by a bell.

- If some electrical appliances are still in the room, they should be turned off and the plugs should be pulled from the outlets before the oxygen is started. If a plug is pulled from an outlet while the oxygen is being given, a spark could cause an explosion because there is live electricity in the outlet.

- Remove cigarettes and matches from the bedside table.

- Oil, alcohol, or anything else that might burn readily should not be used for rubbing patients while oxygen is being given.

- Never comb a patient's hair while he is in an oxygen tent. Because of static electricity, combing hair actually can create an electrical spark that could set off an explosion.

- Wool blankets and anything else that could cause static electricity should be removed from the bed when oxygen is being used. Patients must wear cotton hospital gowns. Other fabrics might generate static electricity.

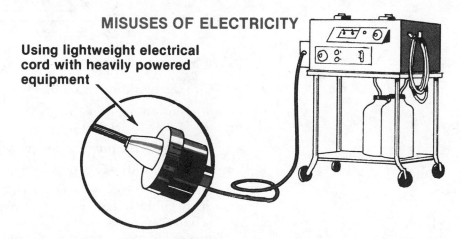

MISUSES OF ELECTRICITY

Using lightweight electrical cord with heavily powered equipment

- Be sure your hands are dry before using electrical equipment. Water should never come in contact with electrical equipment. For example: Placing a glass of water on top of a suction machine can *create* a fire hazard.

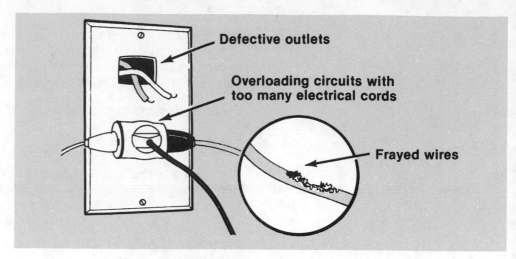

Defective outlets

Overloading circuits with too many electrical cords

Frayed wires

THE MAJOR CAUSES OF FIRE

- SMOKING AND MATCHES
- MISUSE OF ELECTRICITY
- DEFECTS IN HEATING SYSTEMS
- SPONTANEOUS IGNITION
- IMPROPER RUBBISH DISPOSAL

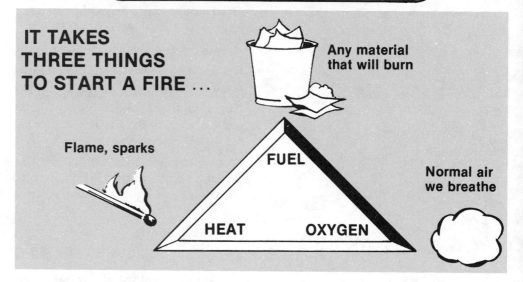

IT TAKES THREE THINGS TO START A FIRE ...

Any material that will burn

Flame, sparks

Normal air we breathe

FUEL

HEAT   OXYGEN

Fire Safety and Prevention

- Fire safety means two things:
    a) Preventing fires.
    b) Doing the right things if a fire breaks out.
- Smoking is the number one cause of fires in health care institutions.
- See that ashtrays are provided and that they are used.
- Never empty ashtrays into plastic bags, plastic wastebaskets, or containers of rubbish that can burn. Smoking materials should be collected in a separate metal container. A pail with water or sand in the bottom should be used to make sure that cigarette and cigar butts are out.
- Smoke only where it is permitted.
- A patient who has been given a sedative should not be allowed to smoke.
- Be familiar with your institution's fire plan.

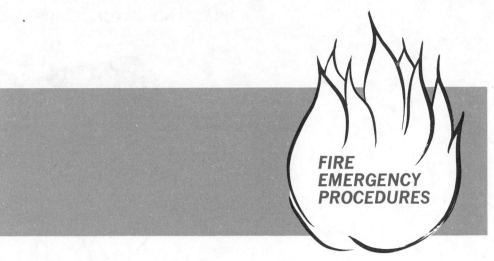

FIRE EMERGENCY PROCEDURES

In Case of a Fire:

- If fire occurs in a patient area, move or assist the patients out of the danger zone by taking them to a safe area.

- Pull the nearest fire alarm box.

- Notify the main switchboard as to the exact location and nature of the fire as soon as possible.

- Follow the fire emergency procedures for your department and health care institution.

- Do not panic—many lives may depend on your actions in an emergency.

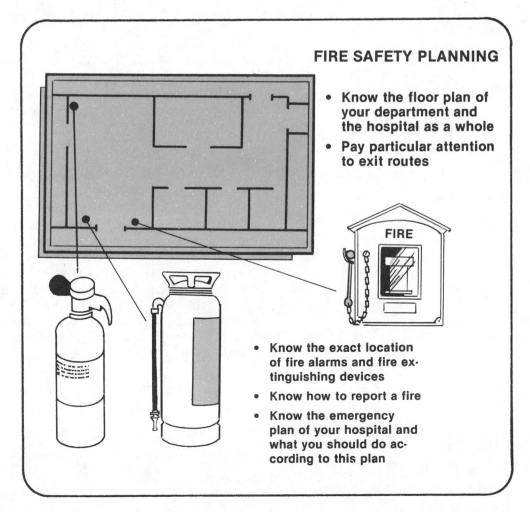

FIRE SAFETY PLANNING

- **Know the floor plan of your department and the hospital as a whole**
- **Pay particular attention to exit routes**

- **Know the exact location of fire alarms and fire extinguishing devices**
- **Know how to report a fire**
- **Know the emergency plan of your hospital and what you should do according to this plan**

SMOKING AND MATCHES

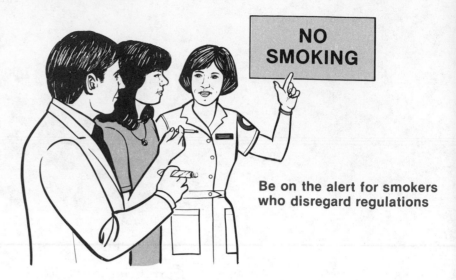

Be on the alert for smokers who disregard regulations

Protective Devices

A protective device is a type of restraint that keeps the patient from harming himself and therefore creates a safe environment for the patient. Protective devices (restraints) are applied only upon the instructions of your head nurse or team leader, or a physician. They will determine the type of restraint to be used and the length of time it is to be left in place. Check your patient frequently when he is in a protective device.

Cardiopulmonary Resuscitation—CPR

The American Red Cross and the American Heart Association offer free classes on this method of saving lives. Most health care institutions require their employees to take this program. The patient is then in a much safer environment. No one is qualified to render CPR to any patient under any conditions unless they have been certified by either the American Red Cross or the American Heart Association.

WHAT YOU HAVE LEARNED

The modern health care institution uses lots of different equipment for patient care and treatment. Much of this equipment is disposable. You must be familiar with the equipment found in the patient's unit, disposable equipment and supplies, and large equipment. Making a bed properly is one of the primary procedures taught to students of nursing. The skill you develop in making beds determines how comfortable the patient will be in bed.

Safety rules are for the protection of everyone, the patient and the entire staff. The rules are the result of years of study and research based on experience. Learn the rules and follow them closely. You will be helping to eliminate accidents.

6 LIFTING, MOVING, AND TRANSPORTING PATIENTS

1. Body Mechanics
2. Transporting the Patient
3. Range of Motion

SECTION 1: BODY MECHANICS

OBJECTIVES: WHAT YOU WILL LEARN

When you have completed this section, you will be able to:

- Lift, hold, or move an object or patient using good body mechanics.
- Lock arms with a patient to raise his head and shoulders.
- Move the helpless patient up in bed.
- Move a patient to the head of the bed with the patient's help.
- Move the mattress to the head of the bed with the patient's help.
- Roll the patient like a log.
- Move a helpless patient to one side of the bed on his back.
- Turn a patient on either side.

**KEY IDEAS:
BODY MECHANICS**

The term body mechanics refers to special ways of standing and moving one's body. The purpose is to make the best use of strength and avoid fatigue. You should understand the rules of good body mechanics and learn to apply them to your work. Then you will find that you will be less tired and will feel better at the end of the day.

Rules to Follow: Good Body Mechanics

- When an action requires physical effort, try to use as many muscles or groups of muscles as possible. For example, use both hands rather than one hand to pick up a heavy piece of equipment.
- Use good posture. Keep you body aligned properly. Keep your back straight. Have your knees bent. Keep your weight evenly balanced on both feet.
- Check your feet when you are going to lift something. They should be 12 inches apart. This will give you a broad base of support and good balance.
- Get close to the load that is being lifted.
- When you have to move a heavy object, it is better to push it, pull it, or roll it rather than lift and carry it.
- Use your arms to support the object. The muscles of your legs actually do the job of lifting, not the muscles of your back.
- When you are doing work such as giving a back rub, making a corner on a bed, or moving the patient, work with the direction of your efforts, not against it. Avoid twisting your body as much as you can.

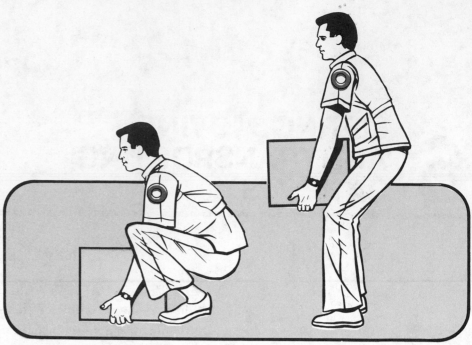

• When you lift an object:

    a)   Squat close to the load.
    b)   Keep your back straight.
    c)   Grip the object firmly.
    d)   Hold the load close to your body.
    e)   Lift by pushing up with your strong leg muscles.

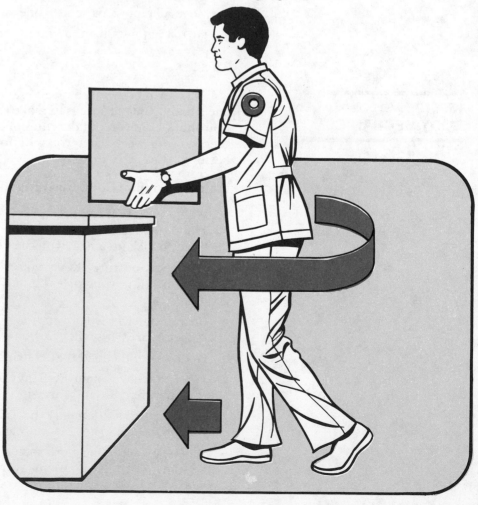

- If you think you may not be able to lift the load, if it seems too large or heavy, then get help.

- Lift smoothly to avoid strain. Always count "ONE, TWO, THREE" with the person you are working with. Or say "READY" and "GO" so you work in unison. Do this with both the patient and with other nursing assistants.

- When you want to change the direction of movement:
  a) Pivot (turn) with your feet.
  b) Turn with short steps.
  c) Turn your whole body without twisting your back and neck.

**KEY IDEAS:
LIFTING AND MOVING
PATIENTS**

Many of your tasks require lifting and moving helpless or nearly helpless patients. A bedridden patient must have his position changed often. Proper support and alignment of the patient's body are important.

The patient's body should be straight and properly supported, otherwise his safety and comfort might be affected. The correct positioning of the patient's body is referred to as body alignment. Body alignment means arrangement or adjustment of the patient's body so that all parts of the body are in their proper positions in relation to each other.

Many conditions and injuries, as well as special patient care treatments, make it difficult or even dangerous for a patient to be in a certain position. As a member of the nursing team, you will be responsible for making sure that a patient you are caring for is in the position ordered by his doctor.

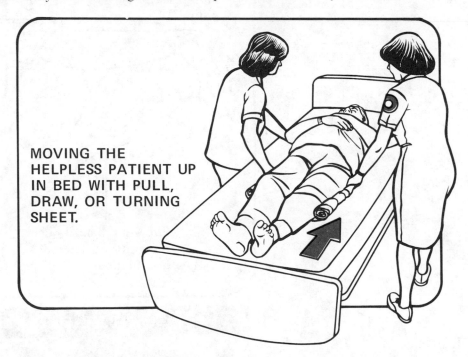

MOVING THE HELPLESS PATIENT UP IN BED WITH PULL, DRAW, OR TURNING SHEET.

A pull sheet can help you move the patient in bed more easily. A regular extra sheet folded over many times and placed under the patient can be used as a pull sheet. The cotton draw sheet can also be used as a pull sheet. When moving the patient, roll the pull sheet up tightly on each side next to the patient's body. Grip the rolled portion to slide the patient into the desired position. By using the pull sheet we avoid friction and irritation to the patient's skin that touches the bedding.

Rules to Follow: Lifting and Moving Patients

- Before you begin each procedure, explain what you are going to do and encourage the patient to participate and help as much as he is able.

- When moving a patient protect all tubing.
- Give the most support to the heaviest parts of the patient's body.
- Hold the patient close to your body for the most support.
- Move the patient with smooth and steady motion. Avoid sudden jerking movements.

Locking Arms with the Patient

To turn the patient's pillow over or to raise the head and shoulders, you should lock arms with the patient who is able to help. For the nonambulatory patient, two nursing assistants should lock arms with the patient to lift him.

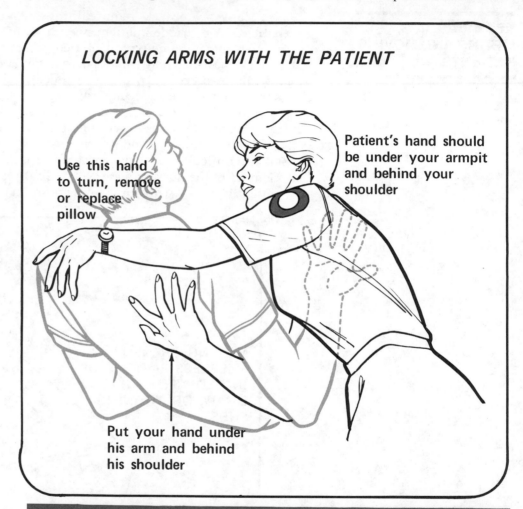

LOCKING ARMS WITH THE PATIENT

Use this hand to turn, remove or replace pillow

Patient's hand should be under your armpit and behind your shoulder

Put your hand under his arm and behind his shoulder

Procedure: Locking Arms with the Patient

1. Wash your hands.
2. Identify the patient by checking the identification bracelet.
3. Ask visitors to step out of the room.
4. Tell the patient you are going to lock arms to raise him.
5. Pull the curtain around the bed for privacy.
6. Lock the wheels on the bed.
7. Face the head of the bed. Bend your knees.
8. Have the patient put his arm under your arm (the arm next to him), and behind your shoulder, with his hand over the top of your shoulder. (If you are standing at his right side, his right hand will be on

(continued next page)

your right shoulder. If you are on his left, you will be locking your left arm with his left arm.)

9. Put your arm under the patient's arm with your hand on his shoulder.

10. When you say "one, two, three" help the patient pull himself up as you support him. This will raise his head and shoulders.

11. Turn or replace the pillow with your free hand. It is this hand that gives support to the back of the shoulders while lifting the patient.

12. To help the patient lie down again, continue supporting him with your locked arm and your free hand. Help the patient gently ease himself down.

13. Make the patient comfortable.

14. Wash your hands.

15. Report to your head nurse or team leader that you have changed the patient's position. Also report your observations of anything unusual.

Procedure: Moving the Non-ambulatory Patient up in Bed

1. Ask another nursing assistant to work with you.

2. Wash your hands.

3. Identify the patient by checking the identification bracelet.

4. Ask visitors to step out of the room.

5. Tell the patient that you and your partner are going to move him up in the bed. Say this even if he appears to be unconscious.

6. Pull the curtain around the bed for privacy.

7. Remove the pillow from the bed. Put it on a chair.

8. Lock the wheels on the bed.

9. Raise the bed to the highest horizontal position.

10. Stand on one side of the bed. The other nursing assistant will stand on the opposite side.

11. Both nursing assistants should stand straight, turned slightly toward the head of the bed. Your feet should be 12 inches apart. The foot closest to the head of the bed should be pointed in that direction. Bend your knees. Keep your back straight.

12. Use of a "draw, pull, or turning sheet" is always preferred for moving a helpless patient up in bed. This is to avoid friction between the patient's skin and bedding. This will prevent irritation of the skin. Roll the sides of the sheet to be used as a pull sheet close to the patient. Each nursing assistant then grasps one side of the rolled portion of the sheet firmly, so that when the patient is moved up, the sheet will stay in place under the patient.

13. You will be sliding the patient's body when you move him up in bed. Straighten your knees as you start to slide the patient. Your body is in the correct position for the direction in which you will move. Therefore, you can shift your weight easily from one foot to the other.

14. When you say "one, two, three" in unison, you and your partner will move together to slide the patient gently and move him toward the head of the bed or to the position he should be in.

(continued next page)

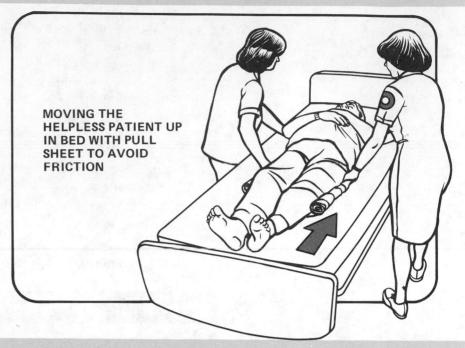

MOVING THE HELPLESS PATIENT UP IN BED WITH PULL SHEET TO AVOID FRICTION

15. Make the patient comfortable. Lower the bed to the lowest horizontal position. Replace the pillow.

16. Wash your hands.

17. Report to your head nurse or team leader that you have changed the patient's position. Also report your observations of anything unusual.

Procedure: Moving a Patient up in Bed with His Help

1. Wash your hands.

2. Identify the patient by checking the identification bracelet.

3. Ask visitors to step out of the room.

4. Tell the patient you are going to move him up in the bed. Before you begin, be sure the patient is allowed to exert himself as much as is

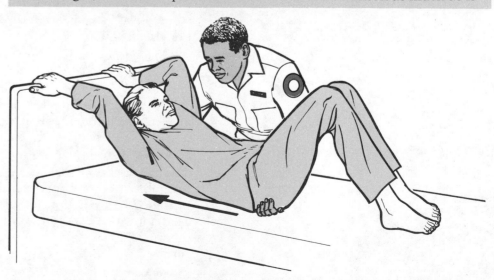

(continued next page)

necessary for this move.

5. Pull the curtain around the bed for privacy.

6. Lock the wheels on the bed.

7. Raise the bed to its highest horizontal position.

8. Lower the backrest, if this is allowed.

9. Lock arms with the patient and remove the pillow with your free hand. Put the pillow on a chair, or at the foot of the bed.

10. Put the side rails in the up position on the far side of the bed.

11. Put one hand under the patient's shoulder. Put your other hand under the patient's buttocks.

12. Ask the patient to bend his knees and brace his feet firmly on the mattress.

13. Ask the patient to grasp the head of the bed.

14. Have your feet 12 inches apart. The foot closest to the head of the bed should be pointed in that direction.

15. Bend your knees. Keep your back straight.

16. Bend your body from your hips facing the patient and turned slightly toward the head of the bed.

17. At the signal "one, two, three" have the patient pull with his hands toward the head of the bed and push with his feet against the mattress.

18. At the same time, help him to move toward the head of the bed by sliding him with your hands and arms.

19. Lock arms with the patient and put the pillow back in place, under his head and shoulders.

20. Make the patient comfortable. Lower the bed to its lowest horizontal position.

21. Wash your hands.

22. Report to your head nurse or team leader that you have changed the patient's position. Also report your observations of anything unusual.

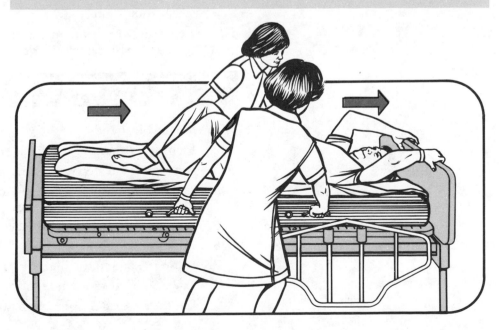

Procedure: Moving the Mattress to the Head of the Bed with the Patient's Help

1. Ask another nursing assistant to work with you.
2. Wash your hands.
3. Identify the patient by checking the identification bracelet.
4. Ask visitors to step out of the room.
5. Tell the patient you are going to move his mattress to the head of the bed.
6. Pull the curtain around the bed for privacy.
7. Lock the wheels on the bed.
8. Raise the bed to the highest horizontal position.
9. Lower the backrest, if allowed.
10. Put the side rail in the up position on the far side of the bed.
11. Each nursing assistant stands at a side of the bed. The sheets should be loosened.
12. Lock arms with the patient and remove the pillow. Put the pillow on the chair.
13. Ask the patient to grasp the headboard with both hands.
14. Ask the patient to bend his knees and brace his feet firmly on the mattress.
15. Grasp the mattress loops, or grasp the sides of the mattress if there are no loops.
16. On the signal "one, two three" have the patient pull with his hands toward the head of the bed and push with his feet against the mattress.
17. At the same time both nursing assistants will slide the mattress toward the head of the bed, keeping their knees bent and their backs straight as they move the mattress.
18. Lock arms with the patient and put the pillow back in place.
19. Make the patient comfortable. Lower the bed to its lowest horizontal position.
20. Wash your hands.
21. Report to your head nurse or team leader that you have moved the mattress. Also report your observations of anything unusual.

Procedure: Moving a Helpless Patient to One Side of the Bed on His Back

1. Wash your hands.
2. Identify the patient by checking the identification bracelet.
3. Ask visitors to step out of the room.
4. Tell the patient you are going to move him to one side of the bed on his back without turning him.
5. Pull the curtain around the bed for privacy.
6. Lock the wheels on the bed.
7. Raise the bed to the highest horizontal position.
8. Lower the backrest and footrest, if this is allowed.
9. Put the side rail in the up position on the far side of the bed.

(continued next page)

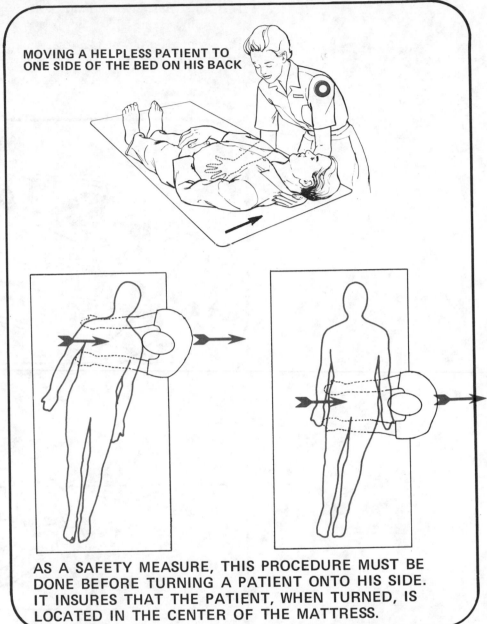

MOVING A HELPLESS PATIENT TO ONE SIDE OF THE BED ON HIS BACK

AS A SAFETY MEASURE, THIS PROCEDURE MUST BE DONE BEFORE TURNING A PATIENT ONTO HIS SIDE. IT INSURES THAT THE PATIENT, WHEN TURNED, IS LOCATED IN THE CENTER OF THE MATTRESS.

10. Loosen the top sheets, but don't expose the patient.

11. Slide both your arms under the patient's back to his far shoulder, then slide the patient's shoulders toward you on your arms.

12. Slide both your arms as far as you can under the patient's buttocks and slide his buttocks toward you. Use a pull (turning) sheet whenever possible.

13. Keep your knees bent and your back straight as you slide the patient.

14. Place both your arms under the patient's feet and slide them toward you on your arms.

15. Lock arms with the patient and adjust the pillow, if necessary.

16. Remake the top of the bed.

(continued next page)

17. Make the patient comfortable. Lower the bed to its lowest horizontal position.
18. Report to your head nurse or team leader that you have changed the patient's position. Also report your observations of anything unusual.

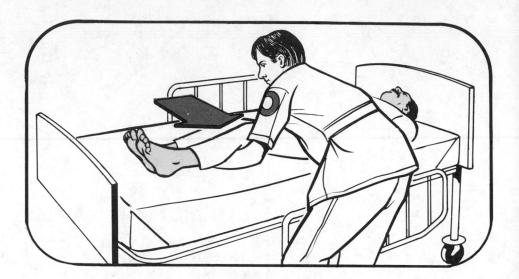

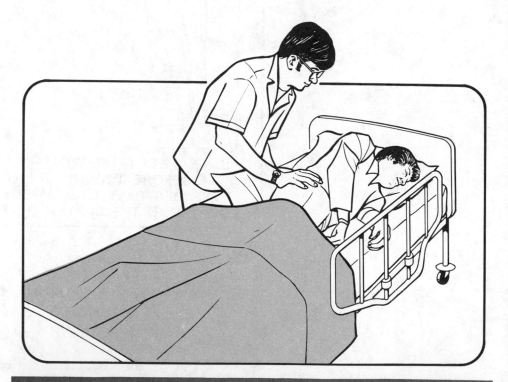

Procedure: Rolling the Patient Like a Log (Log Rolling)

1. Wash your hands.
2. Identify the patient by checking the identification bracelet.
3. Ask visitors to step out of the room.

(continued next page)

4. Tell the patient you are going to roll him to his side as if he were a log.

5. Pull the curtain around the bed for privacy.

6. Get help, if necessary.

7. Lock the wheels on the bed.

8. Raise the bed to the highest horizontal position.

9. Raise the side rail on the far side of the bed.

10. Remove the pillow from under the patient's head, if allowed. Put the pillow at the foot of the bed or on a chair.

11. Slide both your arms under the patient's back to his far shoulder then slide the patient's shoulders toward you on your arms.

12. Slide both your arms as far as you can under the patient's buttocks and slide his buttocks toward you. Use a pull (turning) sheet whenever possible.

13. Keep your knees bent and your back straight as you slide the patient.

14. Place both your arms under the patient's feet and slide them toward you on your arms.

15. Place a pillow between the patient's knees and cross the patient's legs in the direction of movement.

16. Use the pull (turning) sheets when necessary.

17. Keep your knees apart, your back straight, and your weight balanced evenly on both feet.

18. Roll the patient onto his side like a log, turning his body as a whole unit, without bending his joints. Turn him gently.

19. Replace the pillow under the patient's head, if allowed.

20. Use pillows against the patient's back to keep his body in proper alignment.

21. Remake the top of the bed.

22. Reverse the procedure to turn the patient on his opposite side.

23. Make the patient comfortable. Lower the bed to its lowest horizontal position.

24. Wash your hands.

25. Report to your head nurse or team leader that you have changed the patient's position. Also report your observations of anything unusual.

Procedure: Turning a Patient onto His Side Toward You

1. Wash your hands.

2. Identify the patient by checking the identification bracelet.

3. Ask visitors to step out of the room.

4. Tell the patient you are going to turn him on his side.

5. Pull the curtain around the bed for privacy.

6. Lock the wheels on the bed.

7. Raise the bed to its highest horizontal position.

8. Lower the backrest and footrest, if this is allowed.

9. Put the side rail in the up position on the far side of the bed.

(continued next page)

10. Loosen the top sheets, but don't expose the patient.

11. When you are turning the patient toward you, cross the leg furthest from you over the leg closest to you.

12. Cross the patient's arms over his chest.

13. Reach across the patient and put one hand behind his far shoulder.

14. Place your other hand behind his far hip, gently roll him toward you.

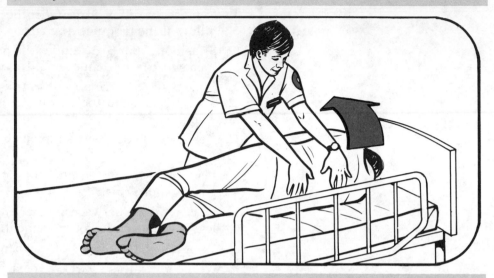

15. Fold a pillow lengthwise and place it against the patient's back for support.

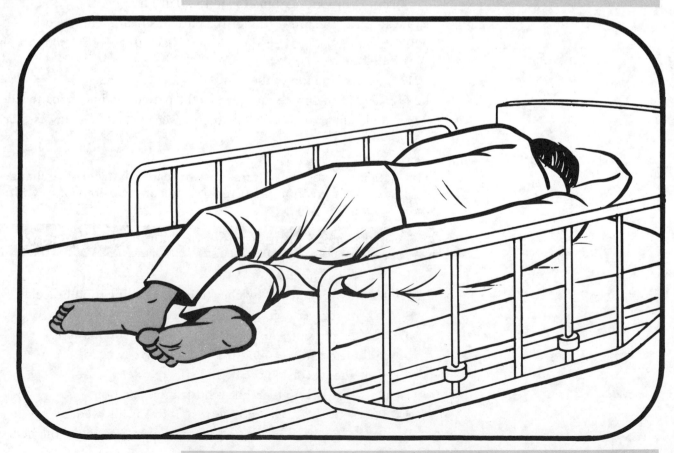

(continued next page)

16. Support the patient's head with the palm of one hand. With your other hand slide a pillow under his head and neck.
17. Place the patient's arms and legs in a comfortable position.
18. Remake the top of the bed.
19. Check to make sure the signal cord is within easy reach of the patient. Be sure both side rails are up.
20. Lower the bed to its lowest horizontal position.
21. Wash your hands.
22. Report to your head nurse or team leader that you have changed the patient's position. Also report your observations of anything unusual.

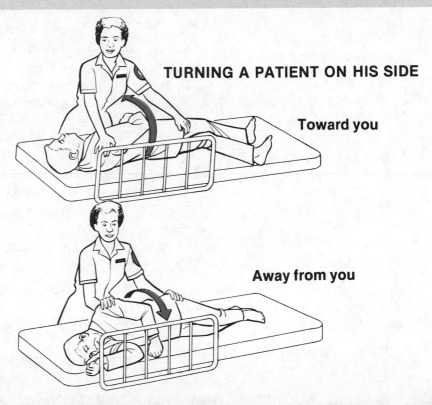

TURNING A PATIENT ON HIS SIDE

Toward you

Away from you

Procedure: Turning a Patient onto His Side Away from you

1. Wash your hands.
2. Identify the patient by checking the identification bracelet.
3. Ask visitors to step out of the room.
4. Tell the patient you are going to turn him onto his other side.
5. Pull the curtain around the bed for privacy.
6. Lock the wheels on the bed.
7. Raise the bed to its highest horizontal position.
8. Lower the backrest and footrest.
9. Put the side rail in the up position on the far side of the bed.
10. Loosen the top sheets, but don't expose the patient.
11. Slide both your arms under the patient's back to his far shoulder, then slide the patient's shoulders toward you on your arms.

(continued next page)

12. Slide both your arms as far as you can under the patient's buttocks and slide his buttocks toward you. Use a pull (turning) sheet whenever possible.

13. Keep your knees bent and your back straight as you slide the patient.

14. Place both your arms under the patient's feet and slide them toward you on your arms.

15. Cross the patient's arms over his chest.

16. When turning a patient away from you, cross the leg closest to you over the leg furthest from you.

17. Place one hand on the patient's shoulder near you.

18. Put your other hand under his buttocks.

19. Turn him gently on his side, facing away from you.

20. Fold a pillow lengthwise. Place it against the patient's back for support.

21. Support the patient's head with the palm of one hand. With your other hand slide a pillow under his head and neck.

22. Make sure the patient's arms and legs are in a comfortable position. Put a pillow between his knees, if this helps to make the patient comfortable.

23. Remake the top of the bed.

24. Lower the bed to its lowest horizontal position.

25. Check to make sure the signal cord is within easy reach of the patient.

26. Raise the side rails to the up position.

27. Wash your hands.

28. Report to your head nurse or team leader that you have changed the patient's position. Also report your observations of anything unusual.

SECTION 2: TRANSPORTING A PATIENT

OBJECTIVES: WHAT YOU WILL LEARN

When you have completed this section, you will be able to:

- Transport a patient by wheelchair or stretcher.
- Move a patient from the bed to a wheelchair and back into bed.
- Move the helpless patient using a portable mechanical patient lift.
- Move a patient from the bed to a stretcher and back into bed.

**KEY IDEAS:
TRANSPORTING A PATIENT
BY WHEELCHAIR**

The patient in a wheelchair should be well covered, if he is not dressed in a robe and slippers. You may cover his feet as well as his shoulders with a sheet or a blanket, making sure it does not get caught in the wheels. The seat of the wheelchair should be covered with a piece of linen, or with a disposable bed protector if the patient is incontinent. The wheelchair must be wiped off with a disinfectant solution after it has been used by each patient.

When you are moving a patient in a wheelchair, you should push the wheelchair from behind, except when going into or out of elevators. When you are entering an elevator, pull the wheelchair into the elevator backwards. When you are leaving an elevator, ask everyone to step out. Push the button

TRANSPORTING THE PATIENT BY WHEELCHAIR

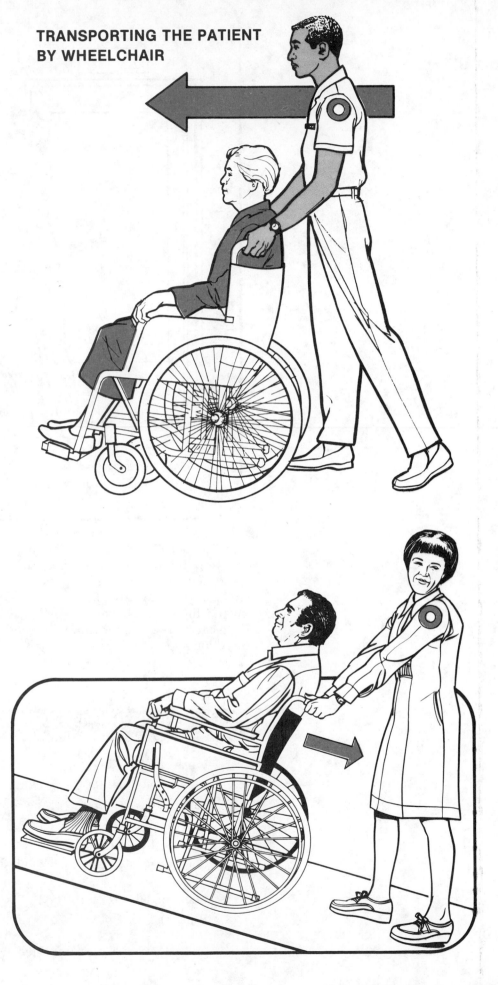

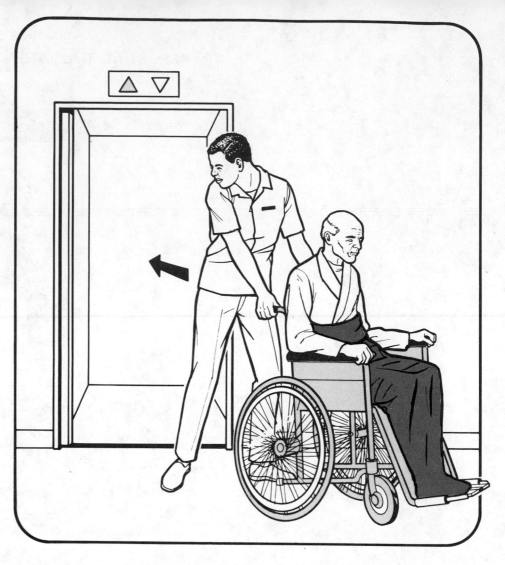

marked "open." Turn the chair around, and pull it out of the elevator backwards. Don't move the wheelchair while the elevator is in motion.

When you are moving a patient down a steep ramp, you should take the chair down backwards. To do this, stand behind the chair with your back facing the direction you want to go. Walk backwards, holding the chair and moving it carefully down the ramp. Glance back now and then to make sure of your direction and to avoid collisions, as if you were driving a car in reverse.

Procedure: Helping a Nonambulatory Patient Back into Bed from a Wheelchair or Arm Chair

1. Wash your hands.
2. Identify the patient by checking the identification bracelet.
3. Ask visitors to step out of the room.
4. Tell the patient you are getting him back into bed.
5. Ask another nursing assistant to help you.
6. Place a pull sheet on the bottom sheets, fan fold the top of the bed to the foot.
7. Lock the wheels on the bed.
8. Raise the head of the bed as high as it will go to a sitting position.

(continued next page)

9. Lower the bed to its lowest horizontal position.

10. Raise the side rail on the far side of the bed.

11. Bring the wheelchair with the patient to the bedside.

12. Position the wheelchair so the back of the chair is in line with the footboard of the bed.

13. Lock the brakes on the wheelchair.

14. Raise the footrests of the wheelchair, lifting the patient's feet off them and onto the floor at the same time.

15. Open up the blanket and safety straps that are on the patient in the wheelchair.

16. Both nursing assistants lock arms with the patient, help him to stand, pivot (turn) and sit on the side of the bed.

17. Rest the patient's head and shoulders on the mattress that is in the highest sitting position.

18. One nursing assistant stands next to the patient's head while the other gently lifts both his feet up onto the mattress.

19. Raise that side rail.

20. Lower the head of the bed.

21. Raise the bed to its highest horizontal position.

22. One nursing assistant goes to the far side of the bed.

23. Lower that side rail.

24. Slide both your arms under the patient's back to his far shoulder, then slide the patient's shoulders toward you on your arms.

25. Slide both your arms as far as you can under the patient's buttocks and slide his buttocks toward you. Use a pull (turning) sheet whenever possible.

26. Keep your knees bent and your back straight as you slide the patient.

27. Place both your arms under the patient's feet and slide them toward you on your arms.

28. Both nursing assistants then roll the pull sheet towards the patient and slide the patient up in bed using the pull sheet.

29. Put a pillow under the patient's head.

30. Remake the top of the bed.

31. Raise both side rails.

32. Make the patient comfortable.

33. Wipe the wheelchair with disinfectant solution and return the chair to its proper place.

34. Wash your hands.

35. Report to your head nurse or team leader that you have put the patient back to bed. Also report your observations of anything unusual.

Procedure: Moving the Nonambulatory Patient into a Wheelchair or Arm Chair From the Bed

1. Assemble your equipment:
   a) Wheelchair or arm chair
   b) Blanket or sheet

(continued next page)

    c)   Mechanical patient lift, if necessary

2. Wash your hands.

3. Identify the patient by checking the identification bracelet.

4. Ask visitors to step out of the room.

5. Tell the patient you are going to help him into a wheelchair.

6. Pull the curtain around the bed for privacy.

7. Lock the wheels on the bed.

8. Place the wheelchair at the bedside with the back of the chair in line with the footboard of the bed. Lock the wheels on the chair.

9. Fold up the footrests of the wheelchair so they are out of the way. If the wheelchair has leg rests, adjust them to hang straight down.

10. Lock the brakes on the wheelchair.

11. Spread a blanket or sheet on the chair. Have the corner of the blanket between the handles over the back so the opposite corner will be at the patient's feet.

12. Ask another nursing assistant to help you.

13. Put the patient's robe and slippers on while he is in bed.

14. Slide both your arms under the patient's back to his far shoulder, then slide the patient's shoulders toward you on your arms.

15. Slide both your arms as far as you can under the patient's buttocks and slide his buttocks toward you. Use a pull (turning) sheet whenever possible.

16. Place both your arms under the patient's feet and slide them toward you on your arms.

17. Raise the side rail.

18. Lower the bed to its lowest horizontal position, so that when you dangle the patient, his feet will touch the floor when he sits up.

19. Raise the backrest so the patient is in a sitting position in bed.

20. Lower the side rail on the side where you and the other nursing assistant will be working.

21. Place both hands under the patient's legs and turn them to the dangling position. His feet should be firmly on the floor. The other nursing assistant supports the patient's back and head and raises them at the same time. The other nursing assistant supports the patient's back while he is in the dangling position with her arm around the patient's shoulders.

22. Each nursing assistant locks arms with the patient. At the count of three they both lift the patient gently to a standing position, pivot (turn) the patient, and sit him in the wheelchair.

23. Fasten the safety straps around the patient to keep him from falling out of the chair.

24. Arrange the blanket snugly but firmly around the patient. Make sure that no part of the blanket can possibly get caught in the wheels.

25. Adjust the footrests so that the patient's feet are resting on them.

26. Observe the patient's color. Use the signal cord to call your team leader or the head nurse and take the patient's pulse if you observe any of the following:

    a)   The patient becomes very pale.

(continued next page)

Procedure continued

b) The patient seems to be perspiring a lot.

c) The patient says something like "I feel weak" or "I feel dizzy" or "I feel faint."

27. Adjust the chair to a comfortable angle.

28. Put a pillow behind the patient's back or shoulders, if needed.

29. Wash your hands.

30. Report to your head nurse or team leader that you have moved the helpless patient out of bed. Also report your observations of anything unusual.

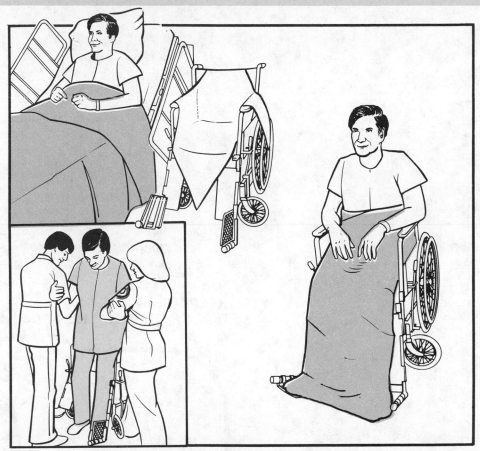

Procedure: Helping a Patient who can Stand and is Ambulatory Back into Bed from a Chair or a Wheelchair

1. Wash your hands.

2. Identify the patient by checking the identification bracelet.

3. Ask visitors to step out of the room.

4. Tell the patient you are getting him back into bed.

5. Pull the curtain around the bed for privacy.

6. Lock the wheels on the bed.

7. Bring the wheelchair very close to the bed.

8. Lock the wheels of the wheelchair.

9. Raise the headrest of the bed to a sitting position.

10. Lower the bed to its lowest horizontal position. If the bed cannot be lowered, bring a footstool to the bedside.

(continued next page)

11. Raise the footrests of the wheelchair, placing the patient's feet on the floor.

12. Open the safety straps on the wheelchair.

13. Help the patient out of the wheelchair to stand, pivot (turn) and sit on the side of the bed. His legs should be resting firmly on the floor.

14. Lean the patient against the backrest.

15. Put one arm around the patient's shoulders for support. Put the other arm under his knees.

16. Swing his body slowly around, helping him to lift his legs onto the bed.

17. Raise the side rail.

18. Lower the head of the bed.

19. Help the patient move to the center of the bed.

20. Put a pillow under the patient's head.

21. Make the patient comfortable. Take off his robe and slippers. Make sure the signal cord is within the patient's easy reach.

22. Remake the top of the bed.

23. Fold the blanket from the wheelchair and put it in its proper place.

24. Wash the wheelchair with an antiseptic or disinfectant solution and return it to its proper place.

25. Report to your head nurse or team leader that you have helped the patient back into bed. Also report your observations of anything unusual.

**HELPING A PATIENT
OUT OF OR INTO THE BED**

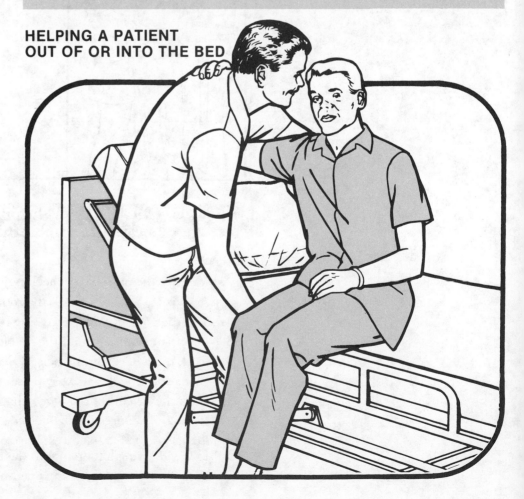

1. Assemble your equipment:
   a. Mechanical patient lift
   b. Sling
2. Wash your hands.
3. Identify the patient by checking the identification bracelet.
4. Ask visitors to step out of the room.
5. Tell the patient that you are going to get him out of bed by using the portable mechanical patient lift. (You may need the help of a second nursing assistant as a partner.)
6. Pull the curtain around the bed for privacy.
7. Position the chair next to the bed with the back of the chair in line with the headboard of the bed.
8. Cover the chair with a blanket or sheet.
9. By turning the patient from side to side on the bed, slide the sling under the patient.
10. Attach the sling to the mechanical lift with the hooks in place through the metal frame.
11. Have the patient fold both arms across his chest, if possible.
12. Using the crank, lift the patient from the bed.
13. Have your partner—a second nursing assistant—guide the patient's legs.
14. Lower the patient into the chair.
15. Remove the hooks from the frame of the portable mechanical patient lift.
16. Wrap the patient with the blanket.
17. Secure the patient to the chair with safety straps, if necessary.
18. Leave the patient safe and comfortable in the chair for the proper amount of time, according to your instructions.
19. To get the patient back to bed, put the hooks through the metal frame of the sling, which is still under the patient.
20. Raise the patient by using the crank on the mechanical patient lift. Lift him from the chair into the bed. Have your partner guide the patient's legs.
21. Lower the patient into the center of the bed.
22. Remove the hooks from the frame.
23. Remove the sling from under the patient by having him turn from side to side on the bed.
24. Put a pillow under the patient's head.
25. Make the patient comfortable. Make sure the signal cord is within the patient's easy reach.
26. Remake the top of the bed.
27. Raise the side rails to the up position.
28. Lower the bed to its lowest horizontal position.
29. Wash the mechanical patient lift with an antiseptic or disinfectant solution and return it to its proper place.
30. Wash your hands.

(continued next page)

31. Report to your head nurse or team leader that the patient was taken out of bed by means of the portable mechanical patient lift, that the patient was left in a chair for the prescribed length of time and that he was put back into bed by means of the mechanical patient lift. Also report your observations of anything unusual.

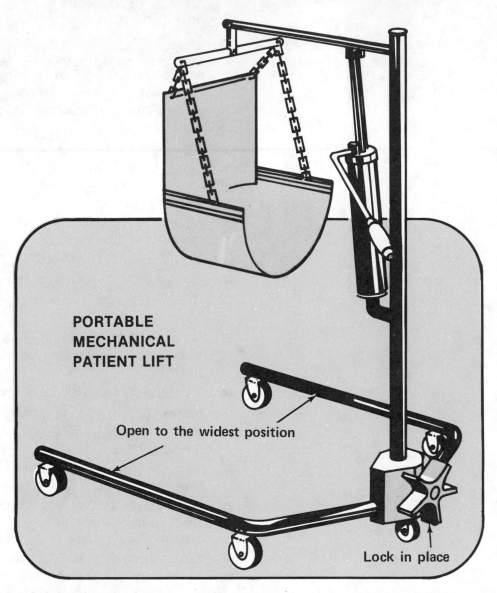

PORTABLE MECHANICAL PATIENT LIFT

Open to the widest position

Lock in place

KEY IDEAS: USING A STRETCHER

A hospital stretcher, sometimes called a litter or gurney, is a wheeled cart on which patients remain lying down while they are moved from one place to another. When moving a helpless patient from his bed to a stretcher, you will need a second nursing assistant working as your partner. Whenever you are moving the stretcher, you should stand at the end where the patient's head is and push the stretcher so the patient's feet are moving first. Be careful to protect the patient's head at all times. When entering an elevator, push the stop button so the doors of the elevator will not close until you are ready. Pull the stretcher into the elevator with the head end first. Stand at the patient's head while the elevator is in motion. When you leave the elevator, press the stop button and push the stretcher out foot end first.

Use restraining straps whenever you move a patient on a stretcher. Check the straps before you move the stretcher. Guide the gurney from the foot end when going down a ramp.

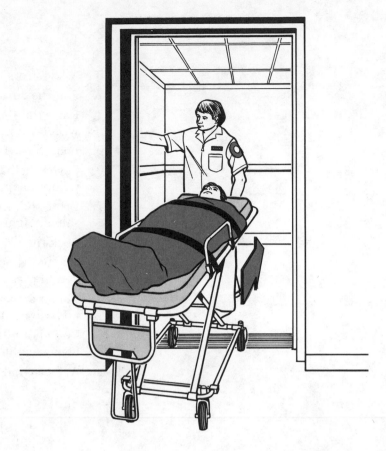

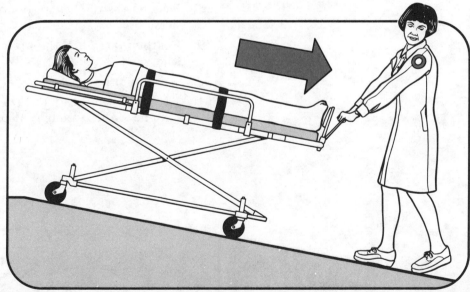

Procedure: Moving a Patient from the Bed to a Stretcher

1. Assemble your equipment:
   a. Stretcher
   b. Sheet or blanket
2. Ask another nursing assistant to help you. The two of you should work in unison to move the patient from the bed to a stretcher.
3. Wash you hands.
4. Identify the patient by checking the identification bracelet.

(continued next page)

5. Tell the patient you are going to move him from the bed to a stretcher.

6. Ask visitors to step out of the room.

7. Pull the curtain around the bed for privacy.

8. Raise the bed so that it is the same height as the stretcher. Lock the wheels on the bed.

9. Loosen the top sheets.

10. Cover the patient with a blanket or sheet. Remove the top sheets without exposing the patient.

11. Bring the stretcher next to the bed. Bed and stretcher should be the same height.

12. Lock the wheels on the stretcher.

13. You will stand on the far side of the bed using your body to hold the bed in place.

14. Your partner will stand on the far side of the stretcher using his body to hold the stretcher in place.

15. You should both have your knees bent, your backs straight, and your weight balanced on both feet.

16. At the signal "one, two, three," push, pull, and slide the patient from the bed to the stretcher. Use a pull (turning) sheet whenever possible.

17. Support the patient's head and feet, keeping his body covered with a loose blanket or sheet.

18. Fasten the stretcher straps around the patient at his hips and shoulders.

19. Put the side rails of the stretcher in the up position for the patient's safety.

20. Wash your hands.

21. Report to your head nurse or team leader that you have moved the patient to the stretcher. Also report your observations of anything unusual.

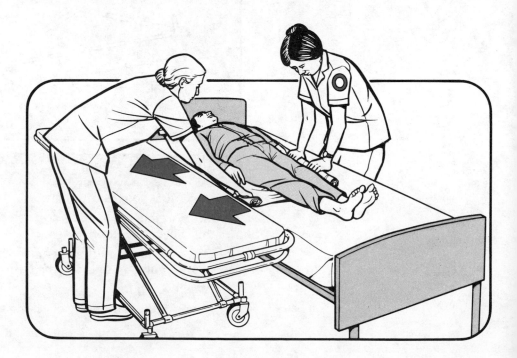

Procedure: Moving a Patient from a Stretcher to the Bed

1. Assemble your equipment:
   a. Stretcher
   b. Sheet or blanket
2. Ask another nursing assistant to help. You should work in unison to move the patient from a stretcher to the bed.
3. Wash your hands.
4. Identify the patient by checking the identification bracelet.
5. Tell the patient you are going to move him from the stretcher to the bed.
6. Ask visitors to step out of the room.
7. Pull the curtain around the bed for privacy.
8. Lock the wheels on the bed.
9. Fan fold the top sheet to the bottom of the bed.
10. Bring the stretcher next to the bed.
11. Raise the bed so that it is even with the stretcher.
12. Lock the wheels on the stretcher.
13. One nursing assistant stands on the far side of the bed using his body to hold the bed in place.
14. The other nursing assistant stands on the far side of the stretcher using his body to hold the stretcher in place.
15. Open the stretcher straps.
16. Both of you should have your knees bent, your backs straight, and your weight balanced on both feet.
17. At the signal "one, two, three," slide the patient from the stretcher to the bed. Use a pull (turning) sheet whenever possible.
18. Keep the patient covered with a loose blanket or sheet and support his head and feet.
19. Slide the patient as comfortable as possible.
21. Make sure the signal cord is within the patient's easy reach.
22. Replace the top sheets, removing the blanket without exposing the patient.
23. Put the side rails in the up position for the patient's safety.
24. Wash your hands.
25. Report to your head nurse or team leader that you have moved the patient from the stretcher to the bed. Also report your observations of anything unusual.

SECTION 3: RANGE OF MOTION

OBJECTIVES: WHAT YOU WILL LEARN

When you have completed this section, you will be able to:

- Perform complete or partial range of motion exercises with a patient.
- Explain the principles of range of motion exercises.
- Define the different joint motions.

A patient who is confined to bed or is unable to get out of bed will not be getting the exercise he needs. Therefore, it may become necessary for the nursing assistant to help the patient exercise his muscles and joints. This is accomplished through range of motion exercises (R.O.M.). These exercises move each muscle and joint through its full range of motion.

The basic movements used in these exercises are:

- Adduction—to move an arm or leg toward the center of the body.
- Abduction—to move an arm or leg away from the center of the body.
- Extension—to straighten an arm or leg.
- Hyperextension—beyond the normal extension.
- Pronation—to bend downward.
- Supination—to bend upward.
- Flexion—to bend a joint (elbow, wrist, knee).
- Dorsiflexion—to bend backward.
- Rotation—to move a joint in a circular motion around its axis.
    Internal—to turn in towards center
    External—to turn out away from center

Rules to Follow: Range of Motion Exercises

- Do each exercise three times. (Follow the head nurse's or team leader's instructions.)
- Follow a logical sequence so that each joint and muscle is exercised. For instance, start at the head and work your way down to the feet.
- If the patient is able to move parts of his body, encourage him to do as much as he can.
- Be gentle—*never bend or extend a body part further than it can go.*
- If a patient complains of unusual pain or discomfort in a particular body part, be sure to report this to your head nurse or team leader.

Procedure: Range of Motion Exercises

1. Assemble your equipment:
    a. Blanket
    b. Extra lighting, if necessary
2. Wash your hands.
3. Identify the patient by checking the identification bracelet.
4. Ask visitors to step out of the room.
5. Explain to the patient that you are going to help him exercise his muscles and joints while he is in bed.
6. Pull the curtain around the bed for privacy.
7. Place the patient in a supine position (on his back) with his knees extended and his arms at his side.
8. Loosen the top sheets but don't expose the patient.
9. Raise the bed to a horizontal position level with your waist.
10. Raise the side rail on the far side of the bed.

(continued next page)

11. Exercise the neck.

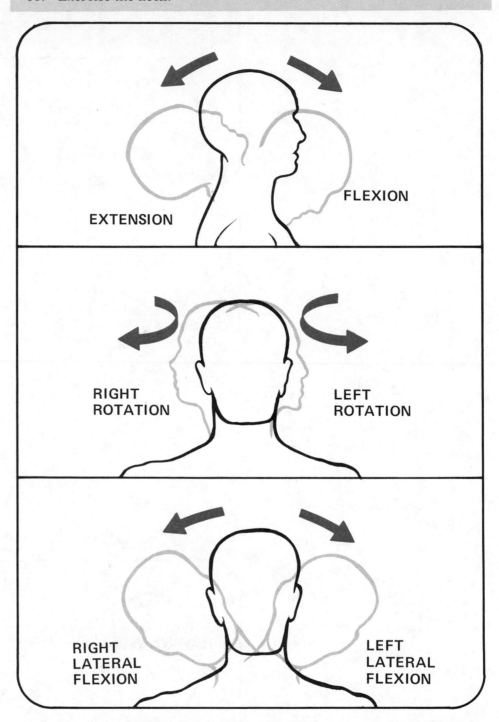

(continued next page)

12. Hold the extremity to be exercised at the joint (i.e., knee, wrist, elbow).

13. Exercise each shoulder.

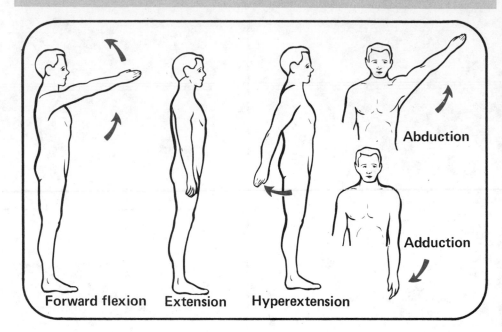

Forward flexion   Extension   Hyperextension   Abduction   Adduction

14. Exercise each elbow.

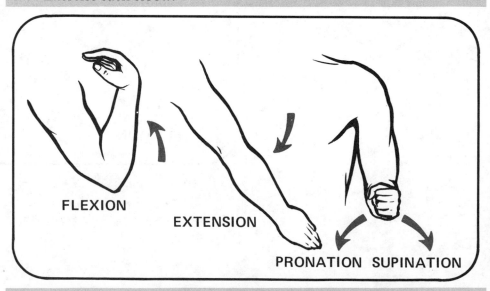

FLEXION   EXTENSION   PRONATION   SUPINATION

(continued next page)

15. Exercise each wrist.

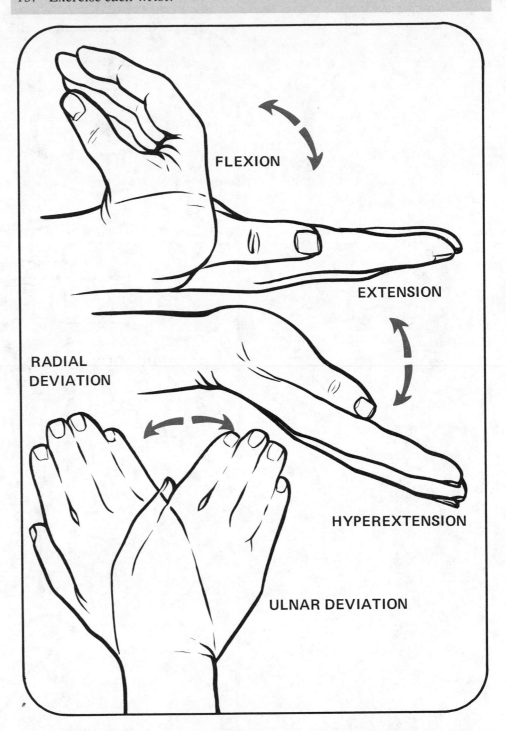

FLEXION

EXTENSION

RADIAL
DEVIATION

HYPEREXTENSION

ULNAR DEVIATION

(continued next page)

16. Exercise each finger.

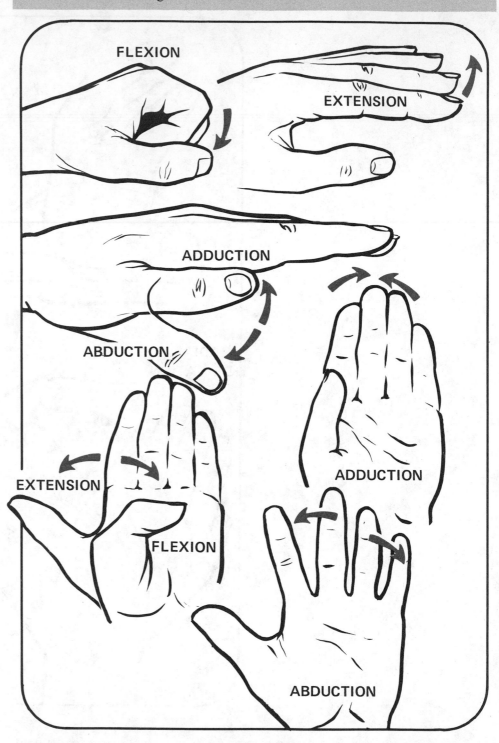

FLEXION

EXTENSION

ADDUCTION

ABDUCTION

EXTENSION

FLEXION

ADDUCTION

ABDUCTION

(continued next page)

17. Exercise each hip.

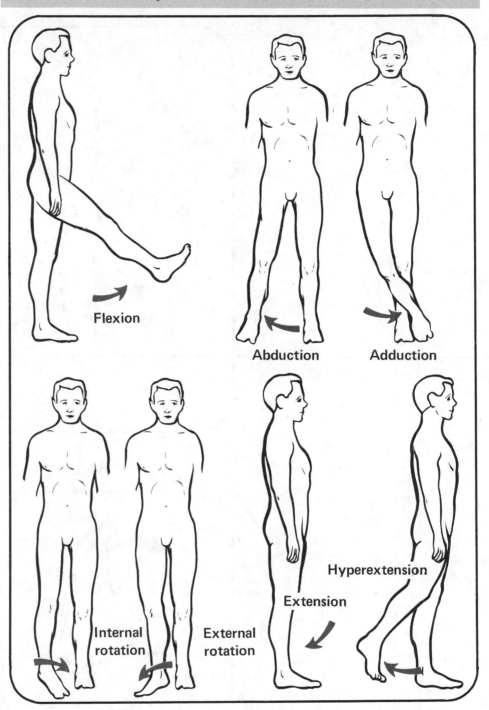

Flexion

Abduction   Adduction

Internal   External
rotation   rotation

Extension   Hyperextension

(continued next page)

18. Exercise each knee.

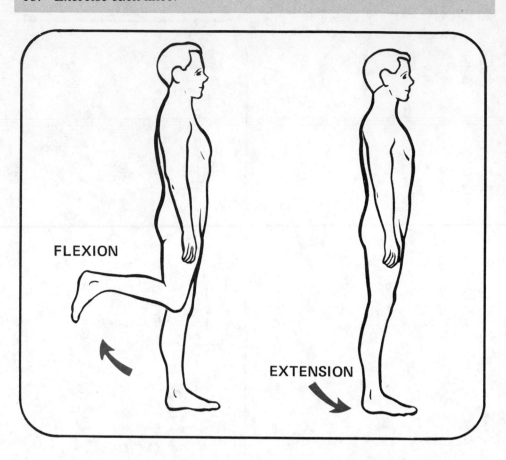

FLEXION

EXTENSION

19. Exercise each ankle.

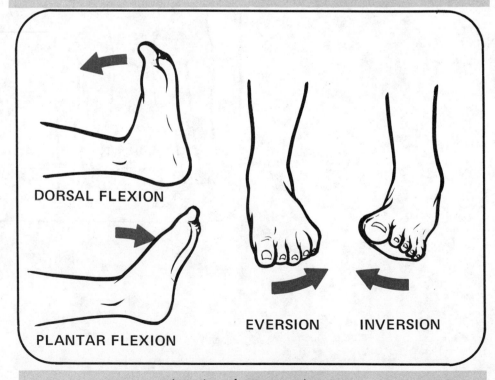

DORSAL FLEXION

PLANTAR FLEXION

EVERSION

INVERSION

(continued next page)

20. Exercise each toe.

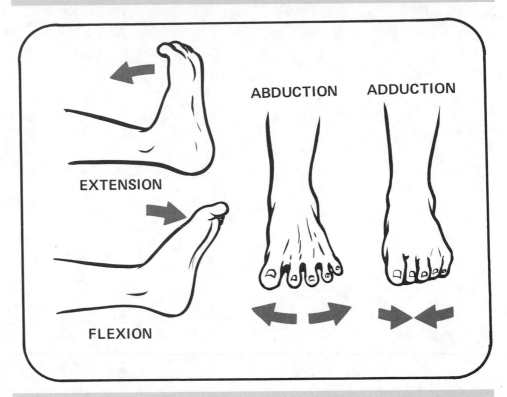

21. Make the patient comfortable.
22. Replace the sheets if a blanket was used. Fold and return the blanket to its proper place.
23. Return the bed to its lowest horizontal position.
24. Be sure the signal cord is within the patient's easy reach.
25. Raise the side rails.
26. Replace any extra lighting to its proper place after washing with an antiseptic or disinfectant solution.
27. Wash your hands.
28. Report to your head nurse or team leader that you have completed range of motion exercises with the patient, the time the exercises were done, and how the patient tolerated the exercise. Also report your observations of anything unusual.

WHAT YOU HAVE LEARNED

Every day in your work you will be doing many different tasks that will require muscular exertion. Understanding and using the principles of good body mechanics will help you in your work. You will save your energy and lessen strain and fatigue. Also, your work will go better—more smoothly and efficiently. You will feel less awkward.

Proper body alignment for the patient can add to his comfort and well-being. Changing the patient's position frequently will reduce the dangers of bed sores caused by pressure, that is, decubitus ulcers.

Range of motion exercises can help the patient who is confined to bed or paralyzed and unable to get out of bed to get the exercise his muscles and joints need.

7

PERSONAL CARE OF THE PATIENT

1. Daily Care of the Patient
2. Bedpan—Urinal—Bedside Commode

SECTION 1: DAILY CARE OF THE PATIENT

OBJECTIVES: WHAT YOU WILL LEARN

When you have completed this section, you will be able to:

- Care for the patient's mouth using good oral hygiene techniques.
- Bathe the patient.
- Give a back rub.
- Change the patient's gown.
- Care for the patient's hair.
- Shave the patient's beard.

KEY IDEAS: SCHEDULE OF DAILY CARE—24 HOUR NEEDS OF THE PATIENT

Early Morning Care—Before Breakfast

- Offer the bedpan or urinal.
- Wash the patient's hands and face.
- Help with oral hygiene.
- Pass fresh drinking water.
- Clean off the overbed table.
- Raise the head of the bed, if permitted.

Morning Care—After Breakfast

- Offer the bedpan or urinal.
- Assist with oral hygiene.
- Help the patient to bathe. Follow instructions from your head nurse or team leader. Give the patient a complete bed bath, partial bed bath, shower, or tub bath.
- Change the patient's gown.
- Help the male patient to shave his face, if allowed.
- Give the patient a back rub, if allowed.
- Help the patient comb his hair.
- Make the bed.
- Straighten the unit.

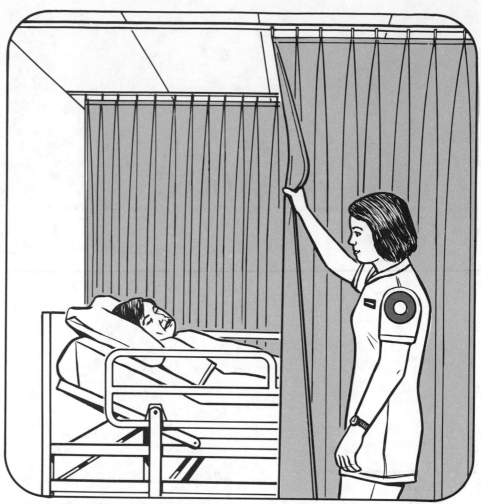

Before giving personal care always pull the curtain around the bed to give the patient privacy.

Afternoon Care—After Lunch—Before Visiting Hours

- Change the patient's gown, if necessary.
- Straighten the unit.
- Pass fresh drinking water.
- Offer the bedpan or urinal.
- Assist with oral hygiene.
- Wash the patient's hands and face.

Evening Care—After Supper—Before Bedtime

- Offer the bedpan or urinal.
- Wash the patient's hands and face.
- Assist with oral hygiene.
- Give each patient a back rub, if allowed.
- Change the draw sheet, if necessary.
- Smooth and tighten the sheets.
- Offer the patient an extra blanket.
- Pass fresh drinking water.

Assisting the Patient with Oral Hygiene

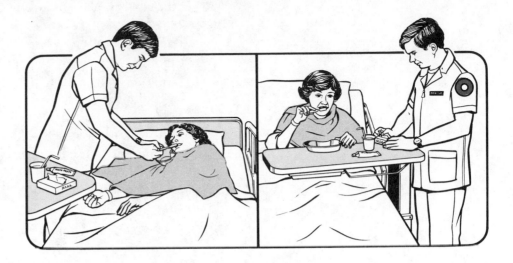

A person's mouth and teeth need even more care when a person is sick than when he is well. This care is called "oral hygiene." A sick person's mouth often has a bad taste. Sometimes the mouth feels "fuzzy" because of an illness. The tongue may be covered with a grayish coating that spoils the appetite. On the other hand, with good care, the patient's mouth will feel fresh and clean. Cleaning the patient's teeth and mouth—that is, giving oral hygiene—is an essential part of daily patient care. Teeth should be brushed every morning and every evening and after each meal. In your work, you will be giving oral hygiene to conscious and unconscious patients. When necessary, you will be cleaning their false teeth (dentures).

Oral hygiene is given to unconscious patients and patients who are N.P.O. (nothing by mouth) every two hours. The purpose is to keep the oral tissues moist. Unless this is done, tissues tend to dry out and develop a mucous coating much more rapidly.

Procedure: Oral Hygiene

1. Assemble your equipment on the bedside table:
   a) Mouthwash
   b) Fresh water
   c) Disposable cup
   d) Straw
   e) Toothbrush
   f) Toothpaste
   g) Emesis basin
   h) Face towel
2. Wash your hands.
3. Identify the patient by checking the identification bracelet.
4. Ask visitors to step out of the room.
5. Tell the patient you will help him clean his teeth and mouth.
6. Pull the curtain around the bed for privacy.
7. Spread the towel across the patient's chest to protect the gown and top sheets.
8. Mix one-half cup of water with one-half cup of mouthwash in the disposable cup.

(continued next page)

9. Let the patient take a mouthful of the mixture and rinse his mouth.

10. Hold the emesis basin under the patient's chin so he can spit out the mouthwash solution.

11. Put toothpaste on the wet toothbrush.

12. If the patient can do it, let him brush his own teeth. If he can't, brush his teeth for him.

13. Help the patient rinse the toothpaste out of his mouth, using the mouthwash solution or fresh water.

14. Clean and put your equipment in its proper place. Discard disposable equipment.

15. Make the patient comfortable.

16. Wash your hands.

17. Report to your head nurse or team leader:

    • That you have given oral hygiene.

    • Your observations of anything unusual.

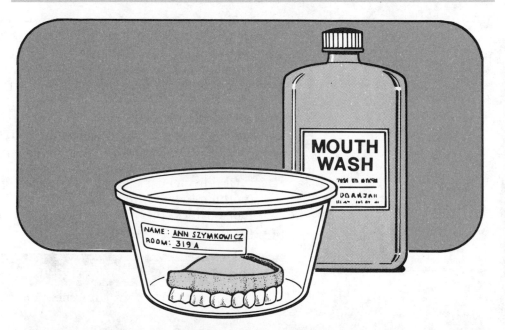

Procedure: Cleaning Dentures (False Teeth)

1. Assemble your equipment on the bedside table:
   a) Tissues
   b) Mouthwash
   c) Disposable denture cup
   d) Emesis basin
   e) Toothbrush or denture brush
   f) Towel
   g) Denture toothpaste

2. Wash your hands.

3. Identify the patient by checking the identification bracelet.

4. Ask visitors to step out of the room.

5. Tell the patient you wish to clean his dentures.

6. Pull the curtain around the bed for privacy.

(continued next page)

7. Spread the towel across the patient's chest to protect the gown and the top sheets.

8. Ask the patient to remove his dentures. Have tissue in the emesis basin ready to receive them. Help the patient who is unable to remove his own dentures.

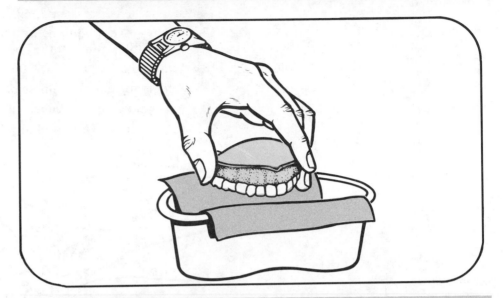

9. Take the dentures to the sink in the lined emesis basin. Hold the dentures securely in the basin.

10. Line the sink with a paper towel or fill the sink with water to guard against breaking the dentures if you drop them accidentally.

11. Apply toothpaste or denture cleanser. With the dentures in the palm of your hand, brush them until they are clean.

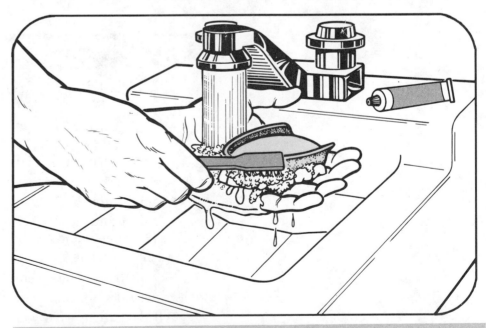

12. Rinse them thoroughly under cool running water.

13. Fill the clean denture cup with half cool water and half mouthwash. Or use water and salt—a saline solution. Place the dentures in the cup.

(continued next page)

14. Help the patient to rinse his mouth with the mouthwash and water solution.

15. Have the patient replace the dentures in his mouth if that is what he wants. Be sure dentures are moist before replacing them.

16. Leave the labeled denture cup with the clean solution on the bedside table where the patient can reach it easily.

17. Clean all your equipment and put it in the proper place. Discard disposable equipment in the proper container.

18. Wash your hands.

19. Report to your head nurse or team leader:

    • That you have cleaned the patient's dentures.

    • Your observations of anything unusual.

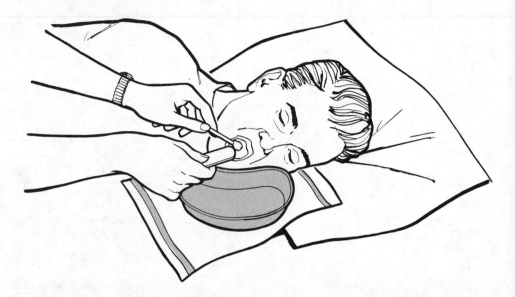

Procedure: Oral Hygiene for the Unconscious Patient (Special Mouth Care)

1. Assemble your equipment on the bedside table:
   a) Towel
   b) Emesis basin
   c) Special disposable mouth care kit of commercially prepared swabs. Or if such a kit is not available:
   • Tongue depressor
   • Applicators or gauze sponges
   • Lubricant such as glycerine, petroleum jelly, or a solution of lemon juice and glycerine

2. Wash your hands.

3. Identify the patient by checking the identification bracelet.

4. Ask visitors to step out of the room.

5. Tell the patient what you are going to do. Even though a patient seems to be unconscious, he still may be able to hear you.

6. Pull the curtain around the bed for privacy.

7. Stand at the side of the bed. Turn the patient's head to the side facing you.

(continued next page)

8. Put a towel on the pillow under the patient's head and partly under his face.

9. Put the emesis basin on the towel under the patient's chin.

10. Ask the patient to open his mouth. If he is in a coma, he will not be able to respond. In this case you will have to hold his mouth open. Press on his cheeks and hold his tongue in place with a tongue depressor.

11. Open the commercial package of swabs. Wipe the patient's entire mouth (roof, tongue, and inside the cheeks and lips) with the prepared swabs.

12. Put used swabs into the emesis basin. Some commercial swabs leave a coating of glycerine solution on the entire inside of the mouth, tongue, and teeth.

13. If a disposable mouth care kit of commercially prepared swabs is not available:

    a) Moisten the applicators with mouthwash solution.
    b) Use your free hand to insert the applicators in the patient's mouth.
    c) Thoroughly wipe the roof of the mouth, the teeth, and the tongue.
    d) Change applicators frequently.
    e) Place the used applicators and other supplies in the emesis basin.
    f) Use clear water on more applicators to rinse out the patient's mouth.

14. Dry the patient's face with the towel.

15. Using an applicator, put a small amount of the lubricant on the patient's lips and tongue and the inside of his mouth.

16. Clean your equipment and put it back in the proper place. Discard disposable equipment in the proper container.

17. Make the patient comfortable.

18. Wash your hands.

19. Report to your head nurse or team leader.:

    ● That you have given the patient special oral hygiene.

    ● Your observations of anything unusual.

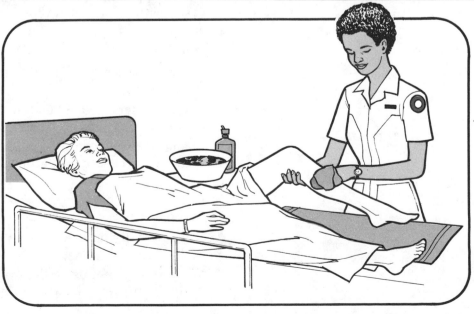

There are several important reasons for bathing the patient. Bathing gets rid of dirt on the patient's body. It eliminates body odors and cools and refreshes the patient. The bath stimulates circulation and helps to prevent bedsores. Bathing requires movements of certain parts of the body: the patient's legs and arms are lifted and his head and torso are turned. This activity exercises muscles that might otherwise remained unused. At this time the nursing assistant has the opportunity to observe the patient for any unusual body changes, such as skin rashes, decubitus ulcers, reddened areas, etc.

A patient may be bathed in one of four ways, depending on his condition. He may be given a complete bed bath, a partial bed bath, a tub bath, or a shower.

Types of Baths

- *The Complete Bed Bath:* The patient who is too weak or sick is given a complete bed bath. When you are giving this bath, you will get little or no help from the patient. Sometimes the doctor will write an order placing the patient on complete bed or body rest. In this case, the patient is not permitted to do anything.

- *The Partial Bed Bath:* A patient may be able to take care of most of his own bathing needs. In this case you bathe only the areas that are hard for him to reach, such as his back or his feet.

- *The Tub Bath:* The tub bath might be ordered by the doctor for therapeutic reasons.

- *The Shower:* Showers may be permitted for convalescent patients—patients who are recovering from their illness. These patients have been judged by their doctor to be strong enough to get out of bed and walk around.

Rules to Follow: Bathing the Patient

- Usually the complete bed bath is given as part of morning care. After the bath, the occupied bed is made, the hair is combed, and the gown is changed.

- Take everything you will need to the bedside before you start the bath. Clear off the bedside table and put the items you will be using on it.

- Always cover the patient with a bath blanket before giving the complete bed bath.

- Have the patient move or help him move close to you, so you can work easily without strain on your back.

- Use good body mechanics. Keep your feet separated, stand firmly, bend your knees, and keep your back straight.

- Raise the patient's bed to its highest position with the side rails up on the far side of the bed.

- Make a mitten for your hand out of the washcloth. This will prevent it from dragging roughly across the patient's skin.

- Change the water during the bed bath as necessary. For example, change the water whenever it becomes soapy, dirty, or cold. Change it before washing the patient's legs and before washing his back.

- Only one part of the body is washed at a time. Wash, rinse, and dry each part or area very well. Then cover it right away with the bath blanket.

- Soap has a drying effect on the patient's skin. Be sure to rinse off all of the soap.

- When you are not using the soap, keep it in the soap dish instead of the basin. In this way, the water will not dissolve the soap and get too soapy.

- Putting the patient's hands and feet into the water makes the patient feel relaxed.
- Observe the condition of the patient's skin when you are giving the bath. Report any redness, rashes, broken skin, or tender places you see on the patient's body.
- Never trim or cut toenails without special instructions from your head nurse or team leader.
- At the beginning of the bath, put the bottle of lotion for the back rub in the basin of water to keep it warm.
- Deodorant should be used only if the patient asks for it. It should be applied after the bath has been completed and before the clean bed has been made.
- Check the patient's gown for personal items or valuables before putting it in the laundry hamper and return them to the patient.

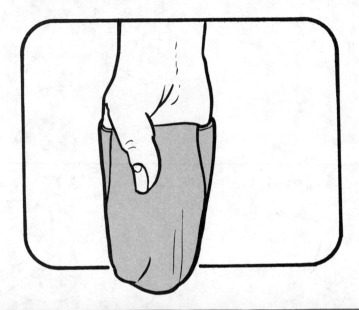

Procedure: The Complete Bed Bath

1. Assemble your equipment on the bedside table:
   a) Soap and soap dish
   b) Washcloth
   c) Wash basin
   d) Bath thermometer, if available
   e) Face and bath towels
   f) Talcum powder or corn starch (optional)
   g) Clean gown
   h) Bath blanket
   i) Orange stick for nail care, if used by your health care institution
   j) Lotion
   k) Comb or hair brush
   l) Disposable plastic laundry bags for dirty linen, if used in your institution, or linen laundry bag. A pillow case is sometimes used for dirty linen.
   m) Clean bed linen, stacked on the chair in order of use, if the bed is to be made following the bed bath.
   n) Disposable gloves, optional
2. Wash your hands.

(continued next page)

3. Identify the patient by checking the identification bracelet.

4. Ask visitors to step out of the room.

5. Tell the patient you are going to give him a bed bath.

6. Pull the curtains around the bed for privacy.

7. Assist the patient with oral hygiene.

8. Offer the bedpan or urinal.

9. Place the laundry bag on a chair near the bed.

10. Pull out all the bedding from under the mattress. Leave it hanging loosely at all four sides of the bed.

11. Take the bedspread and regular blanket off the bed. Fold them loosely over the back of the chair, leaving the patient covered with the top sheet.

12. Place the bath blanket over the top sheet. Ask the patient to hold the blanket in place.

13. Remove the top sheet from underneath without uncovering (exposing) the patient. Fold the sheet loosely over the back of the chair if it is to be used again; if not put it in the laundry bag.

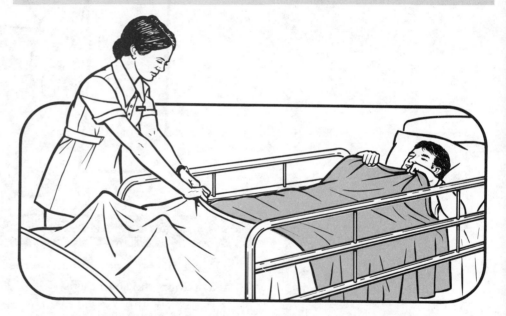

14. Lower the headrest and kneerest of the bed, if permitted. The patient should be in a flat position, as flat as is comfortable for him and as is permitted.

15. Raise the bed to its highest horizontal position, and lock it in place.

16. Remove the patient's gown and jewelry. Keep the patient covered with the bath blanket. If the gown belongs to the patient, put it away as requested. Place the hospital gown into the laundry bag. Put the jewelry into the drawer of the bedside table.

17. Fill the wash basin two-thirds full of water at 115°F (46.1°C). Use the bath thermometer to test the temperature of the water.

18. Help the patient to move to the side of the bed closest to you. Use good body mechanics.

19. Put a towel across the patient's chest and make a mitten with the washcloth. Wash the patient's eyes from the nose to the outside of the face. Ask the patient if he wants soap used on his face. Wash the

(continued next page)

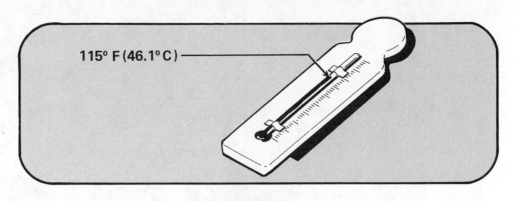

115° F (46.1° C)

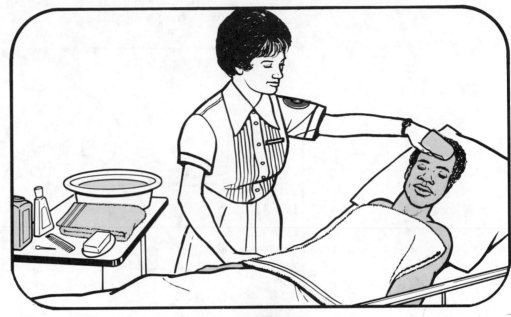

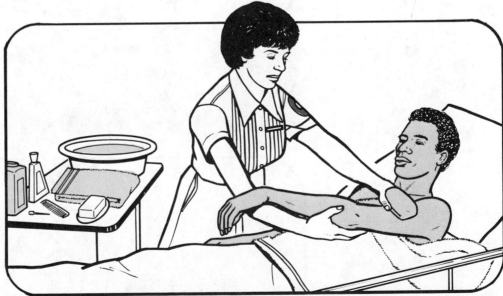

Procedure continued

face. Be careful not to get soap in his eyes. Rinse and dry by patting gently with the bath towel.

20. Put a towel lengthwise under the patient's arm farthest from you. This will keep the bed from getting wet. Support the patient's arm with the palm of your hand under his elbow. Then wash his shoulder, armpit (axilla), and arm. Use long, firm, circular strokes. Rinse and dry the area well.

(continued next page)

Procedure continued

21. Place the basin of water on the towel. Put the patient's hand into the water. Wash, rinse, and dry the hand well. Place it under the bath blanket.

22. Wash, rinse, and dry the arm, hand, axilla, and shoulder closest to you in the same way.

23. Clean the patient's fingernails with an orange stick, if used by your health care institution.

24. Place a towel across the patient's chest. Fold the bath blanket down to the patient's abdomen. Wash and rinse the patient's ears, neck, and chest. Take note of the condition of the skin under the female patient's breasts. Dry the area thoroughly.

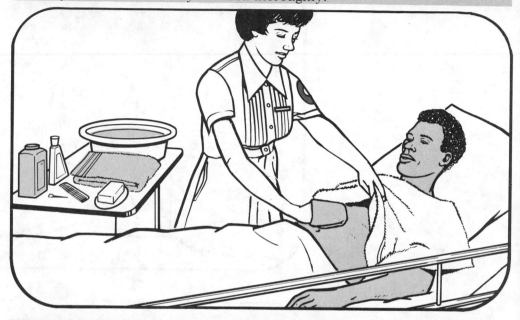

25. Cover the patient's entire chest with the towel. Fold the bath blanket down to the pubic area. Wash the patient's abdomen. Be sure to wash the navel (umbilicus) and in any creases of the skin. Dry the patient's abdomen. Then pull the bath blanket up over the abdomen and chest and remove the towels.

(continued next page)

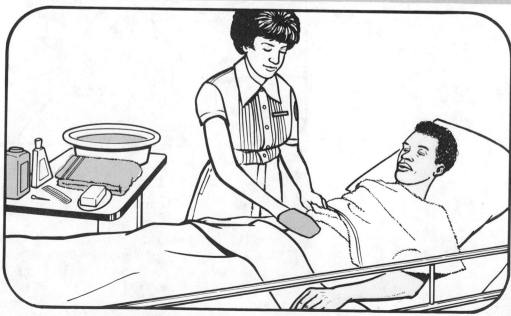

26. Empty the dirty water. Rinse the basin. Fill the basin with clean water at 115°F (46.1°C).

27. Fold the bath blanket back from the patient's leg farthest from you.

28. Put a towel lengthwise under that leg and foot.

29. Bend the knee and wash, rinse, and dry the leg and foot. Take hold of the heel for more support when flexing the knee. If the patient can easily bend his knee, put the wash basin on the towel. Then put the patient's foot directly into the basin to wash it.

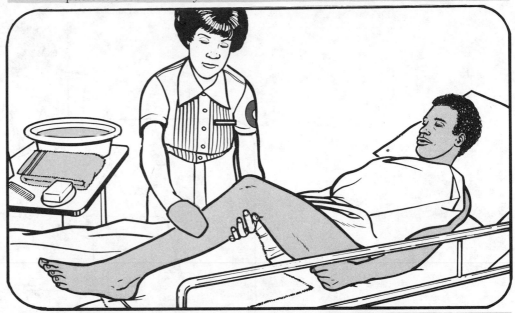

30. Observe the toenails and the skin between the toes for general appearance and condition. Look especially for redness and cracking of the skin. Take away the basin. Dry the patient's leg and foot and between the toes. Cover the leg and foot with the bath blanket and remove the towel.

31. Repeat the entire procedure for the leg and foot closest to you. Empty the basin, rinse and refill it with clean water at 115°F (46.1°C).

32. Ask the patient to turn on his side with his back toward you. If he needs help in turning, assist him. Raise the side rail to the up position so the patient is safe. Return to your working side of the bed.

(continued next page)

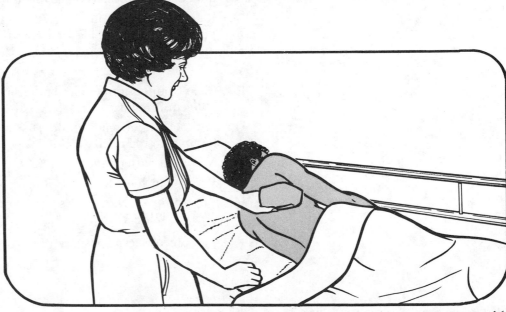

33. Put the towel lengthwise on the bottom sheet near the patient's back. Wash, rinse, and dry his back, buttocks, and back of the neck behind the ears with long, firm, circular strokes. Give the patient a back rub with warm lotion. The patient's back should be rubbed for at least a minute and a half. Give special attention to bony areas (for example, shoulder blades, hips, and elbows). Look for red areas. Dry the patient's back, remove the towel, and turn him on his back.

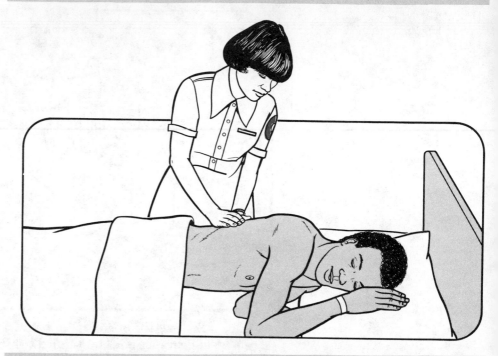

34. Offer the patient a soapy washcloth to wash his genital area. Give him a clean wet washcloth to rinse himself well. Give him a dry towel for drying himself. If he is unable to do this for himself, put on the disposable gloves and wash the patient's genital area. Allow for privacy at all times.

35. Put a clean gown on the patient.

36. Comb the patient's hair if he cannot do this for himself.

37. Make the patient's bed. Straighten the bedside table. Remove any unneeded articles. Replace the items the patient wants on the table.

38. Raise the backrest and kneerest to suit the patient, if this is allowed. Lower the bed to its lowest horizontal position.

39. Place the signal cord in its proper place where the patient can reach it easily.

40. Clean your equipment and put it in its proper place. Discard disposable equipment.

41. Wipe off the bedside table. Discard soiled linen in the dirty linen hamper in the utility room.

42. Make the patient comfortable.

43. Wash your hands.

44. Report to your head nurse or team leader:
    - That you have given the patient a bed bath.
    - Your observations of anything unusual.

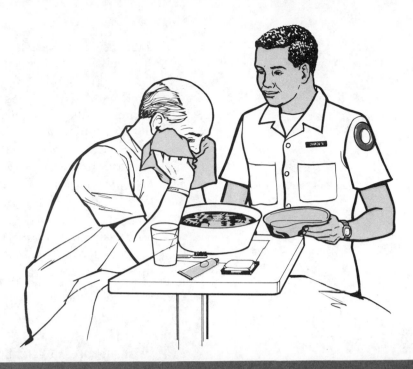

Procedure: The Partial Bed Bath

1. Assemble your equipment on the bedside table:

   a) Soap and soap dish
   b) Washcloth
   c) Wash basin
   d) Bath thermometer
   e) Face and bath towels
   f) Talcum powder or corn starch
   g) Clean gown
   h) Bath blanket
   i) Orange stick for nail care, if used in your health care institution
   j) Lotion for back rub
   k) Comb or hair brush
   l) Disposable plastic laundry bag for dirty linen or a linen laundry bag
   m) Clean bed linen, stacked on the chair in order of use, if the bed is to be made following the bed bath

2. Wash your hands.

3. Identify the patient by checking the identification bracelet.

4. Ask visitors to step out of the room.

5. Tell the patient you are going to help him with a bath.

6. Pull the curtains around the bed for privacy.

7. Assist the patient with oral hygiene.

8. Offer the bedpan or urinal.

9. Place the laundry bag on a chair near the bed.

10. Pull out all of the bedding from under the mattress. Leave it hanging loosely at all four sides of the bed.

11. Take the bedspread and regular blanket off the bed. Fold them loosely over the back of the chair, leaving the patient covered with the top sheet.

12. Place the bath blanket over the top sheet. Ask the patient to hold the blanket in place. Remove the top sheet from underneath without

(continued next page)

uncovering the patient. Fold the sheet loosely over the back of the chair if it is to be used again. Or put it into the laundry bag.

13. Take off the patient's gown and jewelry, keeping him covered with the bath blanket. If the gown belongs to the patient, put it away as requested. Place the jewelry in the drawer of the bedside table. Put the hospital gown into the laundry bag.

14. Fill the wash basin two thirds full of water at 115°F (46.1°C). Use the bath thermometer to test the temperature.

15. Ask the patient to wash the areas of his body that he can reach easily.

16. Place the signal cord where the patient can easily reach it. Instruct him to signal when he is finished washing himself.

17. Wash your hands and leave the room.

18. When the patient signals that he is finished, go back into the room.

19. Wash your hands.

20. Empty the water, rinse the basin and fill it with clean water at 115°F (46.1°C).

21. Wash the areas of the body that the patient was unable to reach. Follow the procedure you learned for a complete bed bath. The body parts washed by the patient plus the body parts washed for the patient by the nursing assistant should equal a complete bed bath.

22. Put a clean gown on the patient without exposing him.

23. If the patient is allowed out of bed, assist him to a chair.

24. Make the empty bed.

25. Place the signal cord in its proper place.

26. Clean your equipment and put it in its proper place. Discard disposable equipment.

27. Wipe off the bedside table. Discard all soiled linen in the dirty linen hamper in the utility room.

28. Make the patient comfortable.

29. Wash your hands.

30. Report to your head nurse or team leader:
    - That you have given the patient a partial bath.
    - Your observations of anything unusual.

Procedure: The Tub Bath

1. Assemble your equipment on a chair near the bathtub.
   a) Bath towels
   b) Washcloths
   c) Soap
   d) Bath thermometer
   e) Chair (place this near the bathtub)
   f) Clean gown
   g) Disinfectant solution

2. Wash your hands.

3. Identify the patient by checking the identification bracelet.

4. Ask visitors to step out of the room.

5. Tell the patient that you are going to give him a tub bath.

6. Pull the curtain around the bed for privacy.

(continued next page)

7. Help the patient out of bed. Get him into a bathrobe and slippers and to the room with the bathtub, either walking or by wheelchair.

8. For safety, remove all electrical appliances from the room with the bathtub.

9. Place the chair next to the bathtub. Assist the patient into the chair.

10. Wash the bathtub with the disinfectant solution.

11. Fill the bathtub half full of water at 105°F (40.5°C). Test the temperature with a bath thermometer.

12. Place one towel in the bathtub for the patient to sit on.

13. Place one towel on the floor where the patient will step out of the tub. This will prevent him from slipping.

14. Assist the patient to get undressed and into the bathtub.

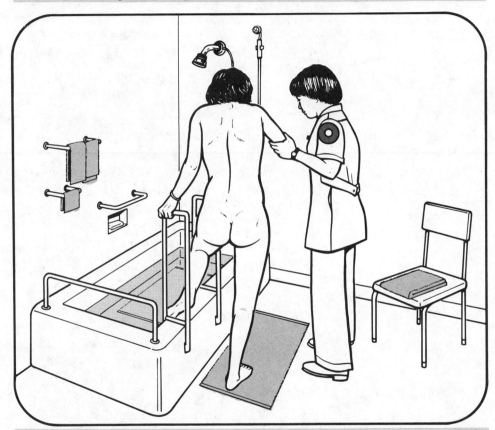

15. Let the patient stay in the bathtub as long as permitted, according to your instructions.

16. Help the patient wash himself, if help is needed.

17. Put one towel across the chair.

18. Help the patient out of the bathtub. Seat him on the towel-covered chair, if he needs assistance.

19. Dry the patient well by patting gently with a towel. Help him put on pajamas or gown, bathrobe and slippers.

20. Help the patient return to his room and into bed.

21. Make the patient comfortable.

22. Return to the tub room. Clean the bathtub with disinfectant solution.

23. Remove all used linen. Put it in the dirty linen hamper in the utility room.

(continued next page)

24. Wash your hands.
25. Report to your head nurse or team leader:
    - That you have given the patient a tub bath.
    - Your observations of anything unusual.

Procedure: Helping the Patient Take a Shower

1. Assemble your equipment on a chair near the shower.
    a) Towels
    b) Soap
    c) Shower cap
    d) Washcloth
    e) Clean gown
    f) Disinfectant solution
2. Wash your hands.
3. Identify the patient by checking the identification bracelet.
4. Ask visitors to step out of the room.
5. Tell the patient that you will assist him with taking a shower.
6. Pull the curtain around the bed for privacy.
7. Help the patient out of bed. Help him into a bathrobe and slippers. Help him to the bathroom with shower, as necessary.
8. For safety, remove all electrical appliances from the shower room.
9. Place one towel on the floor outside the shower.
10. Place one towel on a chair close to the shower. Assist the patient into the chair.
11. Wash the floor of the shower with disinfectant solution.
12. Turn on the shower and adjust the water temperature.
13. Assist the patient into the shower.
14. Give the patient soap and washcloth so he can wash himself, but wait beside the shower in case the patient needs assistance.
15. Turn off the water and assist the patient out of the shower when he is finished washing himself. Seat him on the towel-covered chair.
16. Dry the patient well by patting gently with the towel.
17. Assist him with putting on pajamas or nightgown, bathrobe and slippers.
18. Help the patient back to his room and into bed.
19. Make the patient comfortable.
20. Return to the shower room. Remove all used linen and put it in the dirty linen hamper in the dirty utility room.
21. Wash your hands.
22. Report to the head nurse or team leader:
    - That you have helped the patient with a shower.
    - Your observations of anything unusual.

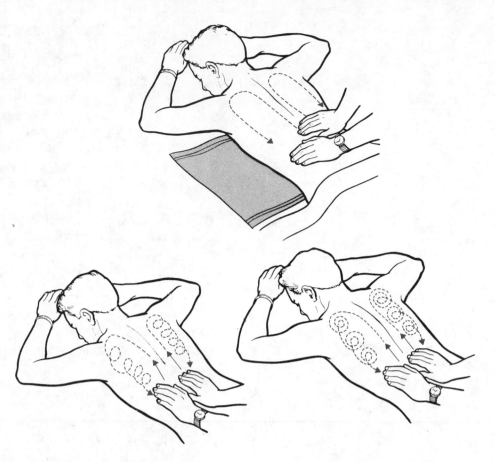

Rubbing a patient's back refreshes him, relaxes his muscles, and stimulates circulation. Because of pressure caused by the bedclothes and the lack of movement to stimulate circulation, the skin of a bedridden patient needs special care.

Back rubs are usually given during morning care, right after the patient's bath. They also are given: a) as part of evening care, b) when changing the position of a helpless patient, c) for very restless patients who need relaxing, and d) on doctor's orders for "special back care."

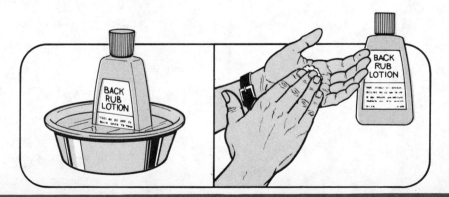

Procedure: Giving the Patient a Back Rub

1. Assemble your equipment on the bedside table:
   a) Towels
   b) Lotion
   c) Basin of warm water at 115°F (46.1°C)

2. Wash your hands.
3. Identify the patient by checking the identification bracelet.

(continued next page)

4. Ask visitors to step out of the room.

5. Tell the patient you are going to give him a back rub.

6. Pull the curtain around the bed for privacy.

7. Ask the patient to turn on his side so his back is toward you. Or have him turn on his abdomen. Use the position that is most comfortable for the patient and for yourself.

8. The side rail should be in the up position on the far side of the bed. Raise the bed to its highest horizontal position.

9. Lotion should be warmed by placing the container in a basin of warm water 115°F (46.1°C). Also, warm your hands by running warm water over them.

10. Open the ties on the patient's gown. Put a towel lengthwise on the mattress close to the patient's back.

11. Pour a small amount of lotion into the palm of your hand.

12. Rub your hands together using friction to warm the lotion.

13. Apply lotion to the entire back with the palms of your hands. Use firm long strokes from the buttocks to the shoulders and back of the neck.

14. Keep your knees slightly bent and your back straight.

15. Exert firm pressure as you stroke upward from the buttocks toward the shoulders. Use gentle pressure as you stroke downward from shoulders to buttocks.

16. Use a circular motion on each bony area.

17. This rhythmic rubbing motion should be continued for from one and one-half minutes to three minutes.

18. Dry the patient's back by patting gently with a towel.

19. Close and retie the gown.

20. Remove the towels.

21. Assist the patient to turn back to a comfortable position.

22. Arrange the top sheets of the bed neatly.

23. Put your equipment back in its proper place. Discard disposable equipment.

24. Lower the bed to its lowest horizontal position.

25. Make the patient comfortable.

26. Wash your hands.

27. Report to your head nurse or team leader:
    - That you have given the patient a back rub.
    - The time it was given.
    - Your observations of anything unusual.

KEY IDEAS: CHANGING THE PATIENT'S GOWN

It is important when you change a patient's gown not to expose his body unnecessarily. In this way you avoid chills caused by drafts. You will also prevent embarrassment for the patient.

Procedure: Changing the Patient's Gown

1. Assemble your equipment on the bedside table:
   a) A clean gown

(continued next page)

Procedure continued

2. Wash your hands.
3. Identify your patient by checking the identification bracelet.
4. Ask visitors to step out of the room.
5. Tell the patient you are going to change his gown.
6. Pull the curtain around the bed for privacy.
7. Have the patient turn on his side with his back toward you so you can untie the tapes.
8. If the patient cannot be turned, you will have to reach under his neck to untie the tapes.
9. Loosen the soiled gown around the patient's body.
10. Get the clean gown ready to put on the patient. Unfold it and lay it across the patient's chest on top of the bath blanket or top sheets.
11. Take off one sleeve at a time, leaving the old gown in place on the patient.
12. Slide each arm through one sleeve of the clean gown.

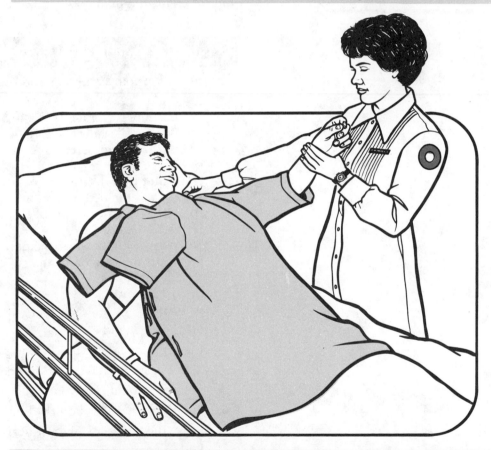

13. If the patient cannot hold his arm up, put your hand through the sleeve. Take his hand in yours and slip the sleeve up the patient's wrist and arm. Do this for both arms. Then pull the gown down over the patient's chest. If the patient has a sore arm, remove the sleeve on the well arm first. Then remove the sleeve on the sore arm. To put the clean gown on, put the sleeve on the sore arm first. Then slide the well arm through the second sleeve.

(continued next page)

14. Remove the soiled gown from under the bath blanket or top sheets.

15. Tie the tapes on the clean gown. Some patients want only the tapes at the neck tied so they will not be lying on the knots.

16. Put the soiled gown in the dirty linen hamper in the dirty utility room.

17. Make the patient comfortable.

18. Wash your hands.

19. Report to your head nurse or team leader:
    - That you have replaced the patient's soiled gown with a clean one.
    - Your observations of anything unusual.

KEY IDEAS: SHAMPOOING THE PATIENT'S HAIR

Patients who will be in the health care institution for a long time may need to have their hair shampooed from time to time. The doctor must write the order for a shampoo. Your head nurse or team leader must give you instructions for giving the shampoo. The patient must be in bed when the shampoo is given.

Procedure: Shampooing the Patient's Hair

1. Assemble your equipment on the bedside table:
   a) Chair
   b) Basin of water at 105°F (40.5°C)
   c) Pitcher of water at 115°F (46.1°C)
   d) Bath thermometer
   e) Large basin
   f) Water trough (tray) or plastic sheet
   g) Disposable bed protector
   h) Pillow with waterproof case
   i) Bath towels
   j) Washcloth, to cover the patient's eyes
   k) Paper or styrofoam cup
   l) Bath blanket
   m) Small towel
   n) Cotton

2. Wash your hands.

3. Identify the patient by checking the identification bracelet.

4. Ask visitors to step out of the room.

5. Tell the patient that you will give him a shampoo.

6. Pull the curtain around the bed for privacy.

7. Raise the bed to its highest horizontal position.

8. Place a chair at the side of the bed near the patient's head. The chair should be lower than the mattress. The back of the chair should be touching the mattress.

(continued next page)

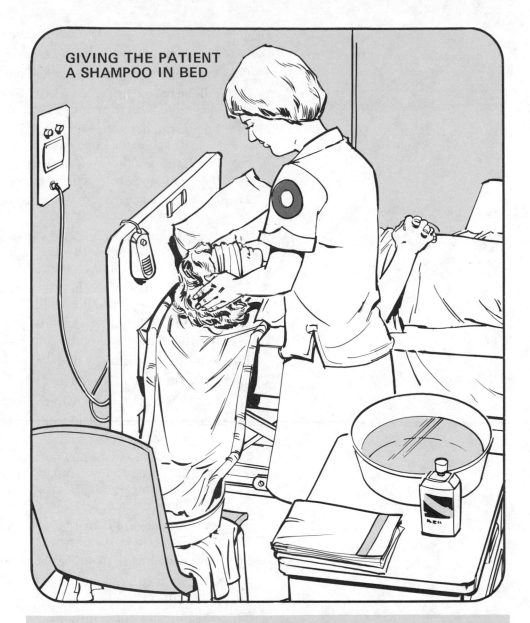

**GIVING THE PATIENT
A SHAMPOO IN BED**

Procedure continued

9. Place the small towel on the chair. Put the large basin on the chair.

10. Put small amounts of cotton in the patient's ears for protection.

11. Ask the patient to move across the bed so that his head is close to where you are standing.

12. Remove the pillow from under the patient's head. Cover the pillow with the waterproof case. Have the pillow under the small of the patient's back, so that when he lies down, his head is tilted back.

13. Put the bath blanket on the bed. From underneath, fan fold the top sheets to the foot of the bed without exposing the patient.

14. Place the disposable bed protector on the mattress under the patient's head.

15. Place the shampoo trough under the patient's head. A trough can be made by rolling up the sides of the plastic sheet. This makes a channel for the water to run off. Three sides must be rolled over three times to make the channel. Put the end of the channel under the patient's head. Have the other open end hanging over the side of the bed. This free end of the plastic sheet should be put into the large basin on the chair.

(continued next page)

16. Loosen the patient's gown at the neck and turn the neckband under.

17. Ask the patient to hold the washcloth over his eyes.

18. Fill the basin with water at 105°F (40.5°C). Put the basin on the bedside table with the paper or styrofoam cup.

19. Fill the pitcher with water at 115°F (46.1°C). Have the pitcher on the bedside table, for extra water, if needed.

20. Brush the patient's hair. Have him turn his head from side to side so the hair can be brushed one exposed side at a time.

21. Fill the paper cup with water from the basin. Pour it over the hair, repeat until completely wet.

22. Apply shampoo and, using both hands, wash the hair and massage the patient's scalp with your fingertips. Avoid using fingernails as they could scratch the scalp.

23. Rinse the soap off the hair by pouring water from the cup over the hair. Have the patient turn his head from side to side. Repeat this until the hair is clear of shampoo.

24. Dry the patient's forehead and ears with the face towel.

25. Remove the cotton from the ears.

26. Raise the patient's head and wrap the head with a bath towel.

27. Rub the patient's hair with the towel to dry it as much as possible.

28. Remove your equipment from the bed. Change the patient's gown, if necessary.

29. Comb the patient's hair. Then leave a towel wrapped around the head. Or spread a towel out over the pillow under the head until the hair is completely dry. If a dryer is available, use it to dry the patient's hair.

30. Remove the bath blanket and at the same time bring the top sheets back up to cover the patient.

31. Lower the bed to its lowest horizontal position.

32. Clean your equipment and put it in its proper place. Discard disposable equipment.

33. Make the patient comfortable.

34. Wash your hands.

35. Report to your head nurse or team leader:
    - That you have given the patient a shampoo.
    - Your observations of anything unusual.

**KEY IDEAS:
COMBING THE
PATIENT'S HAIR**

As with other types of personal care, a patient may be too weak or sick to take care of his own hair. It may be difficult for him to raise his arms. Almost always, however, combing and brushing a patient's hair, which makes him look better, will also make him feel better.

Procedure: Combing the Patient's Hair

1. Assemble your equipment on the bedside table:
   a) Towel
   b) Comb or brush
   c) Hand mirror, if available

2. Wash your hands.

(continued next page)

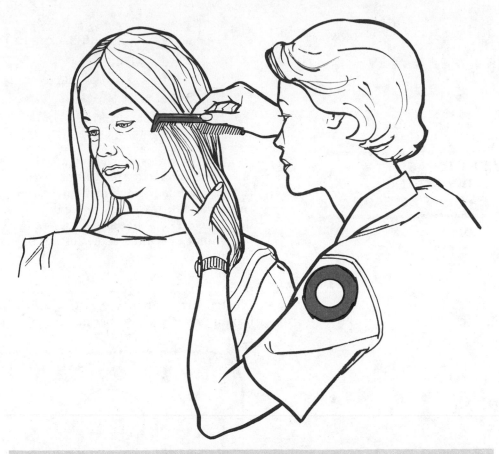

Procedure continued

3. Identify the patient by checking his identification bracelet.

4. Ask visitors to step out of the room.

5. Tell the patient you are going to brush or comb his hair.

6. Pull the curtain around the bed for privacy.

7. If possible, comb the patient's hair after the bath and before you make the bed.

8. Lay a towel across the pillow, under the patient's head. If the patient can sit up in bed, drape the towel around his shoulders.

9. If the patient wears glasses, ask him to take them off before you begin. Be sure to put the glasses in a safe place.

10. Part the hair down the middle to make it easier to comb.

11. Brush or comb the patient's hair carefully, gently, and thoroughly in his usual style.

12. For the patient who cannot sit up, separate the hair into small sections. Then comb each section separately, using a downward motion. Ask the patient to turn his head from side to side. Or turn it for him so you can reach the entire head.

13. Arrange the patient's hair the way he wants you to.

14. If the patient has very long hair, suggest braiding it to keep it from getting tangled.

15. Be sure you brush the back of the head.

16. Remove the towel when you are finished.

17. Let the patient use the mirror.

(continued next page)

18. Put your equipment back in its proper place.
19. Wash your hands.
20. Report to your head nurse or team leader:
    - That you have combed the patient's hair.
    - Your observations of anything unusual.

A regular morning activity for most men is shaving the beard. A patient is often well enough to shave himself. In this case, you will give him only the help that is necessary, such as being sure he has the equipment he needs. Sometimes patients are too ill or weak to shave themselves. In such cases, you will do it. Before shaving any patient's face, be sure to get permission from the head nurse or team leader. Certain patients may not be permitted to shave or be shaved.

Shaving can be done with an electric razor or a safety razor. Often, the patient will have his own electric razor. You will be able to use it to shave him. Electric razors are never used while the patient is receiving oxygen. If oxygen is being given to any other patient in the room, electric razors cannot be used.

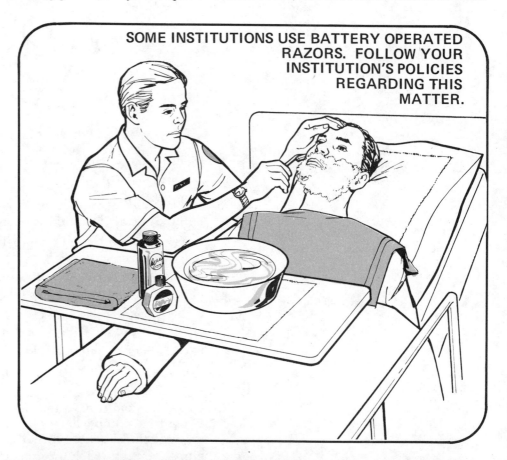

SOME INSTITUTIONS USE BATTERY OPERATED RAZORS. FOLLOW YOUR INSTITUTION'S POLICIES REGARDING THIS MATTER.

Procedure: Shaving the Patient's Beard

1. Assemble your equipment on the bedside table:
   a) Basin of water at 115°F (46.1°C).
   b) Shaving brush and shaving cream
   c) Safety razor

(continued next page)

d) Face towel
e) Mirror
f) Tissues
g) After-shave lotion, if available
h) Face powder, if available
i) Washcloth

2. Wash your hands.
3. Identify the patient by checking the identification bracelet.
4. Ask visitors to step out of the room.
5. Tell the patient that you are going to shave his beard.
6. Pull the curtain around the bed for privacy.
7. Adjust a light so that it shines on the patient's face.
8. Raise the head of the bed, if allowed.
9. Spread the face towel under the patient's chin. If the patient has dentures, be sure they are in his mouth.
10. Pat some warm water or use a damp warm washcloth on the patient's face to soften his beard.
11. Apply shaving soap generously to the face.
12. With the fingers of one hand, hold the skin taut (tight) as you shave in the direction that the hairs grow. Start under the sideburns and work downward over the cheeks. Continue carefully over the chin. Work upward on the neck under the chin. Use short firm strokes.
13. Rinse the razor often.
14. Areas under the nose and around the lips are sensitive. Take special care in these areas.
15. If you nick the patient's skin, report this to your head nurse or team leader.
16. Wash off the remaining soap when you have finished.
17. Apply after-shave lotion or powder as the patient prefers.
18. Clean your equipment and put it in its proper place. Discard disposable equipment.
19. Make the patient comfortable.
20. Wash your hands.
21. Report to your head nurse or team leader:
    - That you have shaved the patient's beard.
    - Your observations of anything unusual.

SECTION 2: BEDPAN—URINAL—BEDSIDE COMMODE

OBJECTIVES: WHAT YOU WILL LEARN

When you have completed this section, you will be able to:

- Help the patient use a bedpan.
- Help the patient use a urinal.
- Help the patient use the bedside commode.

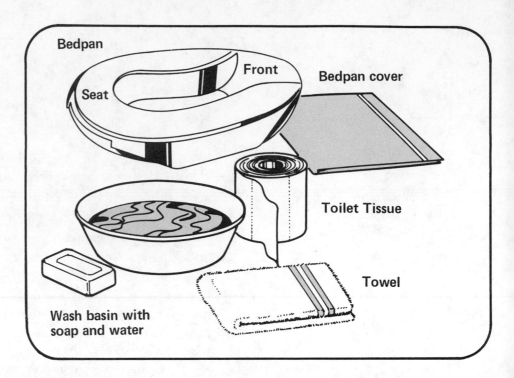

Bedpan · Front · Seat · **Bedpan cover** · **Toilet Tissue** · **Towel** · **Wash basin with soap and water**

Some patients are unable to get out of bed to use the bathroom. For these patients a urinal and a bedpan are required. The urinal is a container into which the male patient urinates. The bedpan is a pan into which he defecates (moves his bowels). The female patient uses the bedpan for urination and defecation. You should always cover the bedpan and remove it from the patient's bedside to the bathroom as quickly as possible after use. At this time you would collect a specimen if required. You would also measure the urine if the patient is on intake and output.

Procedure: Offering the Bedpan

1. Assemble your equipment on the bedside table:
   a) Bedpan and cover, or fracture bedpan and cover
   b) Toilet tissue
   c) Wash basin with water at 115°F (46.1°C)
   d) Soap
   e) Hand towel
   f) Disposable gloves, optional
2. Wash your hands.
3. Identify the patient by checking the identification bracelet.
4. Ask visitors to step out of the room.
5. Ask the patient if he would like to use the bedpan.
6. Pull the curtain around the bed for privacy.
7. Take the bedpan out of the bedside table. Warm the bedpan by running warm water inside it and along the rim. Dry the outside of the bedpan with paper towels.
8. Fold back the top sheets so that they are out of the way.
9. Raise the patient's gown, but keep the lower part of his body covered with the top sheets.
10. Ask the patient to bend his knees and put his feet flat on the mattress. Then ask the patient to raise his hips. If necessary, help the patient to raise his buttocks by slipping your hand under the lower part of his back. Place the bedpan in position with the seat of the bedpan under the buttocks.

(continued next page)

BEDPANS

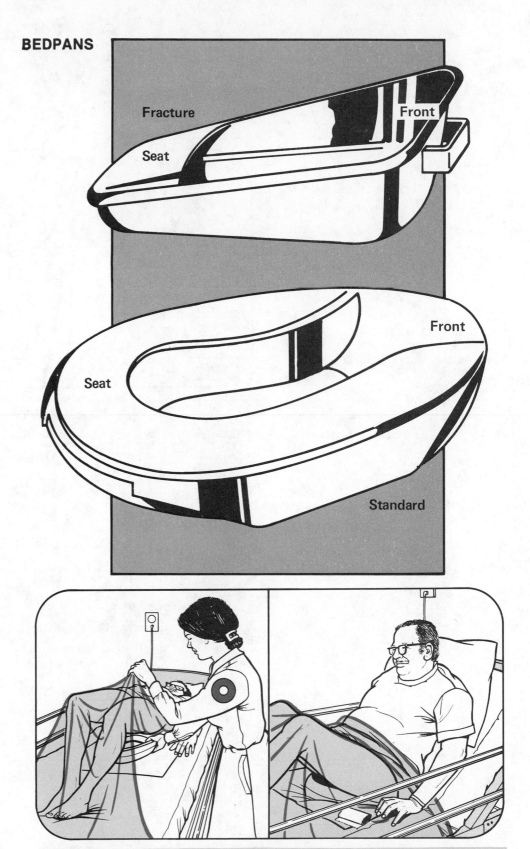

Fracture

Seat

Front

Seat

Front

Standard

Procedure continued

11. Sometimes the patient is unable to lift his buttocks to get on or off the bedpan. In this case, turn the patient on his side with his back to you. Put the bedpan against the buttocks. Then turn the patient back onto the bedpan.

(continued next page)

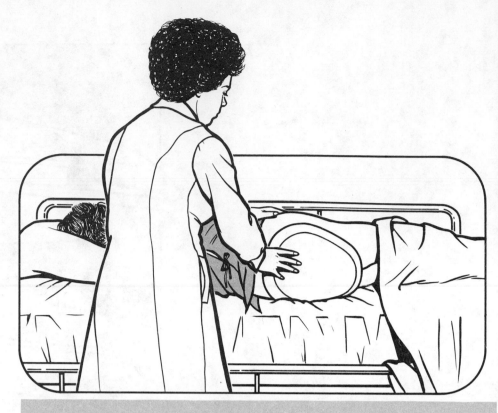

Procedure continued

12. Replace the covers over the patient.

13. Raise the backrest and kneerest, if allowed, so the .patient is in a sitting position.

14. Put toilet tissue and the signal cord where the patient can reach them easily.

15. Ask the patient to signal when he is finished.

16. Raise the side rails to the up position.

17. Wash your hands. Leave the room to give the patient privacy.

18. When the patient signals, return to the room.

19. Wash your hands.

20. Help the patient to raise his hips so you can remove the bedpan.

21. Cover the bedpan immediately. You can use a disposable pad or a paper towel if no cover is available.

22. Help the patient if he is unable to clean himself. Turn the patient on his side. Clean the anal area with toilet tissue.

23. Take the bedpan to the patient's bathroom.

24. If a specimen is required, collect it at this time. Measure the urine if the patient is on intake and output.

25. Check the excreta (feces or urine) for abnormal (unusual) appearance.

26. Empty the bedpan into the patient's toilet.

27. Every institution has different equipment in the bathroom for cleaning the bedpan. Follow your instructions for cleaning the bedpan in your institution. Cold water is always used to rinse the bedpan.

28. Put the clean bedpan and cover back into the bedside table.

29. Help the patient wash his hands in the basin of water.

(continued next page)

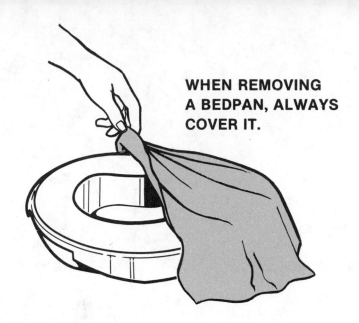

WHEN REMOVING A BEDPAN, ALWAYS COVER IT.

Procedure continued

30. Make the patient comfortable. Lower the backrest as necessary. Pull back the curtains to the open position.
31. Wash your hands.
32. Report to your head nurse or team leader:
    - That the patient has urinated or defecated.
    - If a specimen was collected.
    - Your observations of anything unusual.

Procedure: Offering the Urinal

1. Assemble your equipment on the bedside table:
   a) Urinal and cover
   b) Basin of water at 115°F (46.1°C)
   c) Soap
   d) Towel
   e) Disposable gloves, optional
2. Wash your hands.
3. Identify the patient by checking the identification bracelet.
4. Ask visitors to step out of the room.
5. Ask the patient if he would like to use the urinal.
6. Pull the curtain around the bed for privacy.
7. Give the urinal to the patient.
8. Place the signal cord within easy reach.
9. Ask the patient to signal when he is finished.
10. Wash your hands. Leave the room to give the patient privacy.
11. When the patient signals, return to the room and wash your hands.
12. Cover the urinal and take it to the patient's bathroom.
13. Check urine for abnormal (unusual) appearance.
14. Measure the urine if the patient is on intake and output. Collect a specimen at this time, if required.
15. Empty the urinal into the toilet. Rinse with cold water.
16. Put the clean urinal back in the patient's bedside table.

(continued next page)

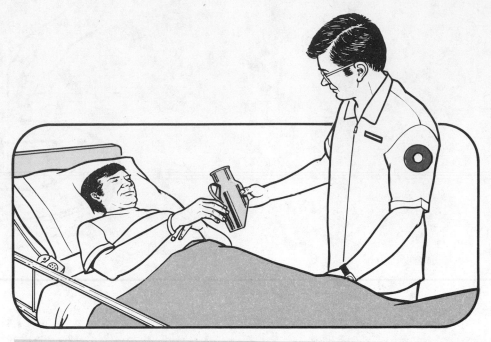

Procedure continued

17. Help the patient wash his hands in the basin of water.
18. Make the patient comfortable.
19. Wash your hands.
20. Report to your head nurse or team leader:
    - That the patient has voided.
    - If a specimen has been collected.
    - Your observations of anything unusual.

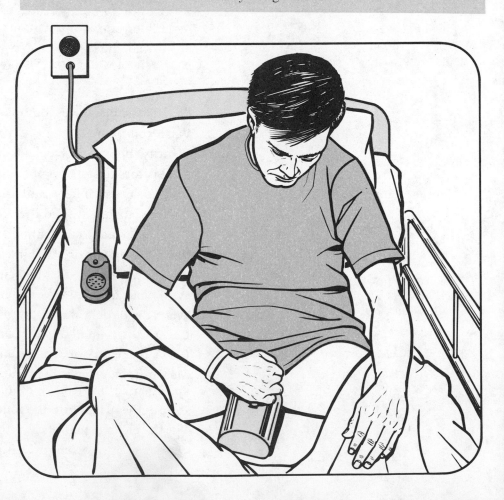

Procedure: Offering the Portable Bedside Commode

1. Assemble your equipment on the bedside table:
   a) Portable bedside commode next to the bed
   b) Bedpan and cover, or the container used in your institution
   c) Toilet tissue
   d) Basin of water at 115°F (46.1°C)
   e) Soap
   f) Towel
   g) Disposable gloves, optional
2. Wash your hands.
3. Identify the patient by checking the identification bracelet.
4. Ask visitors to step out of the room.
5. Tell the patient you will assist him onto the bedside commode.
6. Pull the curtain around the bed for privacy.
7. Put the commode next to the patient's bed. Open the cover and insert a bedpan under the toilet seat.
8. Help the patient put on his slippers and then help him out of bed and onto the commode.
9. Put toilet tissue and the signal cord where the patient can reach them easily.
10. Ask the patient to signal when he is finished.
11. Wash your hands. Leave the room to give the patient privacy.
12. When the patient signals, return to the room. Wash your hands.
13. Help the patient if he is unable to clean himself.
14. Assist the patient back to bed.
15. Close the cover on the commode.
16. Help the patient to wash his hands in the basin of water.
17. Make the patient comfortable.
18. Remove the bedpan from under the commode. Cover it and carry it to the patient's bathroom.
19. Check the excreta (feces or urine) for abnormal (unusual) appearance.
20. Measure output if patient is on intake and output. If a specimen is required, collect it at this time.
21. Empty the bedpan into the toilet.
22. Every institution has different equipment in the bathroom for cleaning the bedpan. Follow your instructions for cleaning the bedpan in your institution. Cold water is always used to rinse the bedpan.
23. Put the clean bedpan back in the bedside table. Put the commode in its proper place.
24. Wash your hands.
25. Report to your head nurse or team leader.
    - That the patient has voided or defecated.
    - If a specimen was collected.
    - Your observations of anything unusual.

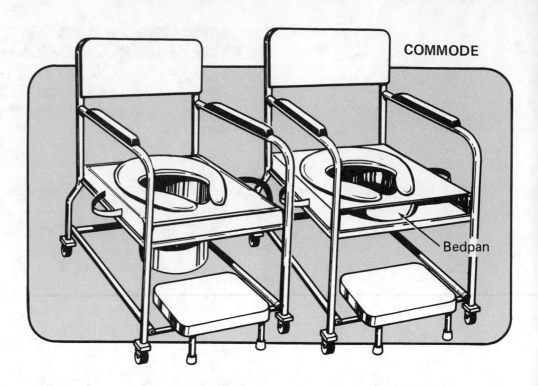

COMMODE

Bedpan

WHAT YOU HAVE LEARNED

Daily personal care of patients is an essential part of your duties as a nursing assistant. Patients should be encouraged to help as much as possible with their daily care, if this is allowed.

You will be giving oral hygiene, bathing the patient, and offering bedpans and urinals. In giving this care, it is important to respect the patient's privacy. These tasks should be performed with tender loving care and careful, regular observations to note any pattern of change in the patient's condition.

8 NUTRITION AND FOOD SERVICE

1. Therapeutic Diets
2. Nutrition for the Patient

SECTION 1: THERAPEUTIC DIETS

OBJECTIVES: WHAT YOU WILL LEARN

When you have completed this section, you will be able to:

- Define a well-balanced diet.
- Name the four basic food groups.
- List some foods included in each group.
- Explain what is meant by a therapeutic diet.
- List various types of therapeutic diets.
- Describe each type of therapeutic diet.
- Explain the purpose of each type of therapeutic diet.

**KEY IDEAS:
A WELL-BALANCED DIET**

The key to a healthy, well-balanced diet lies in eating a variety of foods, and in not eating too much. The foods that are essential for keeping the body well are divided into four groups. Everybody needs the nutrients contained in all of the four groups. If you eat one or more portions of food from each of these four groups every day, your diet will be adequate for good health. The number of servings and the size of portions will depend on the age, size, and activities of the individual. Following are the four basic food groups, along with suggestions for a good diet for the average person. Check your own eating habits to be sure you are eating a well-balanced diet.

A. *Dairy Products:* Milk or milk products are needed to supply protein, calcium, and other minerals, and to supply vitamins and carbohydrates. Every day a small child should have at least three to four 8-ounce glasses of milk. A teenager should have four or more glasses. An adult should have a glass or two daily, but pregnant women and nursing mothers need milk in greater quantity. Other forms of milk and milk products also acceptable include concentrated, evaporated, skim, and dry milk, yogurt, buttermilk, cream, and cheese.

B. *Vegetables and Fruits:* Four servings from this group are needed every day to supply an adequate amount of certain vitamins and minerals, and to provide roughage. One of the servings should be from the citrus fruits—oranges, lemons, grapefruit—that are high in vitamin C. At least four meals a week should include a dark green or yellow vegetable for vitamin A.

C. *Meat and Meat Substitutes:* These include meat, fish, poultry, eggs, cheese, dried beans, peas, and nuts. Three servings daily from this group are recommended for a good diet. At least one serving should be meat, fish, or

THE FOUR BASIC FOOD GROUPS

EAT VITAL FOODS • EVERY MEAL • EVERY DAY
A SELECTED VARIETY FROM EACH GROUP

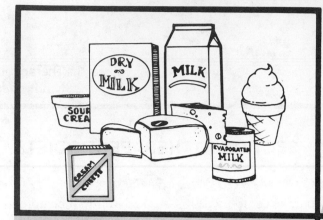

Group 1: Dairy Products

Milk

- 3 to 4 cups (Children)
- 4 or more cups (Teenagers)
- 2 or more cups (Adults)

Cheese, ice cream and other milk-made foods can be substituted for part of the milk requirement

Group 2: Vegetables and Fruit

- **4 or more servings**

Include dark green or deep yellow vegetables: citrus fruit or tomatoes

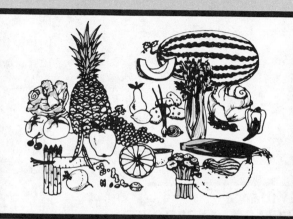

Group 3: Meat and Fish

- **3 servings**

Meats, fish, poultry, eggs or cheese, with dry beans, peas, nuts as alternates

Group 4: Breads, Cereals, and Potatoes

- **6 or more servings**

Enriched or whole grain. Added milk improves nutritional value

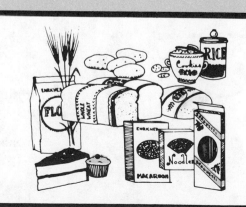

poultry. One serving might be an egg, a slice of cheese, or a small serving of split peas or baked beans.

D. *Breads, Cereals, and Potatoes:* Whole grain or enriched bread and cereals are necessary for the body's nutrition because they provide carbohydrates for energy. Six servings every day from this group are recommended.

Food is able to give nourishment to the body because it contains various chemical substances called nutrients. Some 50 individual nutrients are needed to build the body. Many others are useful although they may not be required. Scientists also have discovered that nutrients work better together than alone. For instance, you may get enough calcium from milk but it is wasted if you do not get enough vitamin C or D from other foods to help the calcium develop the bones.

Many foods we eat contain combinations of various nutrients that are responsible for body functions. For example, whole-grain cereals are high in carbohydrates, but they also contain some protein, minerals, and vitamins. Foods help the body perform its functions only if they contain the right nutrients.

How Nutrients Are Made

The first step in making nutrients takes place in green plants. They take water and minerals from the soil, and water and carbon dioxide from the air. With the help of the sun's energy, these substances are built into nutrients.

How Nutrients Are Used

When people eat plants they get the nutrients from them. Also when people eat meat they get the nutrients animals have taken from green plants.

After food is eaten it enters the digestive tract where the nutrients are changed into simple forms. These simple forms then are carried by the blood to the body cells where the special functions of each are carried out.

There are six classes of nutrients: carbohydrates, fats, minerals, proteins, vitamins, and water. Because there are several kinds of each class of nutrients except water, it is clearer to speak of the classes instead of the individual nutrients. The chart on the following pages gives a brief description of each nutrient class and its bodily function.

Eating properly is very important when you are healthy and feeling well. Good nourishment is even more important when a person is ill. The food service department or dietary department in your institution will be preparing a well-balanced diet of good nourishing meals for many different patients. This basic balanced diet is often called by different names:

- Normal diet
- Regular diet
- House diet
- Full diet

A well-balanced diet is one that contains a variety of food from each of the four basic food groups at every meal.

The normal diet is sometimes changed to meet a patient's special nutritional needs. This modified diet is also known by several names:

- Therapeutic diet
- Special diet
- Restricted diet
- Modified diet

NUTRIENT CLASS	BODILY FUNCTION	FOOD SOURCES
CARBOHYDRATES	Provides work energy for body activities, and heat energy for maintenance of body temperature.	Cereal grains and their products (bread, breakfast cereals, macaroni products), potatoes, sugar, syrups, fruits, milk, vegetables, nuts
PROTEINS	Build and renew body tissues; regulate body functions and supply energy. Complete proteins: maintain life and provide growth. Incomplete proteins: maintain life but do not provide for growth.	Complete proteins: Derived from animal foods — meat, milk, eggs, fish, cheese, poultry. Incomplete proteins: Derived from vegetable foods — soybeans, dry beans, peas, some nuts and whole-grain products.
FATS	Give work energy for body activities and heat energy for maintenance of body temperature. Carrier of vitamins A and D, provide fatty acids necessary for growth and maintenance of body tissues.	Some foods are chiefly fat, such as lard, vegetable fats and oils, and butter. Many other foods contain smaller proportions of fats — nuts, meats, fish, poultry, cream, whole milk.
MINERALS Calcium	Builds and renews bones, teeth, and other tissues; regulates the activity of the muscles, heart. nerves; and controls the clotting of blood.	Milk and milk products, except butter; most dark green vegetables; canned salmon.
Phosphorus	Associated with calcium in some functions needed to build and renew bones and teeth. Influences the oxidation of foods in the body cells; important in nerve tissue.	Widely distributed in foods; especially cheese, oat cereals, whole-wheat products, dry beans and peas, meat, fish, poultry, nuts.

NUTRIENT CLASS	BODILY FUNCTIONS	FOOD SOURCES
MINERALS (continued) **Iron**	Builds and renews hemoglobin, the red pigment in blood which carries oxygen from the lungs to the cells.	Eggs, meat, especially liver and kidney; deep-yellow and dark green vegetables; potatoes, dried fruits, whole-grain products; enriched flour, bread, breakfast cereals.
Iodine	Enables the thyroid gland to perform its function of controlling the rate at which foods are oxidized in the cells.	Fish (obtained from the sea), some plant-foods grown in soils containing iodine; table salt fortified with iodine (iodized).
VITAMINS **A**	Necessary for normal functioning of the eyes, prevents night blindness. Ensures a healthy condition of the skin, hair, and mucous membranes. Maintains a state of resistance to infections of the eyes, mouth, and respiratory tract.	One form of Vitamin A is yellow and one form is colorless. Apricots, cantaloupe, milk, cheese, eggs, meat organs, (especially liver and kidney), fortified margarine, butter, fish-liver oils, dark green and deep yellow vegetables.
B Complex **B₁ (Thiamine)**	Maintains a healthy condition of the nerves. Fosters a good appetite. Helps the body cells use carbohydrates.	Whole-grain and enriched grain products; meats (especially pork, liver and kidney). dry beans and peas.
B₂ (Riboflavin)	Keeps the skin, mouth, and eyes in a healthy condition. Acts with other nutrients to form enzymes and control oxidation in cells.	Milk, cheese, eggs, meat (especially liver and kidney), whole grain and enriched grain products, dark green vegetables.

NUTRIENT CLASS	BODILY FUNCTIONS	FOOD SOURCES
VITAMINS (Continued) Niacin	Influences the oxidation of carbohydrates and proteins in the body cells.	Liver, meat, fish, poultry, eggs, peanuts; dark green vegetables, whole-grain and enriched cereal products.
B₁₂	Regulates specific processes in digestion. Helps maintain normal functions of muscles, nerves, heart, blood — general body metabolism.	Liver, other organ meats, cheese, eggs, milk, leafy green vegetables.
C (Ascorbic Acid)	Acts as a cement between body cells, and helps them work together to carry out their special functions. Maintains a sound condition of bones, teeth, and gums. Not stored in the body.	Fresh, raw citrus fruits and vegetables — oranges, grapefruit, cantaloupe, strawberries, tomatoes, raw onions, cabbage, green and sweet red peppers, dark green vegetables.
D	Enables the growing body to use calcium and phosphorus in a normal way to build bones and teeth.	Provided by Vitamin D fortification of certain foods, such as milk and margarine. Also fish-liver oils and eggs. Sunshine is also a source of Vitamin D.
WATER	Regulates body processes. Aids in regulating body temperature. Carries nutrients to body cells and carries waste products away from them. Helps to lubricate joints. Water has no food value, although most water contains mineral elements. More immediately necessary to life than food — second only to oxygen.	Drinking water, and other beverages; all foods except those made up of a single nutrient, as sugar and some fats. Milk milk drinks, soups, vegetables, fruit juices. Ice cream, watermelon, strawberries, lettuce, tomatoes, cereals, other dry products.

Types of Diets Given to Patients; What They Are and Why They Are Used

Type of diet	Description	Common purpose
Normal regular	Provides all essentials of good nourishment in normal forms	For patients who do not need special diets
Clear liquid (Hospital surgical)	Broth, tea, ginger ale, gelatin	Usually for patients who have had surgery or are very ill
Full liquid	Broth, tea, coffee, ginger ale, gelatin, strained fruit juices, liquids, custard, junket, ice cream, sherbet, soft-cooked eggs	For those unable to chew or swallow solid food
Light or soft	Foods soft in consistency, no rich or strongly flavored foods that could cause distress	Final stage for postoperative patient before resuming regular diet
Soft (mechanical)	Same foods as on a normal diet, but chopped or strained	For patients who have difficulty in chewing or swallowing
Bland	Foods mild in flavor and easy to digest; omits spicy foods	Avoids irritation of the digestive tract, as with ulcer and colitis patients
Low residue	Foods low in bulk; omits foods difficult to digest	Spares the lower digestive tract, as with patients having rectal diseases
High calorie	Foods high in protein, minerals, and vitamins	For underweight or malnourished patients
Low calorie	Low in cream, butter, cereals, desserts, and fats	For patients who need to lose weight
Diabetic	Precise balance of carbohydrates, protein, and fats, devised according to the needs of individual patients	For diabetic patients; matches food intake with the insulin and nutritional requirements
High protein	Meals supplemented with high protein foods, such as meat, fish, cheese, milk, and eggs	Assists in the growth and repair of tissues wasted by disease
Low fat	Limited amounts of butter, cream, fats, and eggs	For patients who have difficulty digesting fats, as in gallbladder, cardiovascular, and liver disturbances
Low cholesterol	Low in eggs, whole milk, and meats	Helps regulate the amount of cholesterol in the blood
Low sodium (low salt)	Limited amount of foods containing sodium, no salt allowed on tray	For patients whose circulation would be impaired by fluid retention; patients with certain heart or kidney conditions
Salt-free (sodium-free)	Completely without salt	
Tube feeding	Milk formula or liquid forms of meat or vegetables given to the patient through a tube; follow with a glass of water	For patients who, because of a condition such as oral surgery can't eat normally

Therapeutic diets require the preparation of meals that differ from those regularly prepared for patients on the normal diet. The special meals given to patients who cannot be on a normal diet are ordered by the doctor. They are worked out by the dietitian according to the patient's illness and what is needed for his recovery. These special meals help the doctor in treating a patient. For example, a man who has a disorder of his digestive system may be on a soft diet. A diabetic patient may be on a diet in which total calories are limited and the amounts of protein, fat, and carbohydrates are specified. A person with heart disease may be restricted to a low-salt (sodium) diet or a salt-free diet. The doctor may order changes in the normal diet for several reasons. These include:

- Changing the consistency of the patient's food, as in liquid or "soft" diets.
- Changing the caloric intake, as in high- or low-calorie diets.
- Changing the amounts of one or more nutrients, as in a high-protein, low-fat, or low-salt (sodium) diet.
- Changing the amount of bulk, as in a low-residue diet.
- Changing the seasonings in the patient's food, as in a bland diet.
- Omitting foods that the patient is allergic to.
- Changing the time and number of meals.

Whenever the word salt is used it means sodium and when sodium is used it means salt. Therefore, when we refer to a salt-free diet we mean a sodium-free diet and when we refer to a low-sodium diet we mean a low-salt diet.

SECTION 2: NUTRITION FOR THE PATIENT

OBJECTIVES: WHAT YOU WILL LEARN

When you have completed this section, you will be able to:

- Prepare the patient before mealtime.
- Serve the food tray.
- Observe and record information concerning meals.
- Feed the helpless patient.
- Serve extra nourishment.
- Distribute drinking water.

**KEY IDEAS:
PREPARING THE PATIENT
AND SERVING A MEAL**

A poor appetite does not mean that the body's need for food is lowered. The sick person's body is in a weakened condition. The patient needs as much food as ever—if not more—to return to health. The surroundings and the food served should be as cheerful, attractive, and appetizing as possible. The sight and aroma of food often make a person hungry. You often can increase a patient's appetite by showing him what he will be eating. Also, people have a better appetite for foods they especially like. Therefore, if a patient asks for a particular food (and if he is permitted to have it) you should try to arrange for that food to be served to him. You can do this by reporting the patient's request to your team leader or head nurse.

Mealtime often is one of the highlights of the day for a convalescent patient or a patient who is not extremely sick. Mealtime is a break in the often boring routine. It gives the patient something to look forward to. Many patients also enjoy making food selections from the menu, when choices are offered. This is another time when attitude is important. If the patient seems to want you to, look at the menu with him and make suggestions. When the food tray is delivered, do everything you can to make the patient's meal as pleasant and comfortable as possible.

As you know, eating in a pleasant, attractive place helps you enjoy your food. This is also true for the hospital patient. When a patient is going to have a meal, be sure the room is clean, quiet, free of unpleasant odors, and not too warm or cold. Take away things that might spoil the patient's appetite—items such as an emesis basin, urinal, or bedpan.

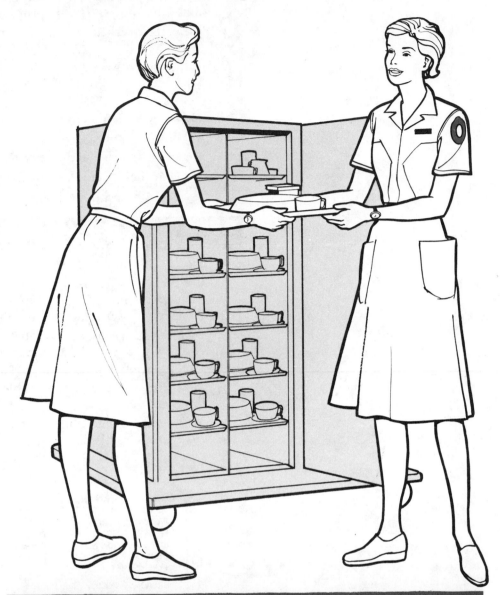

Procedure: Preparing the Patient for a Meal

1. Assemble your equipment on the bedside table:
   a) Bedpan or urinal
   b) Basin of warm water at 115°F (46.1°C)
   c) Washcloth
   d) Towel
   e) Robe and slippers
2. Wash your hands.
3. Identify the patient by checking the identification bracelet.
4. Ask visitors to step out of the room.
5. Tell the patient you are getting him ready for his next meal.
6. Pull the curtain around the bed for privacy.
7. Offer the bedpan or urinal, or assist the patient to the bathroom.
8. Have the patient wash his hands or do this for him.

(continued next page)

Procedure continued

9. Raise the backrest so the patient is in a sitting position, if this is allowed. If not, you might prop up his head by using several pillows.

10. Clear the overbed table. Put it in a convenient position for the patient's meal.

11. If the patient wants to sit in a chair during his meal and if this is allowed, help him into his robe and slippers, and help him out of bed and to the chair.

12. Make the patient comfortable.

13. Wash your hands.

14. Report to your head nurse or team leader:
    - That the patient is ready for his next meal.
    - Your observations of anything unusual.

Procedure: Serving the Food

1. Wash your hands.

2. Check the tray before you give it to a patient. Is everything on it? All the silverware and a napkin? Does the tray look attractive? Was food spilled? Correct anything that is wrong.

3. Be sure you are giving the tray to the right patient. Check the menu card, which will have the patient's name on it, against the identification band to be sure they match.

4. Put the tray on the overbed table. Adjust it to a height comfortable for the patient.

5. Arrange the dishes and silver so the patient can reach everything easily. Be sure his drinking water is handy.

(continued next page)

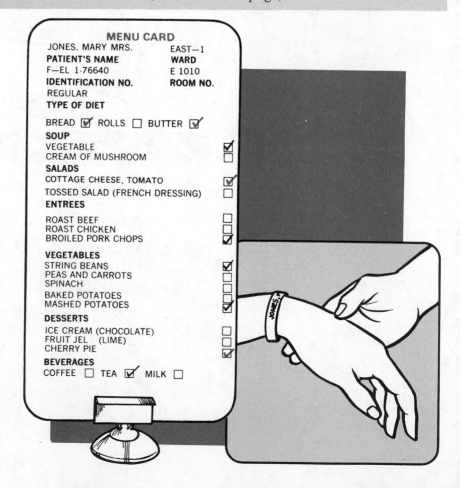

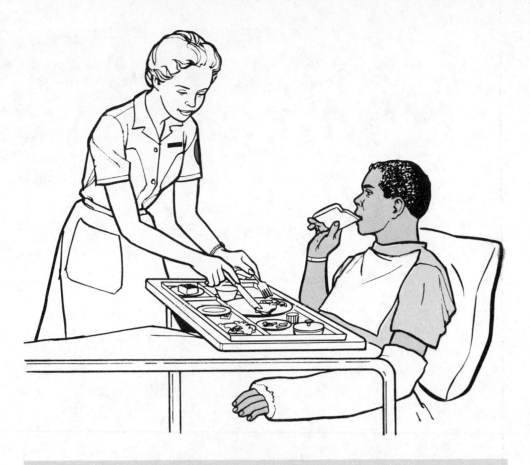

Procedure continued

6. Help any patient who needs it. For example, if a patient seems to be weak or asks for help, you might offer to spread his napkin on his lap or tuck it under his chin. Spread butter on his bread. Cut up his meat. Pour tea or coffee. Do not give him any more help than he really needs. The more a patient can do for himself, the better.

7. A patient may discover that he cannot eat when he is served. If permitted, you may take his tray away and keep the hot food warm for him until he wants to eat.

8. When you are sure the patient can go on with his meal by himself, leave the room.

9. Go back for the food tray when the patient has finished eating.

10. Note how much the patient has eaten and how much he has had to drink.

11. Record fluid intake on the intake and output sheet.

12. Record how the patient has eaten his meal on the daily activity sheet. Record this information separately for breakfast, lunch, and supper:
    a) Did the patient eat all the food served to him?
    b) Did the patient eat about half the food served?
    c) Did the patient eat very little food?
    d) Did the patient refuse to accept the tray and actually eat nothing?

13. Take the tray away and put it in its proper place.

14. If the patient ate sitting in a chair, help him back into bed.

15. Put his personal articles back where the patient wants them.

(continued next page)

16. If the patient ate in bed, brush crumbs from the bed. Smooth out the sheets. Straighten the bedding.
17. Make the patient comfortable.
18. Wash your hands.
19. Report to your head nurse or team leader:
    - That you have served the patient his food.
    - Your observations of anything unusual.

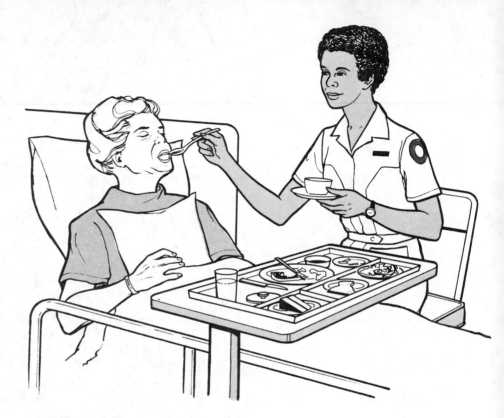

KEY IDEAS: FEEDING THE HELPLESS PATIENT

Some patients are incapable of feeding themselves and, therefore, are considered helpless and will have to be fed. The reason might be:

- The patient cannot use his hands.
- The doctor wants the patient to save his strength and to be on "complete bed rest."
- The patient may be too weak to feed himself.

Usually it is hard for an adult to accept the idea of not being able to feed himself. Because a patient is helpless, he may feel resentful and depressed. Be friendly and natural. Talk pleasantly but not too much. Help the patient overcome his resentment by encouraging him to do as much as he can. Also, remember that because of medical reasons the patient may not always be allowed to help. You will learn how to judge the amount of help a patient can give you when he is being fed. For example, if a patient is strong enough, you might let him hold a piece of bread you have buttered for him.

When feeding a helpless patient, the most important thing is not to rush him through the meal. The time he takes to chew his food, for example, may seem long to you. But he is probably very weak; otherwise he would be feeding himself.

Remember that you should not bring the food tray or have it delivered until you have prepared the patient for his meal and are ready to feed him. Again, make sure you are serving the correct tray to the patient. Preparations before mealtime are the same for the helpless patient as for the patient who can feed himself. Be observant throughout. Watch for signs of choking or anything unusual.

Procedure: Feeding the Helpless Patient or the Patient Who is Unable to Feed Himself

1. Assemble your equipment on the overbed table:
   a) The patient's tray.
2. Wash your hands.
3. Check the name on the name card on the tray against the patient's identification bracelet.
4. Tell the patient you are going to feed him his meal.
5. If you plan to be seated while you feed the patient, bring a chair to a convenient position beside the bed.
6. Check the tray to make sure everything is there. If anything is missing, have it brought in or get it yourself.
7. Tuck a napkin under the patient's chin.
8. Season the food the way the patient likes it. But do this only if his request agrees with the prescribed diet.
9. Always use a spoon when feeding a helpless patient. Fill the spoon only half-full. Give the food to the patient from the tip of the spoon, not the side. Put the food in one side of the patient's mouth so he can chew it more easily. If a patient is paralyzed on one side of his body, make sure you feed him on the side of his mouth that is not paralyzed.
10. If the patient cannot see the tray, name each mouthful of food as you offer it. Offer the different foods in a logical order, soup or juice before the main course. Alternate between liquids and solid foods throughout the meal. Feed the patient as you yourself would want to eat. Or follow the patient's suggestions about how he wants to alternate between various kinds of foods and a beverage.

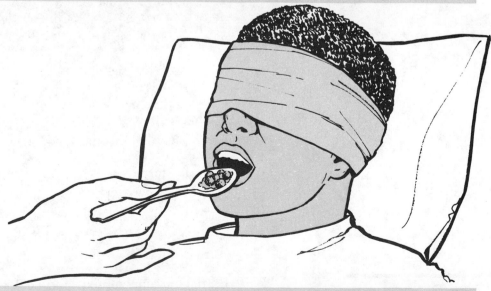

11. If the patient is unable to see and would like to feed himself, you can describe the position of the food on his tray. For example, cold li-

(continued next page)

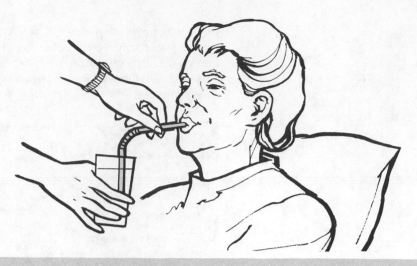

Procedure continued

quids are in the left corner, hot liquids in the right corner. Tell him to picture his plate as the face of a clock, corn at the 3, mashed potatoes at the 6, roast beef at the 12. Try to maintain the patient's independence as much as possible.

12. Warn the patient if you are offering something hot. Use a straw for giving liquids. Use a new straw for each beverage.

13. Feed the patient slowly. Remember that he may chew and swallow very slowly. Allow plenty of time between mouthfuls.

14. Encourage the patient to finish his meal, but do not force him.

15. When the patient has finished eating, help him to wipe his mouth with his napkin, or do this for him.

16. Notice how much the patient has eaten and how much he has had to drink.

17. Record fluid intake on the intake and output sheet.

18. Record how the patient has eaten his meal on the daily activity sheet. Record this information separately for breakfast, lunch, and supper:
    a) Did the patient eat all the food served to him?
    b) Did the patient eat about one-half the food served?
    c) Did the patient eat very little food?
    d) Did the patient refuse to accept the tray and actually eat nothing?

19. As soon as you are sure the patient is finished with the tray, take it away. Put it in its proper place.

20. Adjust the backrest of the bed to make the patient comfortable, if this is allowed.

21. Brush crumbs from the bed. Smooth the sheets. Straighten the bedding.

22. Make the patient comfortable.

23. Wash your hands.

24. Report to your head nurse or team leader:
    ● That you have fed the helpless patient.
    ● Your observations of anything unusual.

KEY IDEAS: BETWEEN-MEAL NOURISHMENTS

Extra nourishment in the form of food or drink is offered to patients during the day. This is a kind of hospital "snack" given to patients to provide quick energy or to break the routine. Patients are often given extra nourishment as part of their medical care. The snack is usually a beverage such as milk, chocolate milk, or fruit juice. Or it may be a portion of food such as gelatin, custard, crackers, or a sandwich. Some patients on special diets are allowed to have only certain kinds and amounts of extra nourishment. Other patients may not be allowed to have anything at all.

In some institutions, extra nourishment is passed out to patients by workers for the food service department. However, you may be assigned this responsibility. If you are, the head nurse or your team leader will give you a list of patients that will show:

- Those who are not to be given anything.

- Those who are allowed to have certain nourishment, such as skim milk or tea.

- Those who have no restrictions on their diet.

A specific time for serving nourishments to patients on special diets may be given on the nourishment chart. Be sure to follow this time schedule carefully.

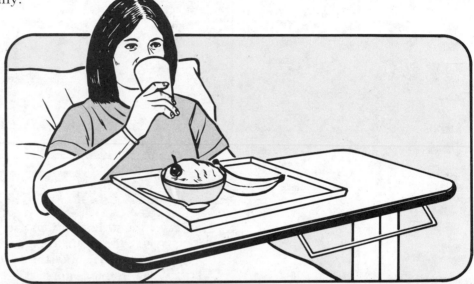

Procedure: Serving Between-Meal Nourishments

1. Wash your hands.
2. Assemble your equipment on a tray or a cart:
   a) Nourishment
   b) Cup, dish, and a spoon or straw
   c) Napkin
3. Identify the patient by checking the identification bracelet.
4. If a patient has a choice of items, ask him what he wants.
5. Prepare the nourishment.
6. Take the nourishment to the patient on a tray or cart.
7. Encourage the patient to take his nourishment. Help him if he needs it. Offer a straw if this is more convenient for him.
8. After the patient has finished, collect the tray.
9. Discard disposable equipment.
10. Record the intake for those patients who are on intake and output.
11. Wash your hands.
12. Report to your head nurse or team leader:
    - That you have served the between-meal nourishment.
    - Your observations of anything unusual.

Part of your job as a nursing assistant will be to see that the patients you are caring for have plenty of fresh water at their bedsides, unless a doctor orders otherwise. Some patients are not allowed to have more than a certain amount of water. Some, for brief periods, may not have water at all.

Fresh water is passed to patients at regular intervals during the day. Your instructor will tell you the schedule of your institution.

Disposable pitchers and cups are used everywhere.

Most patients like ice water. Others want water without ice, straight from the tap. You will be told which patients are allowed to have a choice. If a patient is not allowed to have ice, his water pitcher will be tagged OMIT ICE.

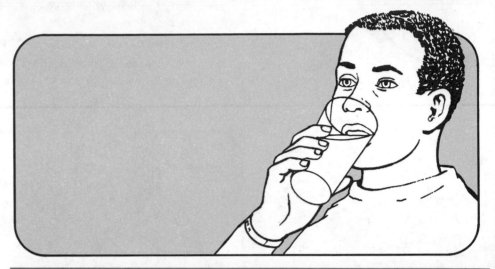

Procedure: Passing Drinking Water

NOTE: In some institutions each water pitcher is taken individually to the clean kitchen or utility room, filled with clean water and ice, and then returned to each individual patient. When this is done, the following procedure is NOT used.

1. Assemble your equipment:
   a) Moving table (cart) with small styrofoam ice chest and cover
   b) Ice cubes
   c) Scoop
   d) Paper or styrofoam cups
   e) Disposable water pitchers
   f) Straws
   g) Paper towels

2. Wash your hands.

3. Fill the ice chest with ice cubes and cover it.

4. Put the equipment on the table.

5. Before you pass drinking water, be sure you know:
   a) Which patients are NPO (nothing by mouth).
   b) Which patients are on restricted fluids and therefore get only a measured amount of water.
   c) Which patients should get only tap water (omit ice).
   d) Which patients may have ice water.

6. Roll the moving table into the hall outside the patient's room.

7. Go into the room and pick up one patient's water pitcher.

8. Empty it in the sink in the room. Fill it half full with tap water.

(continued next page)

9. Walk to the water table in the hall. Fill the pitcher to the brim with ice cubes, being sure the scoop does not touch the water pitcher.

10. Replace the water pitcher on the same patient's table from which it was taken. If the pitcher is labeled with the patient's name, check it against the identification bracelet.

11. Throw away used paper cups.

12. Wipe the table with a clean paper towel. Discard the towel.

13. Place several clean paper cups next to the water pitcher.

14. Place several straws next to the water pitcher.

15. Be sure the patient can reach the water pitcher easily.

16. Offer to pour a fresh glass of water for the patient.

17. Wash your hands.

18. Report to your head nurse or team leader:

    ● That you have passed drinking water to the patient.

    ● Your observations of anything unusual.

WHAT YOU HAVE LEARNED

For good health, every person needs the essential nutrients contained in all four of the basic food groups. Patients on therapeutic diets are permitted only those foods included in their strict prescribed diet. These patients must never be served any other foods. Before you serve any tray, be sure to check the identification bracelet against the name on the tray card. Observe how much the patient has eaten and record this information. Make accurate records of fluid intake on the intake and output sheet. Remember that you should not bring the food tray into a helpless patient's room until you are ready to feed him. When servng between-meal nourishments, check the diet list to be sure each patient is served only those foods permitted on his diet. When passing drinking water, be sure to return the patient's water pitcher to the same patient.

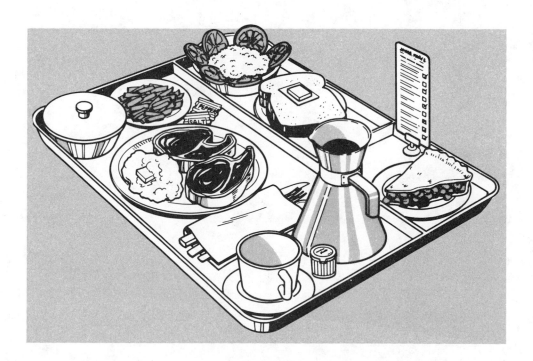

9 INTAKE AND OUTPUT

1. Fluid Balance
2. Fluid Intake
3. Forcing and Restricting Fluids
4. Fluid Output

SECTION 1: FLUID BALANCE

OBJECTIVES: WHAT YOU WILL LEARN

When you have completed this section, you will be able to:

- Explain fluid balance and imbalance.
- List the reasons for making accurate records of fluid intake and output.

Water is essential to human life. Next to oxygen, water is the most important thing the body takes in. A person can be starving, can lose half of his body protein and almost half of his body weight, and he can still live. But losing only one-fifth of the body's fluid will result in death.

Through eating and drinking, the average healthy adult will take in about 3½ quarts of fluid every day. This is his fluid intake. The same adult also will elminate about 3½ quarts of fluid every day. This is his fluid output. Fluid is discharged from the body of a healthy person in several ways:

- Most of the fluid passes through the kidneys and is discharged as urine.
- Some of the fluid is lost from the body through perspiration.
- Some is evaporated from the lungs in breathing.
- The rest is absorbed and discharged through the intestinal system.

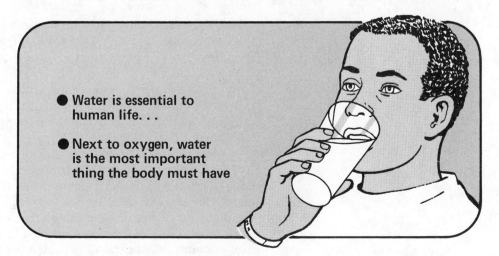

- Water is essential to human life. . .
- Next to oxygen, water is the most important thing the body must have

It is difficult to measure accurately the amount of fluid discharged through evaporation and breathing. Therefore, a person may seem to have a greater fluid intake than output. There is, however, a fluid balance in the normally functioning body. Fluid balance means that just about the same amount of fluid taken in by the body is also eliminated. The fluid taken in is called the fluid intake. The fluid given out, no matter how, is called the fluid output.

An imbalance of fluids in the body occurs when too much fluid is kept in the body or when too much fluid is lost. In some medical conditions, fluid may be held in the body tissues and make them swell. This is called edema. In other conditions, much fluid may be lost by vomiting, bleeding, severe diarrhea, or excessive sweating.

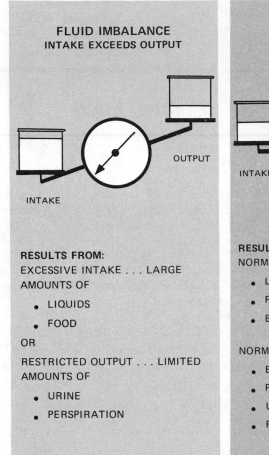

FLUID IMBALANCE
INTAKE EXCEEDS OUTPUT

OUTPUT

INTAKE

RESULTS FROM:
EXCESSIVE INTAKE . . . LARGE AMOUNTS OF

- LIQUIDS
- FOOD

OR

RESTRICTED OUTPUT . . . LIMITED AMOUNTS OF

- URINE
- PERSPIRATION

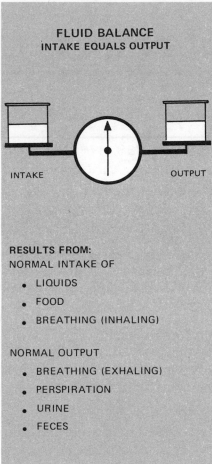

FLUID BALANCE
INTAKE EQUALS OUTPUT

INTAKE

OUTPUT

RESULTS FROM:
NORMAL INTAKE OF

- LIQUIDS
- FOOD
- BREATHING (INHALING)

NORMAL OUTPUT

- BREATHING (EXHALING)
- PERSPIRATION
- URINE
- FECES

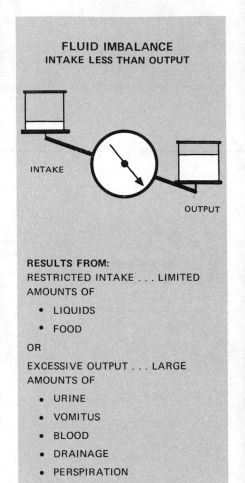

FLUID IMBALANCE
INTAKE LESS THAN OUTPUT

INTAKE

OUTPUT

RESULTS FROM:
RESTRICTED INTAKE . . . LIMITED AMOUNTS OF

- LIQUIDS
- FOOD

OR

EXCESSIVE OUTPUT . . . LARGE AMOUNTS OF

- URINE
- VOMITUS
- BLOOD
- DRAINAGE
- PERSPIRATION

When a patient's body loses more fluid than he is taking in or retains more than he is putting out, his doctor can treat the condition in various ways. A specific method is prescribed to meet the needs of the individual patient. The only way a doctor can know when a patient's balance of fluids is not right is by knowing the patient's measurable intake and output. Therefore, it is very important for members of the nursing staff to keep accurate records of fluid intake and output. The record of the patient's intake and output is kept for a full 24-hour period.

The amounts of intake and output are written on a special sheet of paper. It is called the Intake and Output (I&O) sheet and is kept near the patient's bed. The patient's name, room number, the identification institution number, and the date are recorded at the top of the page. The intake and output sheet is divided into two parts—intake on the left side and output on the right side. After measuring intake or output, you will record the amount and time in the proper columns. At the end of each 8-hour shift, the amounts in each column are totaled and recorded.

INTAKE AND OUTPUT SHEET

Hospital # _____   Patient Name _____

Date _____   Room # _____

Time 7-3	INTAKE			OUTPUT			
	BY MOUTH	TUBE	PARENTERAL	URINE		GASTRIC	
				VOIDED	CATHETER	EMESIS	SUCTION
TOTAL							
Time 3-11							
TOTAL							
Time 11-7							
TOTAL							
24 HOUR TOTAL							
24 Hour Grand Total ● Intake				24 Hour Grand Total ● Output			

SECTION 2: FLUID INTAKE

OBJECTIVES: WHAT YOU WILL LEARN

When you have completed this section, you will be able to:

- Explain the meaning of fluid intake
- Accurately measure fluids, using the metric system
- Show that you can observe exact amounts of fluids consumed by the patient and record them accurately on the intake and output sheet

**KEY IDEAS:
FLUID INTAKE**

A doctor must know exactly how much liquid is taken in every day by certain patients. Although solid foods also contain some liquid, most of the fluids in the body are taken in when a person drinks liquids. Therefore, a patient's fluid intake includes everything he drinks—water, milk, milk drinks, fruit juices, soup, tea, coffee, or anything liquid. Ice cream, junket, and gelatin also are counted as liquids.

Fluid taken in through an intravenous tube and tube feedings are also included in the patient's total fluid intake.

You probably have already noticed that many quantities used in the health care field are measured in cubic centimeters. Because most institutions use this term for measuring intake and output, you should understand what it means.

The term "cc" is an abbreviation for cubic centimeter, a unit of measurement in the metric system. The metric system of measurement is used in many countries of the world. In the United States, we normally use one system for measuring liquids (ounces, pints, quarts) and a different system for measuring lengths (inches, feet, yards, miles). Scientists, engineers, and many health care institution personnel use the metric system for measuring liquids, lengths,

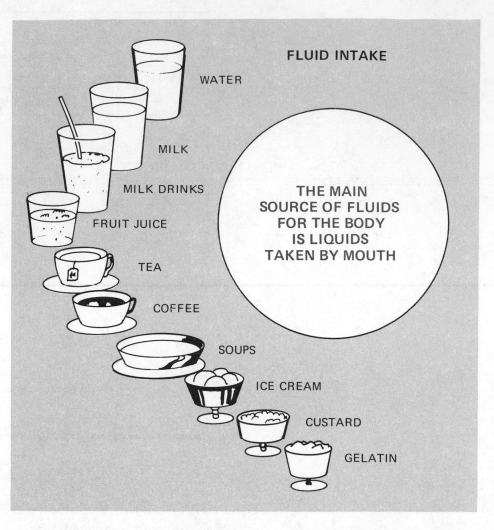

FLUID INTAKE

WATER

MILK

MILK DRINKS

FRUIT JUICE

TEA

COFFEE

SOUPS

ICE CREAM

CUSTARD

GELATIN

THE MAIN
SOURCE OF FLUIDS
FOR THE BODY
IS LIQUIDS
TAKEN BY MOUTH

and weight, as well. The basic unit of measurement is the meter, which is a little longer than the yard. A centimeter (1 one-hundredth (1/100) of a meter) is about four-tenths (4/10) of an inch long.

A cubic centimeter can be thought of as a square block with each edge of the block 1 centimeter long. If we filled this block with water, we would have 1 cubic centimeter (1cc) of water. The list shown here includes liquid amounts that you are probably familiar with. It also gives about the same amounts in cubic centimeters.

The patient's liquid intake is measured in cubic centimeters (cc). A container called a graduate or a measuring cup is used to measure intake and output (I&O). The side of the graduate is marked (calibrated) with a row of short lines and numbers. These show the amount of liquid in both cubic centimeters and ounces. This graduate is like the measuring cup you use at home to measure ingredients for cooking, only larger. Another calibrated graduate used in the home is a baby's milk bottle. This, too, is marked with a row of short lines and numbers. They show the amount of milk in both ounces and cubic centimeters. When full, most baby's bottles contain 8 ounces, or 240 cubic centimeters (cc). To give the baby 4 ounces of milk, or 120 cc, you would fill it half full or to the 4-ounce line.

It is very important that you observe the exact amounts of fluids taken in by the patient and that you record them accurately. You will have to measure the amount of liquid contained in each serving container, bowl, glass, or cup used by the patient. If your institution does not have a list of the amounts contained in each container, bowl, glass, or cup, you will find it helpful to make such a list yourself.

ACTUAL SIZE OF
CUBIC INCH
AND
CUBIC CENTIMETER

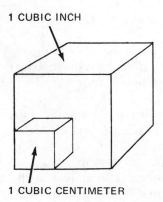

1 CUBIC INCH

1 CUBIC CENTIMETER

U.S. CUSTOMARY
LIQUID MEASURE
WITH EQUIVALENT
METRIC MEASUREMENTS

cc = cubic centimeter
ml = milliliter
oz = ounce
1 cc = 1 ml
¼ teaspoon = 1 cc
1 teaspoon = 4 cc
30 cc = 1 oz
60 cc = 2 oz
90 cc = 3 oz
120 cc = 4 oz
150 cc = 5 oz
180 cc = 6 oz
210 cc = 7 oz
240 cc = 8 oz
270 cc = 9 oz
300 cc = 10 oz

500 cc = 1 pint
1000 cc = 1 quart
4000 cc = 1 gallon

These are three containers used for measuring:

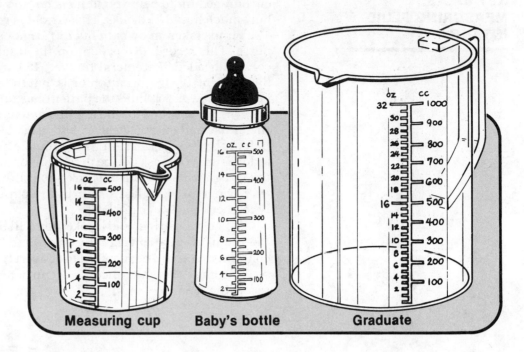

Measuring cup   Baby's bottle   Graduate

- They are all calibrated
- They are made of metal, glass, or plastic
- They are used for measuring liquids in cubic centimeters (cc)
- They are used for measuring liquids in ounces (oz)
- The measuring cup is used to measure liquids in the home
- The baby's bottle is used to measure liquids in the home
- The calibrated graduate is used to measure fluid in the health care institution.

Procedure: Measuring the Capacity of Serving Containers

1. Assemble your equipment in the utility room:
   a) Complete set of dishes, bowls, cups, and glasses used by the patients
   b) Graduate (measuring cup)
   c) Water
   d) Pen and paper
2. Fill the first container with water.
3. Pour this water into the graduate.
4. Look at the level of the water and determine the amount in cc (cubic centimeters).
5. Write this information on the paper. For example, carton of milk = 240 cc.
6. Repeat these steps for each dish, glass, bowl, or cup used by the patients.
7. You will have a complete list to use when measuring intake.

(continued next page)

You should tell the patient that his intake is being measured. You can encourage him to help you, if he is not too ill, by asking him to keep track of how much liquid he drinks. This is not his responsibility, however, it is yours.

Fluids taken in by patients intravenously are recorded by the registered nurse. This record also is kept on the intake and output sheet, in a special column headed "Parenteral Intake." Regardless of how fluids are consumed by a patient, the important thing is that the doctor must know as accurately as possible how much fluid the patient has taken in.

The proper time for the nursing assistant to record the patient's fluids on the intake and output sheet is as soon as the patient has consumed the fluids. Before the end of each shift, the complete amount of intake should be totaled (added) up. Your task will be to remember to record all fluid taken in each time the patient eats or drinks. Think about fluid intake every time you remove a tray, water pitcher, glass, or cup from a patient's bedside. Remember especially to check the water pitcher.

When measuring fluid intake, you will have to note the difference between the amount the patient actually drinks and the amount he leaves in the serving container. You will be required to convert (change) amounts such as ½ bowl of soup, ½ glass of orange juice, or ¼ cup of tea into cc (cubic centimeters) when recording them.

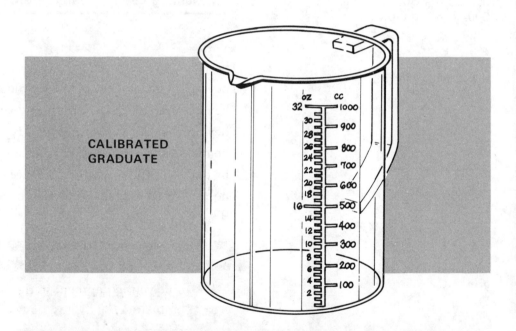

**CALIBRATED
GRADUATE**

Procedure: Determining the Amounts Consumed

1. Assemble your equipment on the bedside table:
   a) Graduate
   b) Pen and paper
   c) Leftover liquids in their serving containers
2. Pour the leftover liquid into the graduate.
3. Look at the level and determine the amount in cc.
4. From your list, determine the amount in the full serving container.
5. Subtract the leftover amount from the full-container amount. This figure is the amount the patient actually drank.
6. Immediately record this amount on the intake side of the intake and output sheet.

SECTION 3: FORCING AND RESTRICTING FLUIDS

OBJECTIVES: WHAT YOU WILL LEARN

When you have completed this section, you will be able to:

- Explain the terms FF and NPO.
- Demonstrate the nursing assistant's role when a patient is on restricted fluids.
- Demonstrate the nursing assistant's role when a patient is on force fluids.
- Demonstrate the nursing assistant's role when a patient is on nothing by mouth.

**KEY IDEAS:
FORCE FLUIDS**

Patients who need to have more fluids added to their normal intake are put on force fluids by the doctor. "FF" is the abbreviation for force fluids. A patient on force fluids often needs encouragement to drink more. Some ways you can persuade the patient to drink more fluids are by:

- Showing enthusiasm and being cheerful.
- Providing different kinds of liquids that the patient prefers as permitted on his therapeutic diet.
- Offering liquids without being asked.
- Offering hot or cold drinks.

Rules to Follow: Force Fluids

- Place a sign on the bed or door.

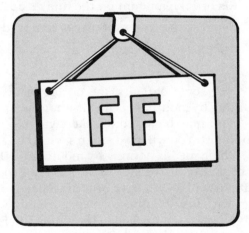

- Check your assignment sheet or card to see if patient is on force fluids.
- If the patient is on force fluids, encourage him to drink the amount required. For example, 800 cc every 8 hours means the patient would have to drink 100 cc every hour. At the end of the 8-hour shift, he would have taken in 800 cc of fluids.
- Use different kinds of fluids as permitted by the patient's therapeutic diet. Examples are hot tea, gelatin, soda, ice cream, milk, juice, broth, coffee, custard, and water.
- Record the amount taken in by the patient in cc on the intake side of the intake and output sheet.

**KEY IDEAS:
RESTRICT FLUIDS**

For some patients, the doctor writes orders to restrict fluids. This means that fluids may be limited to certain amounts. When you are caring for a patient on restrict fluids, it is important to follow orders exactly and to measure accurately. Your calm and reassuring attitude can make a big difference in how the patient feels and reacts.

Rules to Follow: Restrict Fluids

- Check your assignment sheet to see if the patient is on restrict fluids.
- If he is, the patient must stay within the limits stated by your head nurse or team leader.

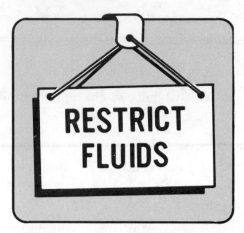

- Place a sign stating restrict fluids on the bed or door.
- Alternate different fluids as permitted by the therapeutic diet. Be sure to limit the patient to the correct amount.
- Record the amount on the intake side of the intake and output sheet.
- Usually, the water pitcher is removed from the bedside.
- Frequent oral hygiene is often necessary.

KEY IDEAS: NOTHING BY MOUTH

For some patients, the doctor writes orders that the patient is to have nothing by mouth. This means that the patient cannot eat or drink anything at all. You may be asked to take away the patient's water pitcher and glass at midnight. You will post a sign saying NPO. NPO is taken from the Latin *nils per os*, which means nothing by mouth. An NPO sign is put at the foot or the head of the bed or on the door of the patient's room. Some institutions do not allow a patient on NPO to have oral hygiene.

Patients often become very irritable when they are not allowed to have anything to eat or drink. They may, therefore, be hard for you to deal with. Calm and reassuring behavior on your part can help the patient go through a very uncomfortable period. A smile and a few kind words will go a long way here.

Rules to Follow: Nothing by Mouth

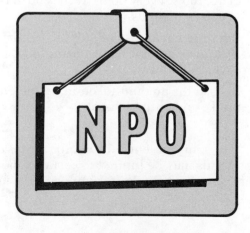

- Check the assignment sheet to see if the patient is on NPO.
- Explain to the patient that he is now on nothing by mouth.
- Remove the water pitcher and anything else by which the patient could take a drink or eat.
- Place a sign stating NPO on the bed or door.
- Do not give any liquids or food to this patient.
- Make a note on the intake side of the intake and output sheet that the patient is NPO.

SECTION 4: FLUID OUTPUT

OBJECTIVES: WHAT YOU WILL LEARN
When you have completed this section, you will be able to:

- Explain fluid output.
- List the ways in which the body loses fluid.
- Use the metric system accurately to measure fluid output.
- Record the amounts accurately on the intake and output sheet.
- Measure the exact amounts of fluid output.

**KEY IDEAS:
MEASURING FLUID
OUTPUT**

Fluid output is the sum total of liquids that come out of the body. To urinate means to discharge urine from the body. Other terms for this body function are:

- To void
- To pass water

The rest of the fluid that is discharged goes out of the body by a process called "insensible loss." This means that the fluid is lost in the air breathed out. Also, from 100 to 200 cc of fluid is discharged from the body in feces. Output also includes emesis (vomitus), drainage from a wound or from the stomach, and loss of blood.

A patient who is on intake and output must have his output as well as his intake measured and recorded. This means that every time the patient uses the urinal, emesis basin, or bedpan, the urine and other liquids must be measured.

You should tell a patient his output is being measured and ask him to cooperate. A female patient must urinate in a bedpan or specipan. The specipan is a disposable container that fits into the toilet bowl under the seat. The specipan can be placed in the patient's toilet bowl, if the patient is allowed out of bed. Ask the patient not to place toilet paper in the bedpan or specipan. Provide a wastepaper basket for her. Then discard tissue into the toilet or hopper. Female patients must also be asked not to let their bowels move while urinating. Male patients on output must be instructed to use a urinal.

Procedure: Measuring Urinary Output

1. Assemble your equipment in the patient's bathroom:
   a) Bedpan, cover, urinal, or specipan
   b) Graduate (measuring container)
   c) Intake and output sheet
   d) Pencil or pen
2. Wash your hands.
3. Pour the urine from the bedpan or urinal into a graduate.

(continued next page)

4. Place the graduate on a flat surface for accuracy in measurement.

5. At eye level, carefully look at the graduate to see the number reached by the level of the urine.

6. Record this amount on the output side of the intake and output sheet.

7. Write down the time and record the amount in cc.

8. Rinse and return the graduate to its proper place.

9. Rinse and return the urinal or bedpan to its proper place.

10. Wash your hands.

11. Report to your head nurse or team leader:

- That you have measured the output for the patient.

- Your observations of anything unusual.

KEY IDEAS: PLASTIC URINE CONTAINER FOR INDWELLING CATHETER

Some patients have a catheter inserted into their urinary bladder by the doctor or professional nurse. This catheter drains all the patient's urine into a plastic urine container. The container hangs on the bed below the level of the urinary bladder. You will empty this container, measure the urine for amount, and record the amount. This will be always done whenever it is full and always before the end of your working shift. The measurement is not taken from the soft expandable plastic urine container. A hard plastic graduate is always used as it is more accurate.

Rules to Follow: Checking Catheters and Containers

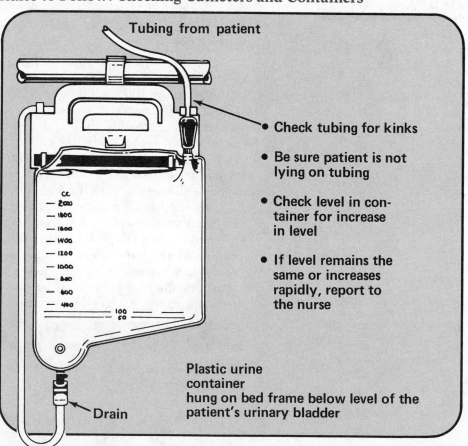

Tubing from patient

- Check tubing for kinks

- Be sure patient is not lying on tubing

- Check level in container for increase in level

- If level remains the same or increases rapidly, report to the nurse

Plastic urine container hung on bed frame below level of the patient's urinary bladder

Drain

Procedure: Emptying a Plastic Urine Container from an Indwelling Catheter

1. Assemble your equipment: A graduate.
2. Wash your hands.
3. Open the drain at the bottom of the plastic urine container and let the urine run into the graduate, then close the drain.
4. Measure the amount of urinary output.
5. Record the amount immediately on the output side of the intake and output sheet.
6. Rinse the graduate and put it in its proper place.
7. Wash your hands.
8. Report to your head nurse or team leader:
   - That you have emptied the urine container and measured the amount of output.
   - That you have recorded the amount on the output side of the intake and output sheet.
   - Your observations of anything unusual.

**KEY IDEAS:
FLUID OUTPUT AND THE
INCONTINENT PATIENT**

If a patient is incontinent of urine, record this on the output side of the I&O sheet each time the patient wets the bed. Even though the urine cannot be measured, the doctor at least knows that the patient's kidney's are functioning.

WHAT YOU HAVE LEARNED

It is important that you observe the exact amount of fluids consumed by the patient and record them accurately. All fluids should be measured in cubic centimeters. Remember to record all fluids taken in each time the patient eats or drinks. Think about fluid intake whenever you remove a tray, water pitcher, glass, or cup from a patient's bedside. Be sure you know which of your patients are on force fluids, restrict fluids, nothing by mouth, and intake and output. Each time the patient who is on intake and output uses the bedpan, urinal, or specipan, measure and record the fluid output accurately on the intake and output sheet.

Remember to drain the urine from a urinary drainage bag into a hard plastic graduate for measuring. The calibrations on the plastic urinary drainage bag are no longer accurate once the bag fills with urine.

10 SPECIMEN COLLECTION

OBJECTIVES: WHAT YOU WILL LEARN

When you have completed this chapter, you will be able to:

- Explain what specimens are.
- Collect specimens correctly and exactly at the time required.
- Label specimens properly.

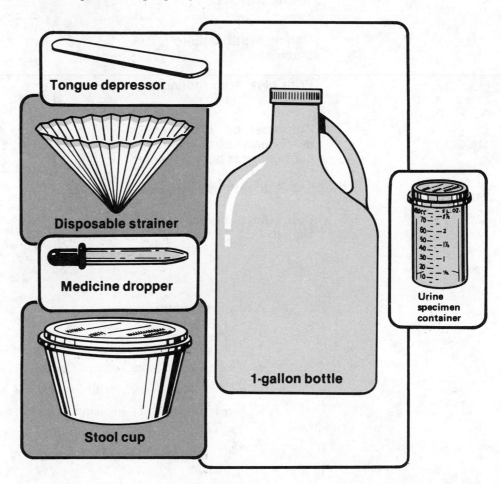

Tongue depressor

Disposable strainer

Medicine dropper

Stool cup

1-gallon bottle

Urine specimen container

**KEY IDEAS:
SPECIMEN COLLECTION**

As one of its natural living functions, the human body regularly gets rid of various waste materials. Most of the body's waste materials are discharged in the urine and feces. The body also gets rid of wastes in the material coughed up and spit out of the mouth (expectorated). This material is called **sputum**.

These body waste materials, when tested in the laboratory, often show changes in the sick person's body. By examining the results of laboratory tests, the doctor gets information that can help him make his diagnosis and decide on appropriate treatment for the patient.

For these reasons, the doctor will sometimes need samples of each of these waste products—urine, feces, and sputum. These samples are called **specimens.** Members of the health care institution nursing staff are responsible for collecting such specimens.

When you are collecting specimens you must be very accurate in following the procedure and labeling the specimen. You have to collect the specimen at exactly the right time, the time that is indicated. You must look at the patient's identification bracelet for the correct name, identification number, and room number when filling out the cover or label on the specimen container. The time and date the specimen was obtained should be printed on the label. The label must be printed clearly so that it can be read easily. It must be attached to the container immediately after the specimen has been collected. Unlabeled specimens should be thrown away so that mistakes will not be made.

BE ACCURATE . . .

Check identification bracelet

Print clearly so the label can be easily read

Put label on specimen immediately after specimen container has been collected

Check identification bracelet

Copy the patient's name from it.

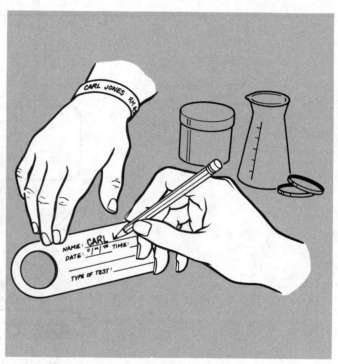

Need for Accuracy

BE SURE YOU FOLLOW ALL THE "RIGHTS" LISTED HERE:

- *The right patient*—from whom the specimen is to be collected.
- *The right specimen*—as ordered by the doctor.
- *The right time*—when the specimen is to be collected.
- *The right amount*—measured exactly for each specimen.
- *The right container*—the cup that is correct for each specimen.
- *The right label*—filled out properly from the patient's identification bracelet.
- *The right requisition or laboratory slip*—lists the kind of laboratory examination or test to be done.
- *The right method*—procedure by which you collect the specimen.
- *The right asepsis*—washing your hands before and after collecting the specimen.
- *The right attitude*—how you approach and speak to the patient.

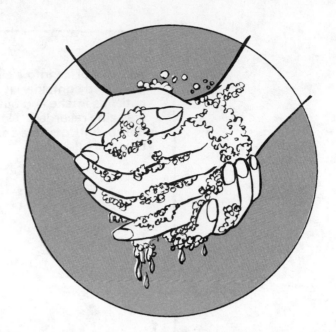

As you learned from the chapter on infection control, asepsis means "free of disease-causing organisms." When collecting specimens, it is very important to use good medical asepsis. You must wash your hands very carefully before and after collecting each specimen to prevent spreading bacteria.

Medical asepsis means preventing the conditions that allow disease-producing bacteria to live, multiply, and spread. As a nursing assistant, you will share the responsibility for preventing the spread of disease and infection by using aseptic technique. Remember especially to wash your hands before and after collecting specimens.

Routine Urine Specimen

The usual single urine specimen collected is called the **routine urine specimen**. This is the specimen that is taken routinely on admission, daily, or preoperatively by the nursing assistant and sent to the laboratory.

Procedure: Collecting a Routine Urine Specimen

1. Assemble your equipment:
   a) Patient's bedpan and cover, or urinal, or specipan
   b) Graduate used for measuring output
   c) Urine specimen container and lid
   d) Label, if your institution's procedure is not to write on the lid
   e) Laboratory request slip, which should be filled out by the head nurse, team leader or ward clerk
   f) Disposable gloves, optional
2. Wash your hands.
3. Identify the patient by checking the identification bracelet.
4. Ask visitors to step out of the room.
5. Tell the patient a urine specimen is needed.
6. Pull the curtain around the bed for privacy, or explain the procedure to the patient. If he is able, he may collect the specimen himself.
7. Have the patient urinate into the bedpan, urinal, or specipan.

(continued next page)

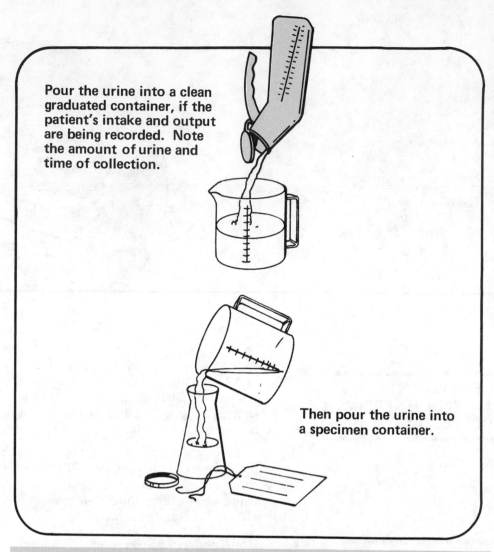

Pour the urine into a clean graduated container, if the patient's intake and output are being recorded. Note the amount of urine and time of collection.

Then pour the urine into a specimen container.

Procedure continued

8. Ask the patient not to put toilet tissue into the bedpan or specipan, but to use the wastebasket temporarily. You will then discard the tissue in the toilet or hopper.

9. Prepare the label immediately by copying all necessary information from the patient's identification bracelet. Record the time and date.

10. Take the bedpan, or urinal if used, to the patient's bathroom or to the dirty utility room.

11. Pour the urine into a clean graduated container.

12. If the patient is on output, note the amount of the urine and record it on the Intake and Output sheet.

13. Pour urine from the graduate into a specimen container and fill it three-fourths full, if possible.

14. Put the lid on the specimen container. Place the correct label on the container for the correct patient.

15. Pour the leftover urine into the toilet or hopper.

16. Clean and rinse out the graduate. Put it in its proper place.

17. Clean the bedpan or urinal and put it in its proper place.

18. Make the patient comfortable.

19. Wash your hands.

20. Send or take the labeled specimen container to the laboratory with a requisition or laboratory request slip.

(continued next page)

21. Report to your head nurse or team leader:
    - That a routine urine specimen has been obtained.
    - That the specimen has been sent to the laboratory.
    - The date and time of collection.
    - Your observations of anything unusual.

KEY IDEAS: MIDSTREAM CLEAN-CATCH URINE SPECIMEN

A special method is used to collect a patient's urine when the specimen must be free from contamination. This special kind of specimen is called a **midstream clean-catch urine specimen.** In most health care facilities, a disposable midstream clean-catch package can be obtained from the CSR (central supply room).

All the equipment and supplies necessary for this specimen are in the kit. Midstream means catching the urine specimen between the time the patient begins to void and the time he stops. Clean catch refers to the fact that the urine is not contaminated by anything outside the patient's body. The procedure requires careful washing of the genital area. This ensures a "clean catch" as the urine itself washes off the body opening.

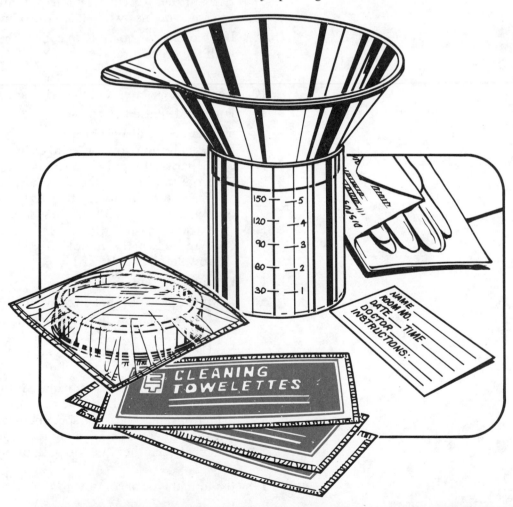

Procedure: Collecting a Midstream Clean-Catch Urine Specimen

1. Assemble your equipment:
   a) Obtain a requisition slip from the ward clerk, team leader, or
   (continued next page)

head nurse for a disposable collection kit for this specimen, or go to the CSR exchange cart, if used in your institution, and get the kit. If your institution does not use disposable equipment, CSR will supply the cotton balls and solution to be used for the cleansing process according to your institution's policy.

b) Label, if your institution's procedure does not call for writing directly on the cover of the urine container.

c) Disposable gloves.

d) Laboratory request slip, which should be filled out by the head nurse, team leader or ward clerk.

e) Patient's bedpan or urinal, if the patient is unable to go to the bathroom.

2. Wash your hands.

3. Identify the patient by checking the identification bracelet.

4. Ask visitors to step out of the room.

5. Tell the patient you need a midstream clean-catch urine specimen.

6. Pull the curtain around the bed for privacy.

7. Explain the procedure. If the patient is able, he may collect this specimen on his own in his bathroom.

8. If the patient is not able to collect the specimen himself, help him with the procedure.

9. Open the disposable kit.

10. Remove towelettes and the urine specimen container from the kit.

11. For female patients:

a) Put on the disposable gloves.

b) Use all three towelettes to cleanse the perineal area.

c) Separate the folds of the labia (lips) and wipe with one towelette from the front to the back (anterior to posterior) on one side. Then throw away the towelette.

d) Wipe the other side with a second towelette, again from front to back. Discard the towelette.

e) Wipe down the middle from front to back, using the third towelette, and discard it.

12. For male patients:

a) If the patient is not circumcised, pull the foreskin back (retract foreskin) on the penis to clean, and hold it back during urination.

b) Use a circular motion to clean the head of the penis. Discard each towelette after each use.

13. Ask the patient to start to urinate into either the bedpan, urinal, or the toilet. After the flow of urine has started, ask the patient to stop urinating. Place the urine specimen container under the patient and ask the patient to start urinating again. But this time catch the urine between the time the patient begins to void and the time he stops.

14. If a funnel type of container is used, remove the funnel and discard it.

15. Cover the urine container immediately with the lid from the kit. Be careful not to touch the inside of the container or the inside of the lid.

16. Label the container right away. Copy all needed information from the patient's identification bracelet. Record the date and time of collection.

(continued next page)

17. Clean the bedpan or urinal. Put it in its proper place.

18. Discard all used disposable equipment.

19. Make the patient comfortable.

20. Wash your hands.

21. The labeled specimen container must be sent or taken to the laboratory with a requisition or laboratory request slip, which is filled out by the head nurse, team leader or ward clerk.

22. Report to your head nurse or team leader:

   • That a midstream clean-catch urine specimen has been obtained.

   • That it has been sent to the laboratory.

   • The date and time of collection.

   • Your observations of anything unusual.

**KEY IDEAS:
24-HOUR URINE
SPECIMEN**

A **24-hour urine specimen** is a collection of all urine voided by a patient over a 24-hour period. All the urine is collected for 24 hours, usually from 7 a.m. on the first day to 7 a.m. the following day.

When you are to obtain a 24-hour urine specimen, it is necessary to ask the patient to void and discard the first voided urine at 7 a.m. This is because this urine has remained in the bladder an unknown length of time. The test should

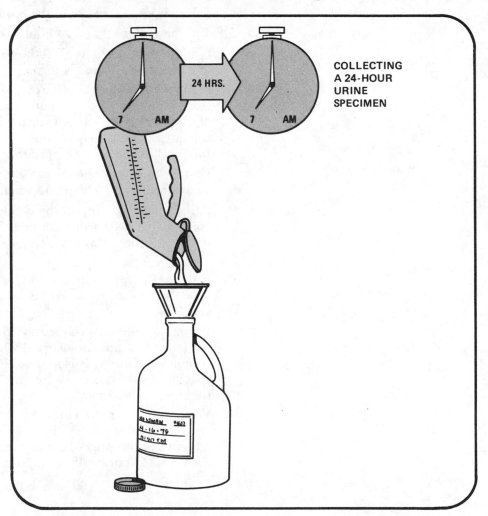

COLLECTING
A 24-HOUR
URINE
SPECIMEN

begin with the bladder empty. For the next 24 hours, save all the urine voided by the patient. On the following day at 7 a.m., ask the patient to void and add this specimen to the previous collection. In this way the doctor can be sure that all of the urine for the test came into the urinary bladder during the 24 hours of the test period.

Procedure: Collecting a 24-Hour Urine Specimen

1. Assemble your equipment:
   a) Large container, usually a 1-gallon plastic disposable bottle
   b) Funnel, if the neck of the bottle is small
   c) Graduate, used for measuring output, if the patient is on intake and output
   d) Patient's bedpan, urinal, or specipan
   e) Label for the container
   f) Laboratory request slip, which should be filled out by the head nurse, team leader, or ward clerk
   g) Tag, to be placed over or on the patient's bed, and in the patient's bathroom to indicate that a 24-hour urine specimen is being collected
   h) Disposable gloves, optional

2. Wash your hands.

3. Identify the patient by checking the identification bracelet.

4. Ask visitors to step out of the room.

5. Tell the patient that a 24-hour urine specimen is needed.

6. Explain the procedure. Tell the patient that you will be placing the large container in his bathroom.

7. Fill in the label for the large container. Copy all needed information from the patient's identification bracelet. Record the date and time of the first collection. Attach the label to the urine specimen container (the large 1-gallon plastic disposable bottle). Place the container in the patient's bathroom.

8. Post the tag over or on the patient's bed. This is so all personnel will be aware that a 24-hour specimen is being collected.

9. Pull the curtain around the bed for privacy each time the patient voids, if he uses a bedpan or urinal rather than a specipan or urinal in the bathroom. Avoid placing tissue in the bedpan with the specimen.

10. If the patient is on intake and output, measure all the urine each time the patient voids. Write the amount on the intake and output sheet.

11. When the collection starts, have the patient void. Throw away (discard) this first amount of urine. This is to be sure that the bladder is completely empty. This first voiding should not be included in the specimen. This is usually done at 7 a.m. The test will continue until the next day at 7 a.m.

12. You may be instructed to refrigerate the urine. If so, fill a large bucket with ice cubes. Keep the large urine container in the ice, in the patient's bathroom. All nursing assistants caring for this patient for the next 24 hours will be responsible for keeping the bucket filled with ice.

(continued next page)

13. For the next 24 hours, save all urine voided by the patient. Pour the urine from each voiding into the large container.

14. At the end of the 24-hour period, have the patient void at 7 a.m. Add this to the collection of urine in the large container. This will be the last time you will collect the urine for this test.

15. The large labeled container with the entire 24-hour collection of urine is taken to the laboratory with a requisition or laboratory request slip that is made out by the head nurse, team leader, or ward clerk.

16. Clean your equipment and put in its proper place. Discard disposable equipment.

17. Remove the 24-hour specimen tag from the patient's bed.

18. Make the patient comfortable.

19. Wash your hands.

20. Report to your head nurse or team leader:

    • That a 24-hour urine specimen has been obtained.

    • That the specimen has been sent to the laboratory.

    • The date and time of collection.

    • Your observations of anything unusual.

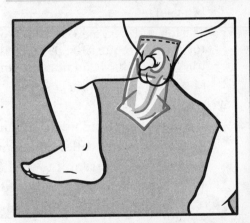 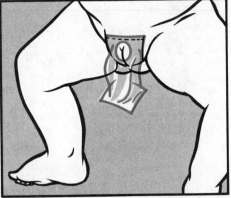

Procedure: Collecting a Routine Urine Specimen from an Infant

1. Assemble your equipment on the bedside table:
   a) Urine specimen bottle or container.
   b) Plastic disposable urine collector.
   c) Label, if your institution's procedure is not to write on the cover.
   d) Laboratory request slip, which should be filled out by the head nurse, team leader, or ward clerk.
   e) Disposable gloves, optional.

2. Wash your hands.

3. Identify the patient by checking the identification bracelet.

4. Ask all visitors except parents or guardian to step out of the room.

5. Tell the parents or guardian and the patient that you want to collect a urine specimen (children who are not yet toilet trained can understand language and are more likely to cooperate, if told).

6. Pull curtains around the bed (even a 2-year-old may be shy about

(continued next page)

having his pants pulled down in front of the strangers who may be visiting the child in the next bed).

7. Take off the child's diaper.

8. Make sure the child's skin is clean and dry in the genital area. This is where you are going to apply the urine collector, which is a small plastic bag.

9. Remove the outside piece that surrounds the opening of the plastic urine collector. This leaves a sticky area, which is placed around the baby boy's penis or the baby girl's vulva. Do not cover the baby's rectum.

10. Put the child's diaper on as usual.

11. Come back and check every half hour to see if the infant has voided. You cannot feel the diaper to find out. You must open the diaper and look at the urine collector.

12. When the infant has voided, remove the plastic urine collector. It comes off easily. Wash off any sticky residue.

13. Replace the child's diaper.

14. Put the specimen in the specimen container and cover it immediately.

15. Label the container properly. Check the patient's identification bracelet.

16. The labeled specimen container must be sent or taken to the laboratory with a requisition or laboratory request slip, which is usually filled out by the head nurse, team leader, or ward clerk.

17. Make the baby comfortable.

18. Wash your hands.

19. Report to your head nurse or team leader:
    - That you have collected a routine urine specimen.
    - That you have sent it to the laboratory.
    - The date and time of collection.
    - Your observations of anything unusual.

KEY IDEAS: SPUTUM SPECIMEN

Sputum is a substance collected from a patient's lungs that contains saliva, mucus, and sometimes pus or blood. It is thicker than ordinary saliva (spit). Most of it is coughed up from the lungs and bronchial tubes. In some health care facilities this procedure is carried out by the Respiratory Department (Pulmonary Medicine).

Usually early morning is the best time to obtain this specimen.

Procedure: Collecting a Sputum Specimen

1. Assemble your equipment:
    a) Sputum container and cover
    b) Label, if your institution's procedure is not to write on the cover
    c) Laboratory request slip, which should be filled out by the head nurse, team leader, or ward clerk
    d) Disposable gloves, optional

2. Wash your hands.

3. Identify the patient by checking the identification bracelet.

4. Tell the patient a sputum specimen is needed.

(continued next page)

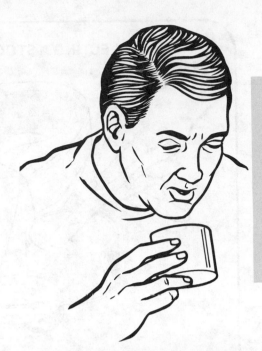

COLLECTING THE SPUTUM SPECIMEN

Procedure continued

5. If the patient has eaten recently, have him rinse out his mouth. If he wants to have oral hygiene at this time, help him as necessary.

6. Give the patient a sputum container. Ask him to take three consecutive deep breaths and on the third exhalation to cough deep from within the lungs to bring up the thick sputum. Explain that saliva (spit) and nose secretions are not adequate for this test.

7. The patient may have to cough several times to bring up enough sputum for the specimen. One to two tablespoons is usually the required amount.

8. Cover the container immediately. Be careful not to touch the inside of either the container or the cover to avoid contamination.

9. Label the container right away. Copy all needed information from the patient's identification bracelet. Record the time of collection and the date.

10. The labeled specimen container must be sent or taken immediately to the laboratory with a requisition or laboratory request slip. This should be filled out by the head nurse, team leader, or ward clerk. The test must be done in the laboratory before the sputum begins to dry.

11. Make the patient comfortable.

12. Wash your hands.

13. Report to your head nurse or team leader:
    - That a sputum specimen has been obtained.
    - That the specimen has been sent to the laboratory.
    - The date and time of collection.
    - Your observations of anything unusual.

**KEY IDEAS:
STOOL SPECIMEN**

Feces, stool, BM, bowel movement, and fecal matter all mean the same thing, the solid waste from a patient's body. The doctor sometimes orders a stool specimen to help him in the diagnosis of a patient's illness. Sometimes a warm specimen is ordered. This means that the specimen must be tested in the laboratory while the specimen is still warm from the patient's body. You will be told whether the specimen is to be warm or cold.

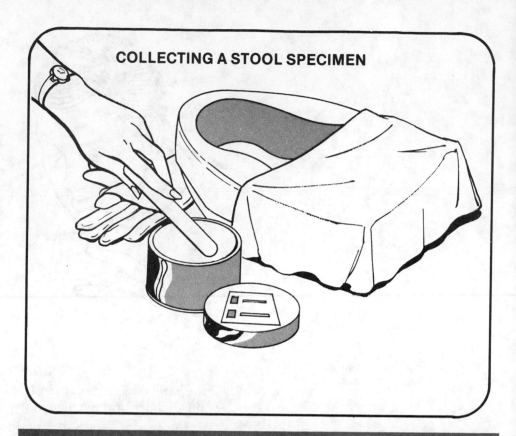

COLLECTING A STOOL SPECIMEN

Procedure: Collecting a Stool Specimen

1. Assemble your equipment:
   a) Patient's bedpan and cover
   b) Stool specimen container
   c) Wooden tongue depressor
   d) Label, if your institution's procedure is not to write on the cover
   e) Laboratory request slip, which should be filled out by the head nurse, team leader, or ward clerk
   f) Plastic bag for warm specimen, if used by your institution
   g) Disposable gloves, optional

2. Wash your hands.

3. Identify the patient by checking the identification bracelet.

4. Ask visitors to step out of the room.

5. Tell the patient that a stool specimen is needed. Explain that whenever he can move his bowels, he is to call you so the specimen can be collected.

6. Pull the curtain around the bed for privacy while the patient is on the bedpan.

7. Have the patient move his bowels into the bedpan.

8. Ask the patient not to urinate into the bedpan and not to put toilet tissue in the bedpan. Provide the patient with a wastepaper basket to temporarily dispose of the toilet tissue. Then discard it in the toilet or hopper.

9. Prepare the label immediately by copying all needed information from the patient's identification bracelet. Record the time of collection and the date.

10. After the patient has had a bowel movement, take the covered bedpan to the patient's bathroom or to the dirty utility room.

(continued next page)

11. Using the wooden tongue depressor, take about 1 to 2 tablespoons of feces from the bedpan and place them in the stool specimen container. Label the specimen container.

12. Cover the container immediately. Be careful not to touch the inside of either the container or the cover to avoid contamination.

13. Wrap the tongue depressor in a paper towel and discard it.

14. Empty the remaining feces into the toilet or hopper.

15. Clean the bedpan and return it to its proper place.

16. Wash your hands.

17. If your head nurse or team leader told you this is a warm specimen, it must be taken to the laboratory for examination while it is still warm from the patient's body. Place the stool specimen container, fully labeled, in the plastic bag (if used by your institution). Attach the laboratory request slip to the bag. Carry it immediately to the laboratory.

18. Make the patient comfortable.

19. Wash your hands.

20. Report to your head nurse or team leader:
    - That a stool specimen has been obtained.
    - That the specimen has been sent to the laboratory.
    - The date and time of collection.
    - Your observations of anything unusual.

KEY IDEAS: STRAINING THE URINE

The urine is strained to determine if a patient has passed **stones** (calculi) or other matter from the kidneys. The doctor may order that all urine passed by the patient is to be strained.

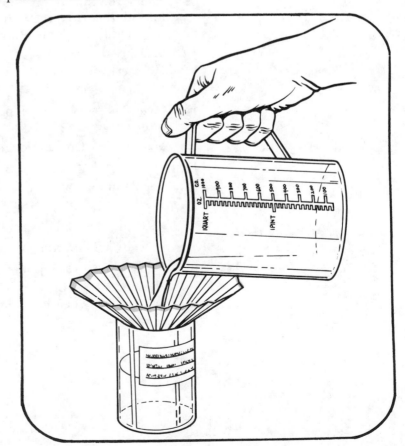

Procedure: Straining the Urine

1. Assemble your equipment in the patient's bathroom:
   a) Paper disposable strainers or gauze squares
   b) Specimen container with cover or a small plastic bag to be used as a specimen container
   c) Label, if your institution's procedure is not to write on the cover
   d) Patient's bedpan and cover, or urinal, or specipan
   e) Laboratory request slip, which should be filled out by the head nurse, team leader, or ward clerk
   f) Tag, to be placed over the bed indicating that all urine must be strained
   g) Disposable gloves, optional

2. Wash your hands.

3. Identify the patient by checking the identification bracelet.

4. Ask visitors to step out of the room.

5. Tell the patient that each time he urinates, it must be into a urinal, bedpan, or specipan, as all urine must be strained. Caution the patient not to put any tissue into the container.

6. Pull the curtain around the bed for privacy whenever the patient voids.

7. When the patient voids, take the bedpan or urinal to the patient's bathroom. Pour the urine through the strainer or gauze into the measuring container.

8. If any particles show up on the gauze or the paper strainer, place the gauze or paper strainer with particles in a plastic bag or specimen container. Do not attempt to remove the particles, because they may be lost or damaged.

9. Label the specimen container immediately. Copy all needed information from the patient's identification bracelet. Record the date and time of collection.

10. Measure the amount of the voiding and record it on the intake and output sheet, if the patient is on intake and output.

11. Discard the urine.

12. Clean and rinse the bedpan and graduate and put them in their proper places.

13. Make the patient comfortable.

14. Wash your hands.

15. Report immediately to your head nurse or team leader:
    - That, in straining the urine, particles were obtained.
    - That a specimen was collected.
    - The date and time of collection.
    - Your observations of anything unusual.

16. The labeled specimen container must be sent or taken to the laboratory with a requisition or laboratory request slip at the head nurse's or team leader's request.

WHAT YOU HAVE LEARNED

A specimen is a sample amount of a substance taken from the patient's body. You will be collecting various specimens. A mistake in collecting or labeling a specimen may cause a mistake in the laboratory report. This might be dangerous to the patient.

Each different kind of specimen that you collect requires a different kind of container. Be sure to use the right one. All specimens must be properly labeled. Never fill the specimen container completely full.

A sputum specimen must be from deep within the lungs, not saliva. Stool specimens usually must still be warm in order to be useful in the laboratory.

11 SPECIAL TREATMENTS

1. Administering Enemas
2. Perineal Care and Indwelling Catheter Care
3. Artificial Eye Care

SECTION 1: ADMINISTERING ENEMAS

OBJECTIVES: WHAT YOU WILL LEARN

When you have completed this section, you will be able to:

- Properly position a patient for an enema
- Administer a cleansing enema
- Administer a retention enema
- Administer a Harris flush or return flow enema
- Use the disposable rectal tube with connected flatus bag

KEY IDEAS:
RECTAL TREATMENTS

Cleansing enemas and oil retention enemas are administered to patients by nursing assistants. A **cleansing enema** washes out waste materials (feces or stool) from the person's lower bowel. An **oil retention enema** inserts oil into the rectum to soften the stool. Retention means that the patient keeps the fluid (oil) in his rectum for 20 minutes. Giving enemas has been made easier in recent years by the use of disposable, prepackaged enema kits. These plastic enema kits contain an enema bag, tubing, and a clamp. The kit should be used once and then thrown away.

If the patient has any complaints before you start giving him an enema, report this to your head nurse or team leader. Do not go ahead with the enema until you are told to do so.

Occasionally a patient may complain of a cramp-like pain after the enema has started. If this happens, stop the flow of solution until the pain goes away. If you stop the flow and then start again when the pain is gone, the full prescribed amount of solution can usually be given without causing the patient very much discomfort.

KEY IDEAS:
POSITIONING THE PATIENT
FOR THE ENEMA

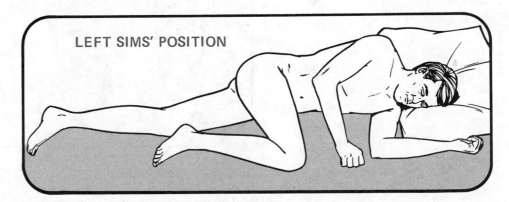

LEFT SIMS' POSITION

233

Left Sims' Position

When the patient is on his left side with his right knee bent toward his chest it is called **left Sims' position**. This is also called the enema position because most patients are given enemas in the left Sims' position.

Paraplegic Enema Position

Sometimes the patient cannot be on his side. He may be unconscious, paralyzed, mentally confused, unable to understand, or very uncooperative. He may be unable to retain the enema fluid. In these cases, the patient lies on his back. His buttocks are raised over the bedpan with the knees separated. The patient should be draped with a small sheet so as not to be exposed. The nursing assistant wears disposable gloves. The rectal tube is inserted into the patient's anus from between the legs. This is sometimes called the paraplegic method.

Rotating Enema Position

The patient is given one-third of the enema while he is lying on his left side. Then one-third more is given while he is lying on his abdomen (prone). The final one-third of the enema is given while the patient is lying on his right side. The reason is so the enema solution will first enter the descending colon. Then it will go to the transverse colon. Last it will enter the ascending colon. This is why it is called a rotating enema position.

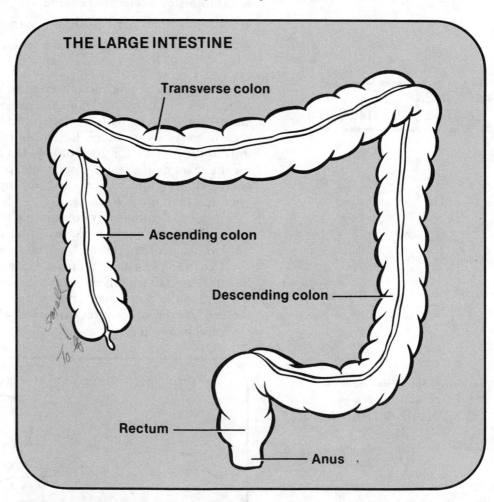

THE LARGE INTESTINE

Transverse colon

Ascending colon

Descending colon

Rectum

Anus

The Cleansing Enema

The cleansing enema is given only when it has been ordered by the patient's physician. This enema is used most often to promote evacuation of the lower bowel, when this does not happen naturally. **Evacuation** means discharge of the contents of the lower bowel through the rectum and anus.

Cleansing enemas may also be given in preparation for certain diagnostic tests. They are frequently used in preparing a patient for an operation or the delivery of a baby.

The solution used in the cleansing enema may be a commercial preparation supplied with a disposable enema kit. Or it may be a solution of salt and water, a weak mixture of soap and water, or sometimes just plain tap water.

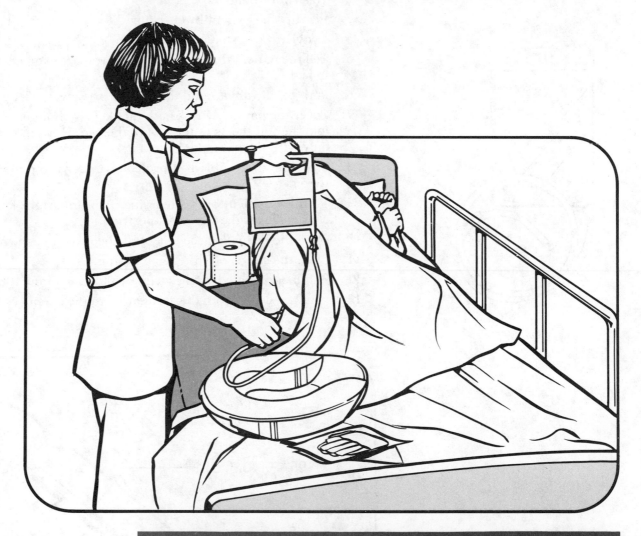

Procedure: The Cleansing Enema

1. Assemble your equipment:

   a) Disposable enema kit (enema container, tubing, and clamp)
   b) Lubricating jelly
   c) Graduated pitcher
   d) Bath thermometer
   e) Solution as instructed by head nurse or team leader:

      • Soapsuds: 1 package enema soap, 1,000 cc water, 105°F (40.5°C)

      • Saline: 2 teaspoons salt, 1,000 cc water, 105°F (40.5°C)

      • Tap water only: 1,000 cc water, 105°F (40.5°C)

   f) Bedpan and cover
   g) Urinal, if necessary

(continued next page)

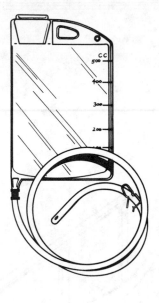

   h)   Emesis basin
   i)   Toilet tissue
   j)   Disposable bed protector
   k)   Paper towel
   l)   Bath blanket
   m) Disposable plastic gloves, optional

2. Wash your hands.

3. Identify the patient by checking the identification bracelet.

4. Ask visitors to step out of the room.

5. Tell the patient that you are going to give him an enema while he is in bed.

6. Pull the curtain around the bed for privacy.

7. Cover the patient with a bath blanket. Without exposing him, fan-fold the top sheets to the foot of the bed. Have the patient covered only with the bath blanket.

8. Place the disposable bed protector under the patient's hips (buttocks).

9. Turn the patient on his left side. Bend his right knee toward his chest. (This is the left Sims' position.)

10. Place the bedpan at the foot of the bed within easy reach.

11. Close the clamp on the enema tubing.

12. Fill the graduated pitcher with 1,000 cc water at 105°F (40.5°C).

13. Pour the water from the graduate into the enema container.

(continued next page)

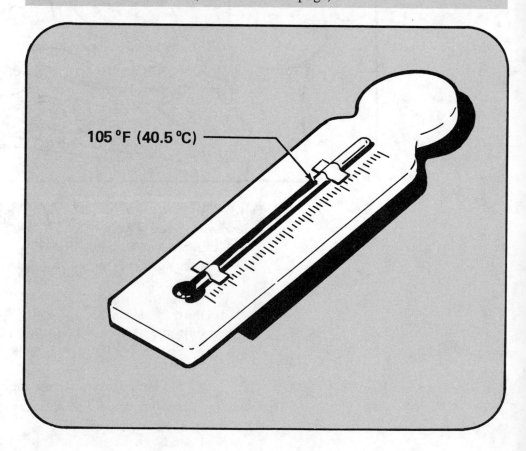

105 °F (40.5 °C)

14. A—If your instructions call for a soapsuds enema, add one package of enema soap to the water in the container. Use the tip of the tubing to mix the solution gently so that no suds form.

    B—If your instructions call for a saline enema, add two teaspoons of salt to the water in the container.

    C—If your instructions call for a tap water enema, do not add anything to the water.

15. Open the clamp on the enema tubing. Let the solution run through the tubing into the bedpan. This will get rid of any air in the tubing, warm the tube, and avoid giving the patient flatus. Then close the clamp.

16. Put the lubricating jelly on a piece of toilet tissue. Lubricate the enema top by rubbing the jelly on it with the tissue, beginning at the end and going up the tube 2-4 inches. Be sure the tip is well lubricated and the opening is not plugged.

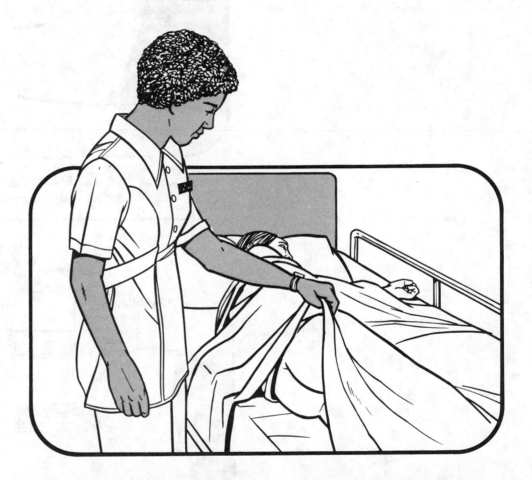

17. Expose the patient's buttocks by raising the blanket in a triangle over the anal area. If you will be using disposable gloves, put them on now.

18. Raise the upper buttocks so you can see the anal area.

(continued next page)

19. Gently insert the enema tip 2 to 4 inches through the anus into the rectum. If you feel resistance or if the patient complains of pain, stop.

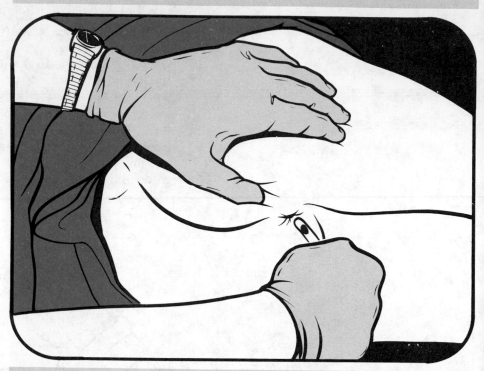

20. Open the clamp and hold the enema container 12 inches above the anus or 18 inches above the mattress.

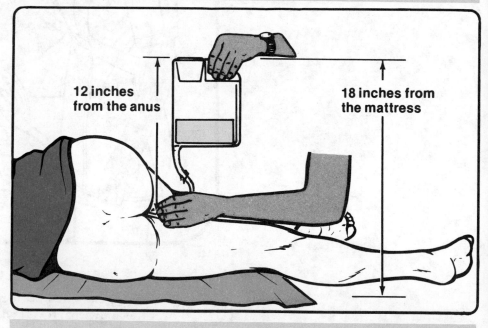

12 inches from the anus

18 inches from the mattress

21. Tell the patient to take slow deep breaths. Explain that this will help relieve the cramps caused by the enema. It will also help the patient to relax.

22. When most of the solution has flowed into the patient's rectum, close the clamp. Slowly withdraw the rectal tubing. Wrap it in the paper towel to avoid contamination. Place the tubing into the enema container.

(continued next page)

23. Help the patient onto the bedpan. Raise the back of the bed, if allowed. Put the toilet tissue where the patient can reach it easily.

24. The patient may be allowed to go the bathroom to expel the enema. If so, you must assist him to the bathroom, and stay near the bathroom, to assist the patient if he needs you. Tell the pateint not to flush the toilet. This is so the results can be observed.

25. Give the patient the signal cord. Check on the patient every few minutes.

26. Dispose of the enema equipment while the patient is on the bedpan.

27. When observing the results of an enema, look for anything that does not appear normal.
    A—Report to your head nurse or team leader if the stool:
    - Is very hard.
    - Is very soft.
    - Is large in amount.
    - Is small in amount.
    - Is accompanied by flatus (gas).

    B—Collect a specimen and report to your head nurse or team leader if the stool:
    - Is completely black.
    - Is streaked with red, white, yellow, or gray.
    - Has a very bad odor.
    - Looks like perked coffee grounds.

28. Empty the bedpan. Clean it and put it in its proper place.

29. Remove the disposable bed protector and discard.

30. Remove the bath blanket. At the same time, raise the top sheets to cover the patient.

31. Wash the patient's hands or have the patient wash his own hands.

32. Make the patient comfortable.

33. Wash your hands.

34. Report to your head nurse or team leader:
    - That you have given the patient a cleansing enema.
    - The time the enema was given.
    - The type of solution used.
    - The results, color of stool, consistency, flatus (gas) expelled, and unusual material noted.
    - Whether or not a specimen was obtained.
    - How the patient tolerated the procedure.
    - Your observations of anything unusual.

The **pre-packaged ready to use enema** is a very effective type of enema that is easy to use. The physician must order this type of enema before it can be administered. This type of enema is used frequently in the home as well as in the health care institution. It is completely disposable and can be purchased in any pharmacy or obtained from the central supply room in a health care institution.

Procedure: Giving the Ready-to-use Cleansing Enema

1. Assemble your equipment:
    a) Disposable prepackaged enema
    b) Bedpan and cover
    c) Urinal, if necessary
    d) Disposable bed protector
    e) Toilet tissue
    f) Disposable plastic gloves, optional
2. Wash your hands.
3. Identify the patient by checking the identification bracelet.
4. Ask visitors to step out of the room.
5. Tell the patient you are going to give him a cleansing enema while he is in bed.
6. Pull the curtain around the bed for privacy.
7. Cover the patient with a bath blanket. Without exposing him, fanfold the top sheets to the foot of the bed. Have the patient covered only with the bath blanket.
8. Place the disposable bed protector under the patient's hips (buttocks).
9. Turn the patient on his left side. Bend his right knee toward his chest. (This is the left Sims' position.)
10. Put the bedpan at the foot of the bed within easy reach.
11. Open the enema package. Take out the disposable enema. Remove the cap. If you will be using disposable gloves, put them on now.

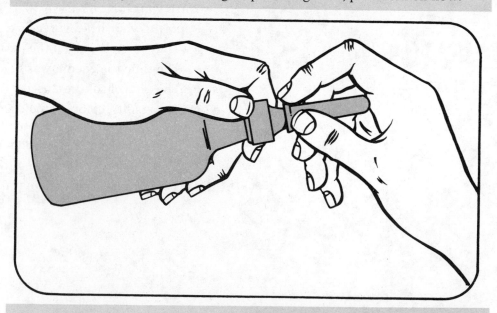

12. Expose the patient's buttocks by raising the blanket in a triangle over the anal area.
13. Raise the upper buttock so you can see the anal area.

(continued next page)

14. Gently insert the enema tip, which is already lubricated, two inches through the anus into the rectum.

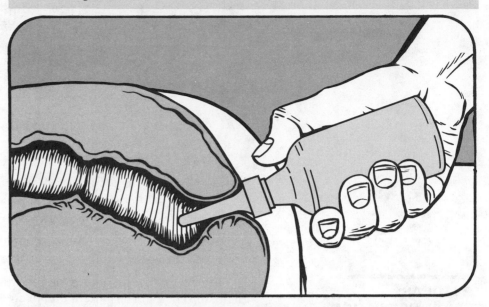

15. Squeeze the plastic bottle until all the liquid goes into the patient's rectum.

16. Remove the tube from the patient's anus. Put the empty plastic bottle back in the box. You will discard it later.

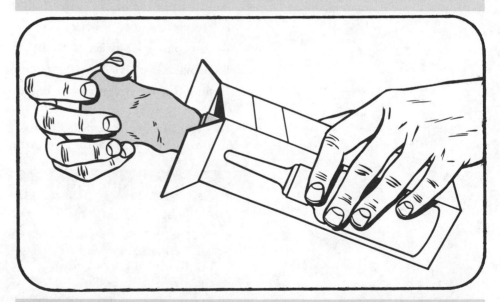

17. Help the patient get on the bedpan. Raise the back of the bed, if allowed. Put the toilet tissue where the patient can reach it easily.

18. The patient may be allowed to go into the bathroom to expel the enema. If so, you must assist him to the bathroom. Tell the patient not to flush the toilet. This is so the results can be observed.

19. Give the patient the signal cord. Check on the patient every few minutes.

20. Discard the disposable enema equipment. Return to the patient when he is finished using the bedpan. Check the contents for color of stool, consistency, amount, unusual material, or anything abnormal. If you observe anything unusual, collect a specimen.

(continued next page)

21. Empty the bedpan, clean it, and put it back in its proper place.
22. Remove the disposable bed protector and discard it.
23. Remove the bath blanket. At the same time, raise the top sheets to cover the patient.
24. Wash the patient's hands.
25. Make the patient comfortable.
26. Wash your own hands.
27. Report to your head nurse or team leader:
    - That you have given the patient a cleansing pre-packaged enema.
    - The time the enema was given.
    - The results, color of stool, consistency, flatus expelled, and unusual material noted.
    - How the patient tolerated this procedure.
    - Your observations of anything unusual.

KEY IDEAS: THE OIL RETENTION ENEMA

The procedure for giving the **retention enema** is different from that for the cleansing enema. The patient is expected to retain (hold in) the enema solution for 10 to 20 minutes. Usually a soapsuds (cleansing) enema is given 20 minutes after the oil retention enema has been expelled.

Retention enemas are given:

- To help soften the feces and gently stimulate evacuation.
- To lubricate the inside surface of the lower intestine.
- To soften the stool, if necessary.
- To ease passage of feces without straining.
- To provide laxative benefits when oral laxatives are not allowed.
- To help the patient eliminate barium sulfate residues after x-ray examinations.
- To soften fecal impaction (hard stool caught in the lower bowel) when straining might be harmful or painful.

Procedure: Giving the Ready-to-Use Oil Retention Enema

1. Assemble your equipment:
    a) Disposable pre-packaged ready-to-use-enema kit
    b) Bedpan and cover
    c) Urinal, if necessary
    d) Disposable bed protector
    e) Equipment for soapsuds enema, if ordered by the physician, 20 minutes after oil retention enema
    f) Toilet tissue
    g) Disposable plastic gloves, optional
2. Wash your hands.
3. Identify the patient by checking the identification bracelet.
4. Ask visitors to step out of the room.
5. Tell the patient that you are going to give him an oil retention enema while he is in bed.
6. Pull the curtain around the bed for privacy.
7. Cover the patient with a bath blanket. Without exposing him, fanfold the top sheets to the foot of the bed. Have the patient covered

(continued next page)

only with the bath blanket.

8. Place the disposable bed protector under the patient's hips (but-tocks).

9. Turn the patient on his left side. Bend his right knee toward his chest. (This is the left Sims' position.)

10. Put the bedpan at the foot of the bed within easy reach.

11. Open the package. Take out the disposable pre-packaged ready-to-use enema bag filled with oil. Remove the cap. If you will be using disposable gloves, put them on now.

12. Expose the patient's buttocks by raising the blanket in a triangle over the anal area.

13. Raise the upper buttock so you can see the anal area.

14. Gently insert the enema tip, which is already lubricated, 2 inches through the anus into the rectum.

15. Squeeze the plastic bottle until all the liquid goes into the patient's rectum.

16. Remove the tube from the patient's anus. Put the empty plastic bot-tle back in the box. You will discard it later.

17. Explain to the patient that he must retain (hold in) the oil for 20 minutes. Encourage the patient to stay in the Sims' position, if at all possible. Check on the patient every few minutes.

18. Your instructions may require you to give a soapsuds enema after the patient has retained the oil for 20 minutes. If so, give the soap-suds enema at this time.

19. Help the patient get on the bedpan. Raise the back of the bed, if allowed. Put the toilet tissue where the patient can reach it easily.

20. The patient may be allowed to go to the bathroom to expel the ene-ma. If so, you must help him get to the bathroom. Tell the patient not to flush the toilet. This is so the results can be observed.

21. Give the patient the signal cord. Check on the patient every few min-utes.

22. Discard the disposable enema equipment.

23. Return to the patient when he is finished using the bedpan. Check the contents for color of stool, consistency, amount, unusual mate-rial, or anything abnormal. If you observe anything unusual, collect a specimen.

24. Empty the bedpan, clean it, and put it back in its proper place.

25. Remove the disposable bed protector and discard it.

26. Remove the bath blanket. At the same time, raise the top sheets to cover the patient.

27. Wash the patient's hands.

28. Make the patient comfortable.

29. Wash your own hands.

30. Report to your head nurse or team leader:
    - That you have given the patient an oil retention enema.
    - The time the oil retention enema was given.
    - The results, color of stool, consistency, flatus expelled, and un-usual material noted.
    - How the patient tolerated the procedure.
    - Your observations of anything unusual.

(continued next page)

The **Harris flush** is an irrigation of the rectum. **Irrigation** means washing out. Clean water runs into the rectum. Gas (flatus) and water run out of the rectum. Again, clean water runs into the rectum. Flatus and water run out of the rectum in the return flow. This procedure is repeated for 10 minutes until the patient is relieved of excess gas.

Procedure: Giving the Harris Flush (Return-flow Enema)

1. Assemble your equipment:
   a) Disposable enema bag, tubing, and clamp
   b) Lubricating jelly
   c) Graduated pitcher
   d) Bath thermometer
   e) Urinal, if necessary
   f) Disposable plastic gloves, optional
   g) Emesis basin
   h) Toilet tissue
   i) Disposable bed protector
   j) Paper towel
   k) Bath blanket
   l) Bedpan

2. Wash your hands.

3. Identify the patient by checking the identification bracelet.

4. Ask visitors to step out of the room.

5. Explain to the patient that you are going to give him a Harris flush, which is a rectal irrigation that will relieve him of gas.

6. Pull the curtain around the bed for privacy.

7. Cover the patient with a bath blanket. Without exposing him, fanfold the top sheets to the foot of the bed. Have the patient covered only with the bath blanket.

8. Place the disposable bed protector under the patient's hips (buttocks).

9. Turn the patient on his left side. Bend his right knee toward his chest. (This is the left Sims' position.)

10. Put the bedpan at the foot of the bed within easy reach.

11. Close the clamp on the enema tubing.

12. Fill the graduated pitcher with 500 cc of water, 105°F (40.5°C). Measure the temperature of the water with the bath thermometer.

13. Pour the water from the graduated pitcher into the enema container.

14. Open the clamp on the enema tubing to let water run through the tubing into the bedpan. This will get rid of any air that may be in the tubing to avoid giving the patient flatus, and will also warm the tube. Then close the clamp.

15. Put the lubricating jelly on a piece of toilet tissue. Lubricate the enema tip by rubbing the jelly on it with the tissue. Be sure the tip is well lubricated and the opening is not plugged.

16. Expose the patient's buttocks by raising the blanket in a triangle over the anal area. If you will be using disposable gloves, put them on now.

17. Raise the upper buttock so you can see the anal area.

18. Gently insert the enema tip 2 inches through the anus into the rectum.

(continued next page)

19. Open the clamp. Hold the enema container 12 inches above the anus. Allow about 200 cc of water to enter the rectum.

20. Lower the enema bag below the bed frame. Let the water run back into the enema bag without removing the tube from the patient's rectum.

21. Hold the enema bag 12 inches above the anus. Let 200 cc of water run into the patient's rectum. Then lower the bag. Allow the water to run back into the enema bag. Keep the tube in the patient's rectum.

22. Continue letting water in and out of the rectum for 10 to 20 minutes as you are instructed.

23. Tell the patient to take slow deep breaths. Explain that this kind of breathing will help relieve the cramps caused by the enema. It will also help him to relax.

24. Observe the amounts (large or small) of flatus the patient expels as the water runs out of the patient into the enema bag.

25. Remove the tubing when the treatment is finished. Wrap the enema tip in the paper towel. This is to avoid contamination. Place it in the disposable enema container.

26. Help the patient get on the bedpan. Raise the back of the bed, if allowed. Put the toilet tissue where the patient can reach it easily. Give the patient the signal cord. Check on the patient every few minutes.

27. The patient may be allowed by the nurse to go to the bathroom to expel more flatus. If so, you must help him to the bathroom. Tell the patient to check the amount of flatus (large or small) that he expels.

28. Dispose of the enema equipment while the patient is on the bedpan.

29. Return to the patient when he is finished using the bedpan. Check the contents of the bedpan for bowel movement, color of stool, consistency, amount, unusual material, or anything abnormal. If you observe anything unusual, collect a specimen. Ask the patient if flatus was expelled.

30. Empty the bedpan, clean it, and put it back in its proper place.

31. Remove the disposable bed protector and discard it.

32. Remove the bath blanket. At the same time, raise the top sheets to cover the patient.

33. Wash the patient's hands.

34. Make the patient comfortable.

35. Wash your own hands.

36. Report to your head nurse or team leader:

    ● That you have given the patient a Harris flush.

    ● The time the Harris flush was given and how long it was continued.

    ● The results, amount of flatus expelled, and unusual material noted.

    ● Whether or not a specimen was obtained.

    ● How the patient tolerated the procedure.

    ● Your observations of anything unusual.

A **rectal tube with connected bag** is used to relieve the accumulation of intestinal gas (flatus) that often accumulates in the patient's lower bowel. You will use the rectal tube only once a day for 20 minutes, unless otherwise instructed. The whole kit—tube and bag—is discarded after one use.

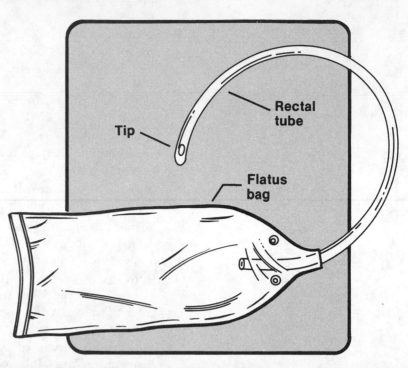

Procedure: Using the Disposable Rectal Tube with Connected Flatus Bag

1. Assemble your equipment:
   a) Disposable rectal tube with connected flatus bag
   b) Small piece of adhesive tape
   c) Tissue
   d) Lubricating jelly
   e) Disposable gloves, optional
2. Wash your hands.
3. Identify the patient by checking the identification bracelet.
4. Ask visitors to step out of the room.
5. Explain to the patient that you are going to insert a rectal tube, for the purpose of relieving him of gas (flatus).
6. Pull the curtain around the bed for privacy.
7. Turn the patient on his left side. Bend his right knee toward his chest. (This is the left Sims' position.)
8. Expose the patient's buttocks by raising the top sheets in a triangle over the anal area. If you will be using disposable gloves, put them on now.
9. Lubricate the tip of the rectal tube. Do this by squeezing lubricating jelly onto the tissue and rubbing the jelly on the tip. Be sure the opening at the end of the tube is not clogged. (If the rectal tube is already pre-lubricated, this step is not necessary.)
10. Raise the patient's upper buttock so you can see the anal area.
11. Gently insert the rectal tube 2 to 4 inches through the anus into the rectum.

(continued next page)

12. Use a small piece of adhesive tape to attach the tube to the patient's buttocks in order to hold the tube in place.

13. Let the tube remain in place for 20 minutes. Then remove and discard the equipment (Usually this procedure is done once in a 24-hour period.

14. Make the patient comfortable.

15. Wash your hands.

16. Report to your head nurse or team leader:

    ● The time the rectal tube was inserted and the time it was removed.

    ● The patient's comments about the amount (small or large) of flatus that he expelled through the tube.

    ● Your observations of anything unusual.

**KEY IDEAS:
RECTAL SUPPOSITORIES**

Rectal suppositories are inserted into the rectum to aid in elimination, to assist in healing, to relieve pain, or to re-toilet train an incontinent patient. A single or double cone shape is used for adults, a long thin one is used for children. Simple, non-medicinal suppositories are made of soap, glycerine, or cocoa butter. Medicinal suppositories that contain drugs are not administered by nursing assistants.

Procedure: Inserting a Rectal Suppository

1. Assemble your equipment on the patient's bedside table:
   a) One suppository as ordered
   b) Disposable gloves
   c) Lubricant
   d) Toilet tissue
   e) Bedpan and cover

2. Wash your hands.

3. Identify the patient by checking the identification bracelet.

4. Ask visitors to step out of the room.

5. Tell the patient that you are going to insert a rectal suppository.

6. Pull the curtain around the bed for privacy.

7. Raise the bed to its highest horizontal position.

8. Ask the patient to turn on his left side and raise his right knee toward his chest (left Sims' position). If he cannot do this, turn him and place the patient into this position.

9. Expose the patient's buttocks by raising the top sheets in a triangle over the patient's buttocks.

10. Put.on the disposable gloves.

11. Put the lubricating jelly on a piece of toilet tissue and lubricate the suppository by gently rubbing the jelly on it with the tissue.

12. Raise the upper buttock so you can see the anal area.

13. Holding the suppository between the thumb and the index finger, gently insert it through the anus into and along the wall of the rectum as far as the index finger will reach (2 inches).

14. Withdraw finger and press folded toilet tissue against the anus briefly.

15. Remove the gloves turning them inside out as you remove them.

16. Replace the top sheets and turn the patient into a position of comfort.

(continued next page)

17. Give the patient the signal cord and instruct him to signal you when he needs a bedpan.

18. If you are re-toilet training the patient, place him on a bedpan.

19. Raise the side rails, and lock them in place if the patient is on the bedpan.

20. Lower the bed to its lowest position.

21. Discard disposable gloves. Wash your hands.

22. Check the patient every 5 minutes.

23. Report to your head nurse or team leader:
    - That you have inserted the rectal suppository.
    - The time you inserted it.
    - The results obtained from inserting the suppository.
    - Your observations of anything unusual.

SECTION 2: PERINEAL CARE AND INDWELLING CATHETER CARE

OBJECTIVES: WHAT YOU WILL LEARN

When you have completed this section, you will be able to:

- Give perineal care
- Give daily indwelling catheter care
- Give the vaginal douche (irrigation)

KEY IDEAS: PERINEAL CARE

Perineal care is always given before daily indwelling catheter care. It provides cleanliness and comfort for the patient. It helps to prevent irritation and infection. Perineal care is also given following childbirth. Follow the instructions of your head nurse or team leader in your institution.

Procedure: Giving Perineal Care

1. Assemble your equipment:
   a) Disposable bed protector
   b) Bedpan and cover
   c) Graduated pitcher
   d) Cotton balls
   e) Disposable gloves, optional

2. Wash your hands.

3. Identify the patient by checking the identification bracelet.

4. Ask visitors to step out of the room.

5. Tell the patient that you are going to clean the genital area.

6. Pull the curtains around the bed for privacy.

7. Be sure there is plenty of light.

8. Cover the patient with a bath blanket. Without exposing him, fan-fold the top sheets to the foot of the bed. Have the patient covered only with the blanket. If you will be using disposable gloves, put them on now.

9. Fill the graduated pitcher with warm water at 100°F (37.7°C), or use the solution provided in your institution.

10. Place the disposable bed protector under the patient's buttocks.

(continued next page)

11. Help the patient to get on the bedpan.

12. Hold pitcher 4-5 inches above pubic area and pour solution over vulva (genital area).

13. Dry the patient gently with the cotton balls. Remove and discard disposable gloves.

14. Remove the bedpan and disposable bed protector. Place them on a chair.

15. Cover the patient with the top sheets. Remove the bath blanket.

16. Make the patient comfortable.

17. Empty, rinse, and put the equipment back where it belongs.

18. Discard disposable equipment.

19. Wash your hands.

20. Report to your head nurse or team leader:
    - That you have given the patient perineal care.
    - The time it was given.
    - Your observations of anything unusual.

**KEY IDEAS:
DAILY INDWELLING
CATHETER CARE**

An **indwelling catheter** is a tube inserted through the patient's urethra into the bladder to allow for urinary drainage. The indwelling catheter is specially made so that it will stay in place within the patient's bladder.

Daily catheter care is very important to prevent infection. Medical aseptic technique should be used at all times when you are handling and caring for the equipment.

The catheter is attached to tubing that should be taped loosely to the inner side of the patient's thigh. This is so it does not pull and irritate the bladder. This tubing leads to a plastic urine container. The container is attached to the bed frame. It is kept lower than the level of the urinary bladder so there is a constant downhill flow from the patient. The urine collects in the plastic container.

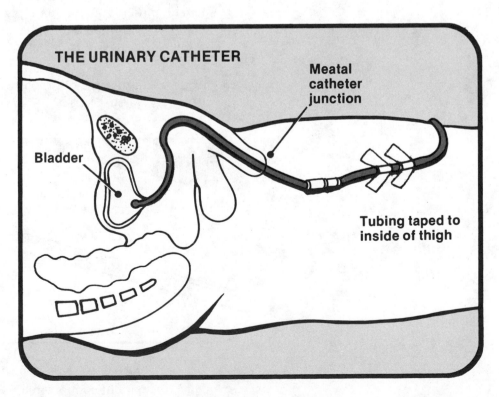

THE URINARY CATHETER

Meatal catheter junction

Bladder

Tubing taped to inside of thigh

This is a closed drainage system. The system must never be opened. If the patient is allowed to get out of bed, the container is carried at a lower level than the patient's bladder. A careful record of urinary output is kept for all patients who have indwelling catheters in place.

Procedure: Giving Daily Indwelling Catheter Care

1. Assemble your equipment:
    a) Disposable catheter care kit
    b) Disposable gloves
    c) Disposable bed protector
2. Wash your hands.
3. Identify the patient by checking the identification bracelet.
4. Ask visitors to step out of the room.
5. Tell the patient you are going to clean the area around his catheter tube. Make sure the patient's genital area has already been washed or that perineal care has been done.
6. Pull the curtains around the bed for privacy.
7. Make sure there is plenty of light. Observe for crusting, lesions, or anything else abnormal.
8. Cover the patient with a bath blanket. Without exposing him, fanfold the top sheets to the foot of the bed. Have the patient covered with only the blanket.
9. Open the catheter kit. Place the disposable bed protector under the patient's buttocks.
10. Put on the disposable gloves.
11. Take the applicators from the kit. The applicators are covered with antiseptic solution. Apply antiseptic solution on the entire area where the catheter enters the patient's body. With your gloved thumb and forefinger (index finger), gently spearate the labia on female patients. If the male patient has a foreskin, gently pull it back to apply antiseptic solution to the entire area.
12. Apply antiseptic solution to the four inches of the tube closest to the patient.
13. Apply the antiseptic ointment where the tube is inserted.
14. Check the tape to be sure the tubing is taped correctly in place.

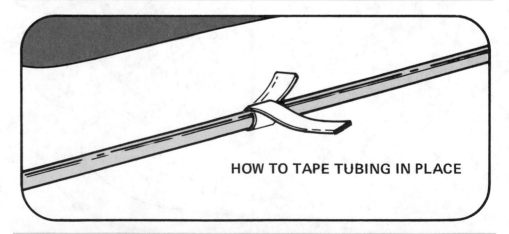

HOW TO TAPE TUBING IN PLACE

15. Cover the patient with the top sheets. Remove the bath blanket.
16. Make the patient comfortable.

(continued next page)

17. Remove the disposable bed protector.
18. Discard disposable equipment.
19. Wash your hands.
20. Report to your head nurse or team leader:
    - That catheter care has been given.
    - The time it was given.
    - Your observations of anything unusual.

KEY IDEAS: VAGINAL DOUCHE/ NONSTERILE (IRRIGATION)

The introduction of solution into the vaginal canal with an immediate return of the solution by gravity is called the **vaginal irrigation** or **douche**. This type of irrigation is usually used for cleansing the vaginal canal (vaginal tract) or to relieve inflammation of the vaginal tract. When used to excess it can wash away normal protective secretions, and never should be done without the physician's order. The doctor may order this treatment to cleanse before surgery, before an examination, to cleanse in cases of severe discharge, to treat an inflammation, or to neutralize secretions in the vaginal canal. The rules of medical asepsis must be followed for this treatment.

Procedure: Giving the Vaginal Douche/Nonsterile Irrigation

1. Assemble your equipment:
   a) Disposable douche kit (irrigating container with tubing, clamp, and douche nozzle)
   b) Graduated pitcher
   c) Bath thermometer
   d) Bedpan and cover
   e) Bath blanket
   f) Disposable waterproof bed protector
   g) Solution as instructed by head nurse or team leader, usually 1,000 cc tap water at 105°F (40.5°C)
   h) Disposable gloves
   i) Emesis basin
   j) Cotton balls and cleansing solution in small disposable container, as ordered by your head nurse or team leader
2. Wash your hands.
3. Identify the patient by checking the identification bracelet.
4. Ask visitors to step out of the room.
5. Tell the patient you are going to give her a vaginal douche.
6. Pull the curtains around the bed for privacy.
7. Offer the patient the bedpan, explaining that her bladder must be empty to insure desired results from the douche.
8. Remove bedpan. Measure output if the patient is on intake and output. Record on the I & O sheet. Empty the contents of the bedpan, wash and place on a chair nearby.
9. Wash the patient's hands.
10. Wash your hands.
11. Cover the patient with a bath blanket. Without exposing her, fanfold the top sheets to the foot of the bed. The patient should have held the bath blanket while you do this. Leave the patient covered with only the bath blanket.
12. Place the disposable bed protector under the patient's hips (buttocks).
13. Raise the bed to its highest horizontal position.

(continued next page)

14. Open the douche kit, close the clamp on the tubing.

15. Fill the graduated pitcher with 1,000 cc of water or solution as ordered at 105°F (40.5°C). Test the temperature of the water with the bath thermometer. Then pour the water into the irrigating douche container.

16. Pour the cleansing solution over cotton balls in a small disposable container to saturate them with solution.

17. Place the patient into the dorsal recumbent position. The head of the bed should be flat. Drape the patient with a small sheet.

18. Place the bedpan under the patient's hips (buttocks).

19. Place emesis basin on the bed to receive the used cotton balls.

20. Put on disposable gloves.

21. To cleanse the vulva using cotton balls saturated with cleansing solution:

    a) Wipe from the front to the back over the large outside lips (labia majora) on one side. Discard in emesis basin.

    b) Wipe from the front to the back over the large outside lips (labia majora) on the other side. Discard in emesis basin.

    c) Wipe from the front to the back over the midline of the large outside lips (labia majora). Discard in emesis basin.

    d) Expose the small inside lips (labia minora) by using thumb and forefinger to separate the large outside lips (labia majora) and cleanse as follows:

    e) Wipe from front to back on the far side of the small lips (labia minora). Discard cotton ball.

    f) Wipe from front to back on the near side of the small lips (labia minora). Discard cotton ball.

    g) Then wipe from front to back in the center (midline) over vaginal orifice (opening).

    h) Repeat until entire area is clean, always using new cotton balls.

22. Open clamp to expel air and allow solution to flow over vulva. Do not touch vulva with nozzle.

23. With solution flowing, insert douche nozzle tip into vagina from 2 to 3 inches with an upward and then downward and backward gentle movement.

24. Allow solution to flow holding the douche container no more than 12 inches above the vulva or 18 inches above the mattress.

25. Rotate the nozzle until all the solution has been given. This will insure cleansing of the vagina.

26. Clamp tubing and remove douche nozzle gently. Wrap in paper towel to prevent contamination. Put the tubing into the douche container. Remove and discard disposable gloves.

27. Help the patient to sit up on the bedpan by raising the back of the bed, if allowed (Fowlers Position). This will help the solution to drain from the vagina.

28. Dry perineum with toilet tissue and discard into bedpan.

29. Remove bedpan and place on chair.

30. Help the patient to turn on her side and dry buttocks with toilet tissue.

31. Remove bed protector.

32. Lower the bed to its lowest horizontal position.

33. Change any linen that has become damp.

(continued next page)

Procedure continued

34. Raise the top sheets over the bath blanket and then remove the bath blanket from under the top sheets.

35. Make the patient comfortable.

36. Observe contents of the bedpan. Collect a specimen if the returned solution is not as clear as when it was inserted.

37. Clean bedpan and emesis basin and return to their proper place.

38. Discard disposable supplies.

39. Wash the patient's hands.

40. Wash your hands.

41. Report to your head nurse or team leader:
    - That you have given the patient a vaginal douche.
    - The time the douche was given.
    - The type of solution used.
    - That a specimen was collected and why.
    - How the patient tolerated the procedure.
    - Your observation of the returned solution and unusual material noted.
    - Your observations of anything unusual.

SECTION 3: ARTIFICIAL EYE CARE

OBJECTIVES: WHAT YOU WILL LEARN

When you have completed this section, you will be able to:

- Care for a patient's artificial eye

**KEY IDEAS:
CARE OF THE ARTIFICIAL
EYE**

Cleaning the patient's artificial eye is part of daily personal hygiene. Often a patient cannot care for it himself. If he has an artificial eye, it must be cared for properly to prevent infection and **encrustation**. (Encrustation means formation of dried mucous material in the eye socket and around the artificial eye.) Assist the patient, but permit him to do as much as he is able.

Procedure: Caring for the Artificial Eye

1. Assemble your equipment on the bedside table:
   a) An eyecup half-filled with lukewarm water at 98°F to 100°F (36.6°C to 37.7°C) and labeled with the patient's name and room number (if no eyecup is available, use a clean denture cup)
   b) Gauze, 4x4 (2 pieces), for the bottom of the cup
   c) Small basin with lukewarm water
   d) Four cotton balls
   e) Optional: any special cleansing solution the doctor orders

2. Wash your hands.

3. Ask visitors to step out of the room.

4. Identify the patient by checking the identification bracelet.

5. Tell the patient you are going to take care of his eye.

6. Pull the curtains around the bed for privacy.

7. Help the patient to lie down on the bed. This is to prevent accidental dropping of the artificial eye.

(continued next page)

8. Have the patient close his eyes. Clean any external secretions from the patient's upper eyelid. Use cotton balls and warm water from the basin. Clean from the inner canthus to the outside of the eye area. If you need to wipe more than once, use a clean (new) cotton ball each time. Use gentle strokes.

9. Remove the artificial eye. To do this, carefully depress the lower eyelid with your thumb. Lift the upper lid gently with your forefinger. The eye should slide out and down, into your hand. Have the patient do this, if he is able.

10. Place the eye in the cup on the 4x4 gauze. Let it soak in the water.

11. Clean the eye socket. Wash off external matter and encrustations with cotton balls and warm water. Using gentle strokes, clean from the inner canthus to the outside of the eye. This means you move from the nose to the outside of the eye.

12. Take the eyecup to the patient's bathroom. Close the drain in the sink. Fill the sink one-half full with water to prevent breakage if the eye is dropped.

13. Take the eye in your hand and wash with running lukewarm water 98°F to 100°F (36.6°C to 37.7°C). Use plain water unless the doctor ordered a special solution. Place the eye in the gauze and rub gently between your thumb and forefinger. DO NOT USE ALCOHOL, ETHER, OR ACETONE. THESE DISSOLVE THE PLASTIC OF THE ARTIFICIAL EYE AND ALSO MAY DULL THE LUSTER.

14. Rinse the eye under running lukewarm water at 98°F to 100°F (36.6°C to 37.7°C), then dry it, using the second 4 x 4 gauze. Discard the water from the eyecup. Place the slightly moistened eye on dry gauze in the eyecup. A slightly moistened eye is easier to insert. Return to the patient's bedside.

15. If the patient cannot wear the eye, store it in the eyecup with water and place in bedside table drawer.

16. Wash your hands thoroughly a second time before inserting the artificial eye. If the patient is to insert the eye, have him wash his hands.

17. Insert the eye in the patient's eye socket. Have the notched edge toward the nose. Raise the upper lid with your forefinger. With your other hand, insert the eye. Place the eye under the upper lid. Then depress the lower lid. The eye should settle in place.

18. Make the patient comfortable.

19. Discard disposable equipment.

20. Report to your head nurse or team leader:
   - That you have completed care of the artificial eye.
   - The time it was done.
   - Your observations of anything unusual.

WHAT YOU HAVE LEARNED

The guiding principles for all forms of special treatments are effectiveness, safety, good aseptic technique, and consideration for the patient's comfort. The disposable, ready-to-use equipment and the correct technique help you meet all these requirements conveniently and efficiently.

12 MEASURING AND RECORDING VITAL SIGNS

1. Vital Signs
2. Measuring the Temperature
3. Measuring the Pulse
4. Measuring Respirations
5. Measuring Blood Pressure

SECTION 1: VITAL SIGNS

OBJECTIVES: WHAT YOU WILL LEARN

When you have completed this section, you will be able to:

- Explain vital signs
- State the average adult normal rates

**KEY IDEAS:
VITAL SIGNS**

When the body is not functioning normally, changes happen in the measurable rates of the vital signs. Everyone who is measuring and recording information about patients' vital signs must be very careful and accurate. When you record the readings, write carefully. Make sure your handwriting is clear and easy to read. If you are not sure of your reading or if the readings seem unusual, tell your head nurse or team leader. Common abbreviations for the vital signs are:

- Temperature = T
- Pulse = P
- Respiration = R
- Blood Pressure = BP
- Vital Signs = TPR & BP

When your head nurse or team leader says:

- "Take temps," she means measure the patient's temperature, pulse, and respiration.
- "Take vital signs," she means measure the patient's temperature, pulse, respiration, and blood pressure.
- "Take blood pressure," she means measure the patient's blood pressure, pulse, and respiration.

Write down the numbers for the patient's temperature, pulse, respiration, and blood pressure right away. If you are using a TPR book, check to find the right column. The columns have certain hours of the day written at the top, for example, 8 a.m. or 12 noon. Check the patient's name. Be sure you are writing the vital signs opposite the right name and at the right time. Report to the head nurse or team leader if there are changes in the patient's temperature, pulse, respiration, or blood pressure. In most institutions this is done by drawing a red circle around the number on the "temp." board or in the TPR book.

Average Normal Adult Rates

TEMPERATURE: 98.6°F or 37°C
PULSE: 72-80 beats per minute
RESPIRATION: 16-20 per minute

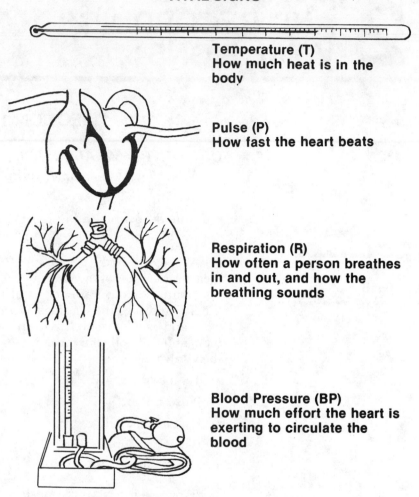

VITAL SIGNS

Temperature (T)
How much heat is in the
body

Pulse (P)
How fast the heart beats

Respiration (R)
How often a person breathes
in and out, and how the
breathing sounds

Blood Pressure (BP)
How much effort the heart is
exerting to circulate the
blood

SECTION 2: MEASURING THE TEMPERATURE

OBJECTIVES: WHAT YOU WILL LEARN

When you have completed this section, you will be able to:

- Read a thermometer accurately
- Demonstrate the procedure for measuring oral temperatures
- Demonstrate the procedure for measuring rectal temperatures
- Demonstrate the procedure for measuring axillary temperatures
- Demonstrate the proper use of a battery-operated electronic thermometer

KEY IDEAS:
BODY TEMPERATURE

Body temperature is a measurement of the amount of heat in the body. The body creates heat in the process of changing food into energy. The body can also lose heat—through perspiration, respiration (breathing), and excretion. The balance between the heat produced and the heat lost is the body temperature. The normal adult body temperature is 98.6°Fahrenheit, or 37°Centigrade. There is a normal range in which a person's body temperature may vary and still be considered normal.

Normal Ranges of Body Temperature

	Fahrenheit	Centigrade
ORAL	97.6 to 99°F	36.4 to 37.2°C
RECTAL	98.6 to 100°F	37.0 to 37.8°C
AXILLARY	96.6 to 98°F	35.9 to 36.7°C

Types of Thermometers

The body temperature is measured with an instrument called a thermometer. There are several different types of thermometers.

- Glass Thermometer—this is a delicate, hollow glass tube with a liquid metal called mercury sealed inside it. Mercury is an element that is very sensitive to temperature. It expands (gets larger) when the temperature goes up. Mercury contracts (gets smaller) when the temperature goes down. Even if the temperature rises only slightly, the mercury will expand and travel up the tube, reflecting the change. The outside of the glass thermometer is marked with lines, or calibrations, and numbers. These markings help us measure exactly the temperature readings displayed by the level of the mercury.

  There are three types of glass thermometers. They are:

  Oral—this type is used to measure the patient's temperature by mouth and is also used in measuring the axillary temperature (in the patient's armpit).

  Rectal—this type is used to measure the patient's temperature by inserting the thermometer into the patient's rectum. This type is used because its construction makes it stronger.

  Security—this type is used for taking an infant's rectal temperature. Many institutions use the security or stubby type with a red knob at the stem for rectal temperatures, and with a green knob at the stem for oral temperatures. Follow your institution's policy.

- Battery-operated electronic thermometers—are being used in many health care institutions. This type of thermometer eliminates the human error and variation in reading a glass thermometer. The electronic thermometers have both a blue (oral) and a red (rectal) attachment called a probe. A disposable plastic cover (sheath) is used over the probe for each patient.

- Chemically treated paper or plastic thermometers—some health care institutions now also use plastic or chemically treated single use paper thermometers that change color to indicate the patient's temperature.

Rules to Follow: Care of Glass Thermometers

- Because glass thermometers break and shatter easily, we must handle them with care. Be especially careful to avoid breaking a thermometer while it is in a patient's mouth or rectum.

- The liquid metal, mercury, inside the thermometer is a poison, that is, it may be harmful if it is ingested (taken into the body by mouth) or if it has contact with the skin for a prolonged period of time.

- Check the containers in which the thermometers are kept. Follow your instructions for cleaning these containers. You are expected to keep the containers filled with the proper disinfectant solution.

- Never clean a glass thermometer with hot water as it will cause the mercury to expand so much that the thermometer will explode.

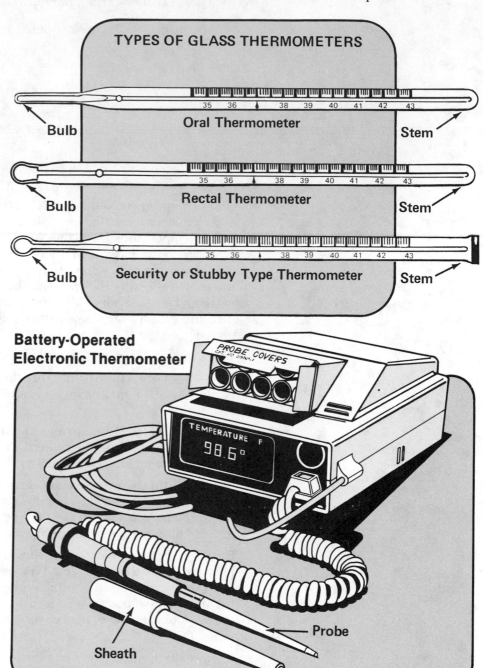

TYPES OF GLASS THERMOMETERS

Bulb Oral Thermometer Stem

Bulb Rectal Thermometer Stem

Bulb Security or Stubby Type Thermometer Stem

Battery-Operated Electronic Thermometer

PROBE COVERS

TEMPERATURE F
98.6°

Sheath Probe

Procedure: Shaking Down the Glass Thermometer

1. Assemble your equipment on the bedside table:
   a) Thermometer in container with proper disinfectant solution as used in your institution.
2. Wash your hands.
3. Before using the thermometer, check to make sure that it is not cracked or that the bulb is not chipped.
4. Hold the thermometer firmly between your fingers and your thumb

(continued next page)

at the stem and farthest from the bulb. The bulb is the end that is inserted into the patient's body.

5. Stand clear of any hard surfaces such as counters and tables to avoid striking and breaking the thermometer while you are shaking it. For practice you might stand with your arm over a pillow or mattress in case you accidentally drop the thermometer.

6. When you are sure that you have a good hold on the thermometer, shake your hand loosely from the wrist. Do it as if you were shaking water from your fingers.

7. Snap your wrist again and again. This will shake down the mercury to the lowest possible point. This should be below the numbers and lines (calibrations).

8. Always do this before and after using a thermometer.

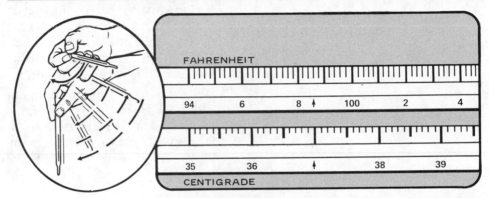

SHAKE THE MERCURY DOWN TO THE LOWEST POINT BELOW THE NUMBERS AND LINES

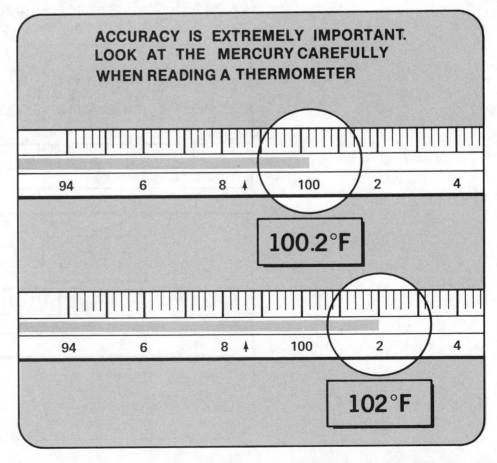

ACCURACY IS EXTREMELY IMPORTANT. LOOK AT THE MERCURY CAREFULLY WHEN READING A THERMOMETER

100.2°F

102°F

Procedure: Reading a Fahrenheit Thermometer

1. With your thumb and first two fingers, hold the thermometer at the stem.

2. Hold the thermometer at eye level. Turn the thermometer back and forth between your fingers until you can clearly see the column of mercury.

3. Notice the scale or calibrations. Each long line stands for 1 degree.

4. There are 4 short lines between each of the long lines. Each short line stands for 2 tenths (or 0.2) of a degree.

5. Between the long lines that represent 98° and 99° look for a longer line with an arrow directly beneath it. This special line points out normal body temperature.

6. Look at the end of the mercury. Notice the line or number where the mercury ends. If it is one of the short lines, notice the previous longer line toward the silver tip that goes into the patient's mouth. The temperature reading is the degree marked by that long line plus 2, 4, 6, or 8 tenths of a degree. Example: If the mercury ends after the 99 line, but on the second short line, the temperature is 99.4°F. If the mercury ends between 2 lines, take the line it is closer to.

7. Write down the patient's temperature right away. If you are using a TPR book, check to find the right column next to the patient's name and the right time of day. Write the patient's temperature using the figure you read on the thermometer. Some institutions will write 99.4°F. Other will write 99⁴. Follow the method used in your institution.

Procedure: Reading a Centigrade (Celsius) Thermometer

1. With your thumb and first two fingers, hold the thermometer at the stem.

(continued next page)

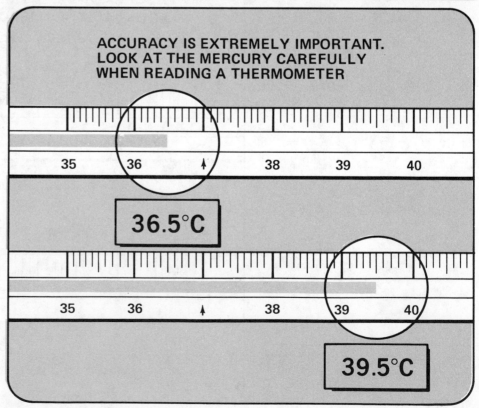

ACCURACY IS EXTREMELY IMPORTANT.
LOOK AT THE MERCURY CAREFULLY
WHEN READING A THERMOMETER

36.5°C

39.5°C

2. Hold it at eye level. Turn the thermometer back and forth between your fingers until you can clearly see the column of mercury.

3. Notice the scale or calibrations. Each long line shows one degree.

4. There are 9 short lines between each number. These short lines are 1, 2, 3, 4, 5, 6, 7, 8, and 9 tenths of a degree. If the mercury ended after the 36 and on the third short line, the temperature would read 36.3°C. If the mercury ended after the long line 37 and on the eighth short line, the temperature would read 37.8°C. If the mercury ends after line 37 on the fifth short line, the temperature would be referred to as 37.5°C.

5. Write down the patient's temperature right away. If you are using a TPR book, check to find the correct column next to the patient's name and the right time of day. Write the patient's temperature using the figure you read on the thermometer. Some facilities write 37°C. Others will write 37. Follow the method used in your facility.

KEY IDEAS: RECORDING THE PATIENT'S TEMPERATURE

For recording the patient's temperature, three symbols are used:

° = degrees

F = Fahrenheit

C = Centigrade or Celsius

You will record the patients' temperatures according to the method used in your institution.

Fahrenheit temperature can be written in two ways:

98.6°F or 98^6°F

If you are using a Centigrade (Celsius) thermometer, the temperature would be written:

37°C or 37.3°C or 37^3°C

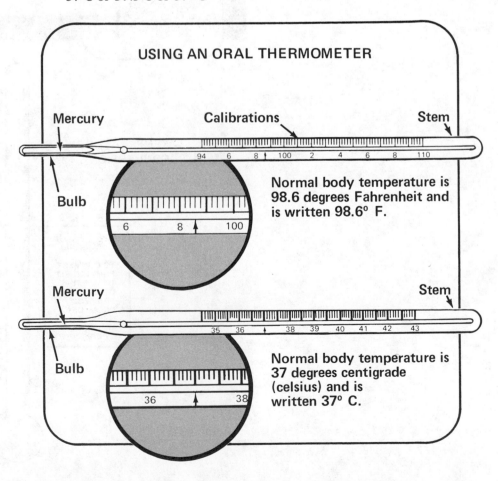

USING AN ORAL THERMOMETER

Mercury   Calibrations   Stem

94 6 8 100 2 4 6 8 110

Bulb

6   8   100

Normal body temperature is 98.6 degrees Fahrenheit and is written 98.6° F.

Mercury   Stem

35 36   38 39 40 41 42 43

Bulb

36   38

Normal body temperature is 37 degrees centigrade (celsius) and is written 37° C.

Write an R with the temperature reading if a rectal temperature was taken. Write an A beside the temperature reading if an axillary temperature was taken.

THE TWO MAJOR SCALES USED FOR MEASURING TEMPERATURE IN THE UNITED STATES

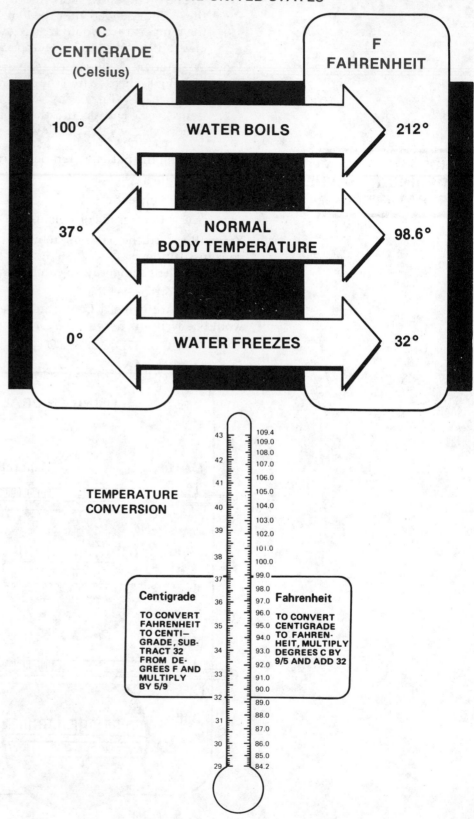

C CENTIGRADE (Celsius)		F FAHRENHEIT
100°	WATER BOILS	212°
37°	NORMAL BODY TEMPERATURE	98.6°
0°	WATER FREEZES	32°

TEMPERATURE CONVERSION

Centigrade

TO CONVERT FAHRENHEIT TO CENTI—GRADE, SUB-TRACT 32 FROM DE-GREES F AND MULTIPLY BY 5/9

Fahrenheit

TO CONVERT CENTIGRADE TO FAHREN-HEIT, MULTIPLY DEGREES C BY 9/5 AND ADD 32

INSERTING THE ORAL THERMOMETER

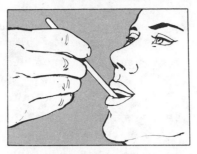

A. Insert the thermometer gently into the patient's mouth under the tongue.

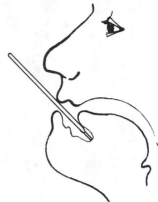

C. Instruct the patient to keep the thermometer under the tongue by gently closing the lips around the thermometer.

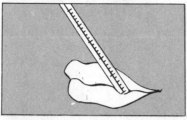

B. Position the thermometer to the side of the mouth.

Procedure: Measuring an Oral Temperature

1. Assemble your equipment:
   a) Oral thermometer in container with proper disinfectant solution
   b) Tissue or paper towel
   c) Temp. board, TPR book, or the form used in your institution
   d) Pen or pencil
2. Wash your hands.
3. Identify the patient by checking the identification bracelet.
4. Tell the patient that you are going to take his temperature.
5. Ask the patient if he has recently had hot or cold fluids or if he has been smoking. If the answer is yes, wait 10 minutes before taking an oral temperature.
6. Ask visitors to step out of the room.
7. Pull the curtain around the bed for privacy.
8. The patient should be in bed or sitting in a chair.
9. Take the thermometer out of its container. Rinse with cool tap water. (This will remove the taste of the disinfectant solution it is kept in.) Dry with paper towel or tissue.
10. Shake the mercury down.
11. Gently put the bulb end in the patient's mouth under the tongue. Ask him to keep his mouth and lips closed.
12. Leave the thermometer in the patient's mouth for 8 minutes. Please Note: The latest research states that oral temperature is more accurate when the oral thermometer remains in the mouth for 8 minutes. However, if in your institution the policy is for 3 to 5 minutes,

(continued next page)

follow the procedure of your institution. Eight minutes will give you the most accurate reading.

13. Take the thermometer out of the patient's mouth. Hold the stem end and wipe the thermometer with the tissue. Wipe from the stem of the thermometer toward the bulb end.

14. Read the thermometer.

15. Record the temperature in the TPR book, temp. board, or the form used in your institution.

16. Shake the mercury down. Replace the thermometer in its container, filled with the proper disinfectant solution.

17. Make the patient comfortable.

18. Wash your hands.

19. Report to your head nurse or team leader:
    - That the oral temperature was above 100°F or 37.8°C. (Many institutions report an oral temperature above 100°F or 37.8°C by circling the figure in red on the temp. board; but be sure to report any elevation.)
    - Your observations of anything unusual.

KEY IDEAS: MEASURING RECTAL TEMPERATURE

Remember that you will always use a rectal thermometer for taking rectal temperatures. Notice that the rectal thermometer has a small round bulb on one end. This bulb prevents the thermometer from injuring the sensitive lining of the patient's rectum. Under the following conditions you would automatically take a rectal temperature:

- When the patient is an infant or a child under 12 years of age.
- When the patient is having warm or cold applications on his face or neck.
- When the patient cannot keep his mouth closed on the thermometer.
- When the patient finds it hard to breathe through his nose.
- When the patient has sneezing or coughing spells.
- When the patient's mouth is dry or inflamed (red).
- When the patient is restless, delirious, unconscious, or confused.
- When the patient is getting oxygen by cannula, catheter, face mask, or oxygen tent.
- When the patient has a nasogastric tube (Levin's tube, NG tube) in place.
- When the patient has had major surgery in the area of his face or neck.
- When the patient's face is partially paralyzed as from a stroke.

Procedure: Measuring Rectal Temperature

1. Assemble your equipment:
    a) Rectal thermometer in container with proper disinfectant solution
    b) Tissue or paper towel
    c) Lubricating jelly
    d) Temp. board, TPR book, or the form used in your institution
    e) Disposable gloves (optional)

2. Wash your hands.

3. Identify the patient by checking the identification bracelet.

4. Ask visitors to step out of the room.

5. Tell the patient that you are going to take his temperature by rectum.

(continued next page)

6. Pull the curtain around the bed for privacy. Lower the backrest on the bed, if allowed.

7. Take the thermometer out of its container. Rinse it off with cool tap water. Hold the thermometer only by the stem. Dry it with a paper towel or tissue.

8. Inspect the bulb of the thermometer carefully for cracks or chipped places. A broken thermometer could seriously injure the patient's rectum. Do not use a chipped, cracked or broken thermometer.

9. Hold the thermometer at the stem end. Shake it down until the mercury is below the numbers and lines.

10. Put a small amount of lubricating jelly on a piece of tissue. Then lubricate the bulb of the thermometer with the lubricated tissue. This makes insertion easier and also makes it more comfortable for the patient.

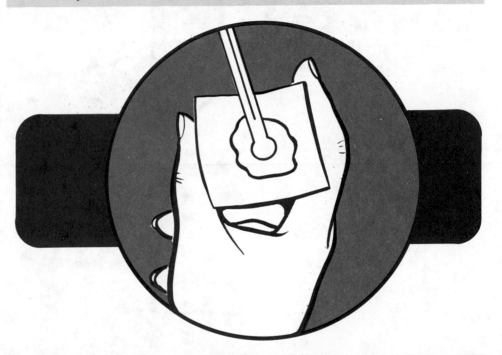

11. Ask the patient to turn on his side. Or turn him yourself, if necessary. Turn back the top covers just enough so that you can see the patient's buttocks. Avoid overexposing him.

12. With one hand, raise the upper buttock until you can see the anus, the opening to the rectum. With the other hand gently insert the bulb one inch through the anus into the rectum.

13. If the patient is an infant, remove the diaper. Lay the baby on his back. Raise his legs with one hand. Insert the themometer with the other hand one-half inch into the rectum. Always hold the thermometer while it is in the child's rectum.

14. Hold the thermometer in place for 3 minutes. Do not leave a patient with a rectal thermometer in the rectum, no matter what his condition. If the patient is able, he may hold it.

15. Remove the thermometer from the patient's rectum. Holding the stem end of the thermometer, wipe it with a tissue from stem to bulb, to remove particles of feces.

16. Read the thermometer.

17. Record the temperature right away in the TPR book, temp. board, or form used in your institution. Note that this is a rectal tempera-

(continued next page)

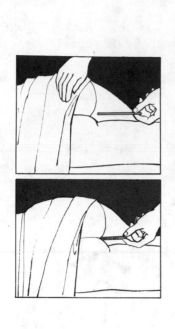

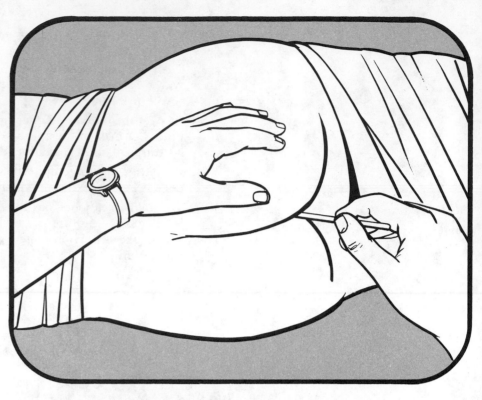

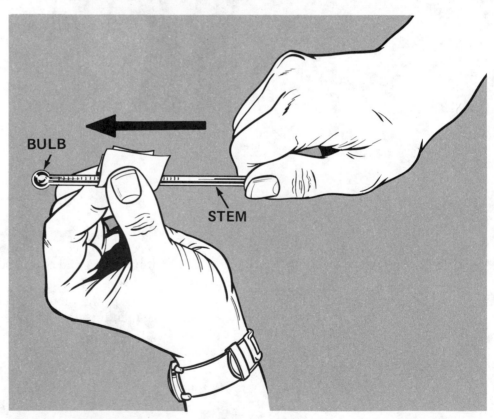

BULB

STEM

Procedure continued

ture by writing an R in front of the figure. This is necessary because an average rectal temperature is slightly higher than an oral one.

18. Shake the mercury down until it is below the numbers and lines.

19. Replace the thermometer in its container filled with the proper disinfectant solution.

(continued next page)

20. Make the patient comfortable.
21. Wash your hands.
22. Report to your head nurse or team leader:
    - If the rectal temperature is higher than 101°F or 38.3°C. Many institutions report the rectal temperature over 101°F or 38.3°C by circling the figure in red on the temp. board, TPR book, or on the form used in your institution.
    - Your observations of anything unusual.

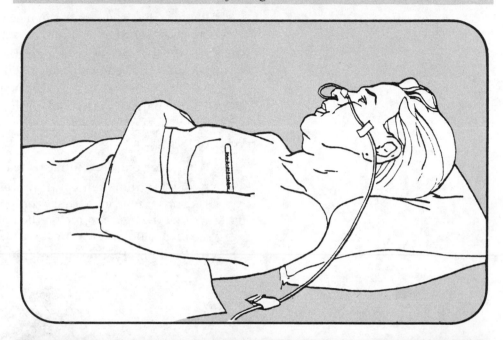

Procedure: Measuring Axillary Temperature

1. Assemble your equipment:
   a) Oral thermometer in container with proper disinfectant solution
   b) Tissue or paper towel
   c) Temp. board, TPR book, or the form used in your institution
   d) Pen or pencil
2. Wash your hands.
3. Identify the patient by checking the identification bracelet.
4. Ask visitors to step out of the room.
5. Tell the patient that you have to take his temperature.
6. Pull the curtain around the bed for privacy.
7. Holding the stem end, remove the oral thermometer from its container.
8. Rinse the thermometer with cool tap water and dry it with tissue. Shake the mercury down.
9. Inspect the bulb of the thermometer carefully for scratches or chipped places. A broken thermometer could seriously injure the patient. Do not use a chipped, cracked or broken thermometer.
10. Remove the patient's arm from the sleeve of his gown. If the axillary region is moist with perspiration, pat it dry with a towel.
11. Place the bulb of the oral thermometer in the center of the armpit (axilla). The thermometer then should be held upright by the arm and the chest. (continued next page)

12. Put the patient's arm across his chest or abdomen.

13. If the patient is unconscious or is too weak to help, you will have to hold the thermometer in place.

14. Leave the thermometer in place 10 minutes. Stay with the patient.

15. Remove the thermometer. Wipe it off with tissue from the stem to the bulb.

16. Read the thermometer.

17. Shake the mercury down until it is below the numbers and lines.

18. Replace the thermometer in its container filled with the proper disinfectant solution.

19. Record the patient's temperatue on the temp. board, in the TPR book, or on the form used in your institution. Note that this is an axillary temperature by writing an "A" in front of the figure.

20. Put the patient's arm back in the sleeve of his gown.

21. Make the patient comfortable.

22. Wash your hands.

23. Report to your head nurse or team leader:
    - If the axillary temperature was over 99°F (37.2°C). Many institutions report an axillary temperature over 99°F (37.2°C) by circling the figure in red on the temp. board, in the TPR book, or on the form used in your institution.
    - Your observations of anything unusual.

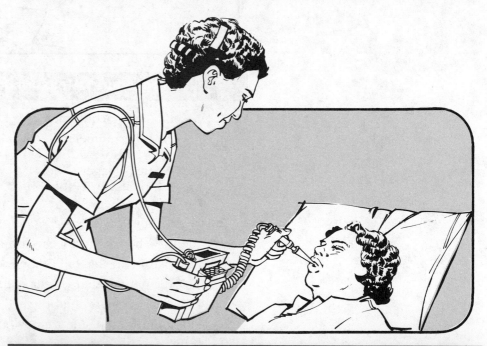

Procedure: Using a Battery-operated Electronic Oral Thermometer

1. Assemble your equipment:
   a) Disposable plastic probe cover
   b) Battery-operated electronic thermometer
   c) Oral (blue) attachment
   d) Temp. board, TPR book, or form used in your institution
   e) Pen or pencil

2. Wash your hands.

(continued next page)

3. Identify the patient by checking the identification bracelet.

4. Ask visitors to step out of the room.

5. Tell the patient that you are going to take his temperature.

6. Pull the curtain around the bed for privacy.

7. Check to be sure that the oral (blue top) probe connector is properly placed in its receptacle on the base of the unit.

8. Remove the probe from its stored position. Insert it into a sheath or probe cover.

9. Insert the covered probe into the patient's mouth slowly until the metal tip is at the base under the tongue to the back of the patient's mouth.

10. Hold the probe in the patient's mouth. It is much heavier than a glass thermometer and some patients are unable to hold it.

11. Wait about 15 seconds for the buzzer to ring for a computed temperature reading. Then remove the probe from the patient's mouth.

12. Record the temperature on the temp. board, in the TPR book, or the form used in your institution. This is very important because when you return the probe to its stored position, the reading automatically returns to zero.

13. Discard the used probe cover (sheath) immediately without touching it.

14. Return the probe to its stored position in the face of the thermometer.

15. Store the thermometer in its charging stand whenever it is not in use.

16. Make the patient comfortable.

17. Wash your hands.

18. Report to your head nurse or team leader:
    - If the oral temperature was over 100°F (37.8°C).
    - Your observations of anything unusual.

Procedure: Using a Battery-Operated Electronic Rectal Thermometer

1. Assemble your equipment:
   a) Plastic disposable probe cover (sheath)
   b) Battery-operated electronic thermometer
   c) Rectal (red) attachment
   d) Temp. board, TPR book, or form used by your institution
   e) Pen or pencil

2. Wash your hands.

3. Identify the patient by checking the identification bracelet.

4. Ask visitors to step out of the room.

5. Tell the patient that you are going to take his temperature.

6. Pull the curtain around the bed for privacy.

7. Check to be sure the rectal (red) probe connector is seated properly in its receptacle on the base of the thermometer.

8. Remove the probe from its stored position and insert it into a probe cover (sheath).

9. Insert the covered probe slowly through the patient's anus into the rectum one-half inch.

(continued next page)

10. Hold the probe in the patient's rectum.

11. Wait for the buzzer to ring for a computed temperature reading. Then remove the probe from the rectum.

12. Record the temperature reading on the temp. board, in the TPR book, or the form used in your institution.

13. Discard the used probe cover immediately without touching it.

14. Return the probe to its stored position in the face of the thermometer.

15. Store the thermometer in its charging stand whenever it is not in use.

16. Make the patient comfortable.

17. Wash your hands.

18. Report to your head nurse or team leader:
    - If the rectal temperature was over 101°F (38.3°C).
    - Your observations of anything unusual.

Procedure: Using a Battery-Operated Electronic Oral Thermometer to Measure Axillary Temperature

1. Assemble your equipment:
   a) Plastic disposable probe cover (sheath)
   b) Battery-operated electronic thermometer
   c) Oral (blue) attachment
   d) Temp. board, TPR book, or form used in your institution
   e) Pen or pencil

2. Wash your hands.

3. Identify the patient by checking the identification bracelet.

4. Ask visitors to step out of the room.

5. Tell the patient that you are going to take his temperature.

6. Pull the curtain around the bed for privacy.

7. Check to be sure the oral (blue) probe connector is properly seated in its receptacle on the base of the unit.

8. Remove the probe from its stored position and insert it into a probe cover (sheath).

9. Place the covered probe in the center of the patient's armpit (axilla).

10. Put the patient's arm across his chest. Hold the probe in place.

11. Wait about 15 seconds for the buzzer to ring for a computed temperature reading. Then remove the probe from the patient's axilla.

12. Record the temperature on the temp. board, TPR book, or on the form used in your institution. This is very important because when you return the probe to its stored position, the reading automatically returns to zero.

13. Discard the used probe cover immediately without touching it.

14. Return the probe to its stored position in the face of the thermometer.

15. Store the thermometer in its charging stand whenever it is not in use.

16. Make the patient comfortable.

17. Wash your hands.

(continued next page)

18. Report to your head nurse or team leader:
    - If the axillary temperature was over 99°F (37.2°C).
    - Your observations of anything unusual.

Normal Readings

Methods of Measuring Temperature	Normals	
	°C	°F
ORAL	37.0°	98.6°
AXILLARY	36.4°	97.6°
RECTAL	37.5°	99.6°

Report any change in temperature to your head nurse or team leader.

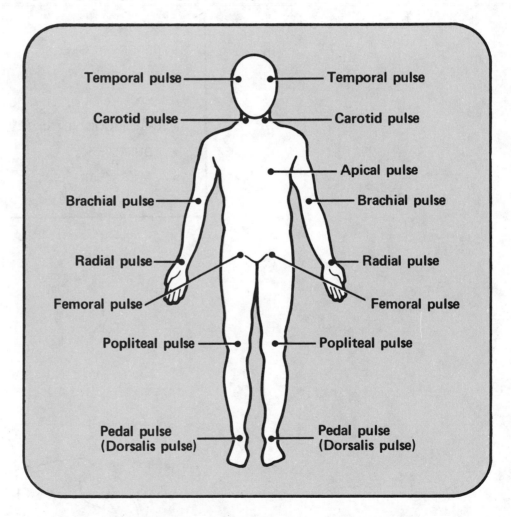

SECTION 3: MEASURING THE PULSE

OBJECTIVES: WHAT YOU WILL LEARN

When you have completed this section, you will be able to:

- Count the pulse
- Report the rate and rhythm of the pulse accurately

Each time the heart beats, it pumps a certain amount of blood into the arteries. This causes the arteries to expand (get bigger). Between heartbeats, the arteries contract and return to their normal size. The heart pumps the blood in a steady rhythm. The rhythmic expansion and contraction of the arteries, which can be measured to show how fast the heart is beating, is called the **pulse**. Measuring the pulse is a simple method of observing how the circulatory system is functioning.

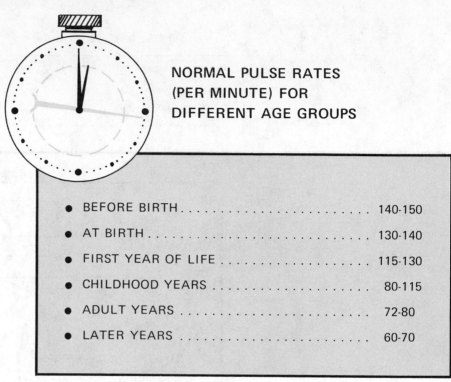

NORMAL PULSE RATES (PER MINUTE) FOR DIFFERENT AGE GROUPS

- BEFORE BIRTH 140-150
- AT BIRTH 130-140
- FIRST YEAR OF LIFE 115-130
- CHILDHOOD YEARS 80-115
- ADULT YEARS 72-80
- LATER YEARS 60-70

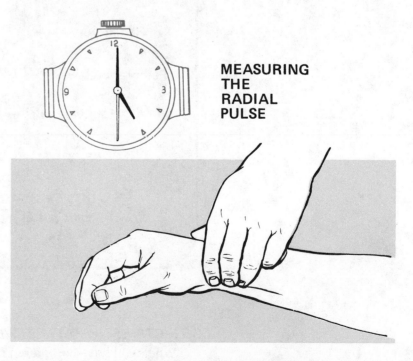

MEASURING THE RADIAL PULSE

The pulse measures how fast the heart is beating. At certain places on the body, the pulse can be felt easily under a person's fingers. One of the easiest places to feel the pulse is at the wrist. This is called a **radial pulse** because you are feeling the radial artery. When taking the pulse, you must be able to report accurately the following:

- Rate—the number of pulse beats per minute.
- Rhythm—the regularity of the pulse beats, that is, whether or not the length of time between the beats is steady and regular.
- Force of the beat (weak or bounding).

The normal average rate of pulse for adults is 72 beats per minute. The range of normal rates for adults is from 72 to 80 beats per minute. Always report a pulse rate of under 60 or over 100 beats per minute.

Procedure: Measuring the Radial Pulse

1. Assemble your equipment:
   a) Watch with a second hand
   b) TPR book, temp. board, or form used in your institution
   c) Pen or pencil
2. Wash your hands.
3. Identify the patient by checking the identification bracelet.
4. Ask visitors to step out of the room.
5. Tell the patient that you are going to take his pulse.
6. If the patient is standing, ask him to sit down. Or have him lying in a comfortable position in bed.
7. The patient's hand and arm should be well supported and resting comfortably.
8. Find the pulse by placing the tips of your middle three fingers on the palm side of the patient's wrist in a line with his thumb directly next to the bone. Press lightly until you feel the beat. If you press too hard, you may stop the flow of blood and obliterate the pulse. Then you would not be able to feel the pulse. Never use your thumb. Your thumb has its own pulse and you would be counting your own pulse instead of the patient's. When you have found the pulse, notice the rhythm. Notice if the beat is steady or irregular. Notice the force of the beat.
9. Look at the position of the second hand on your watch. Then start counting the pulse beats (what you feel) until the second hand comes back to the same number on the clock.
   - *Method A:* Count the pulse beats for one full minute and report the full minute count. This is always done if the patient has an irregular beat.
   - *Method B:* Count for 30 seconds, until the second hand on the watch is opposite its position when you started. Then multiply the number of beats by 2. This is the number you record. For example, if you count 35 for 30 seconds, the count for one full minute is 70.
10. Record the pulse count on the temp. board, in the TPR book, or on the form used in your institution. Be sure you write in the correct column and next to the patient's name.
11. Make the patient comfortable.
12. Wash your hands.
13. Report to your head nurse or team leader:
    - If the pulse rate was under 60 or over 100.
    - If the pulse was irregular by circling in red the number on the

(continued next page)

temp. board, TPR book, or on the form used by your institution. Sometimes irr. is written near the number.

● Your observations of anything unusual.

KEY IDEAS: THE APICAL PULSE AND PULSE DEFICIT

The pulse rate should be the same as the heart rate. However, in some patients the heartbeats are not strong enough to be transmitted along the arteries. This may be because of some forms of heart disease. For these patients, an apical pulse would be taken. An **apical pulse** is a measurement of the heartbeats at the apex of the heart. The apex of the heart is located just under the left breast.

Sometimes the patient has a **"pulse deficit."** This means that there is a difference between the apical heartbeat and the radial pulse rate. To determine this, the apical pulse (heart rate) is counted with a stethoscope over the apex of the heart. At the same time, the pulse rate is counted at the radial pulse. The two figures are compared. The difference between the apical heartbeat and the radial pulse beat is the pulse deficit. This is called the apical pulse deficit. For maximum accuracy, both pulses should be taken at the same time by two nursing assistants. A different method calls for one nursing assistant who first takes the apical pulse and then takes the radial pulse. This second method is not considered as accurate as the first method.

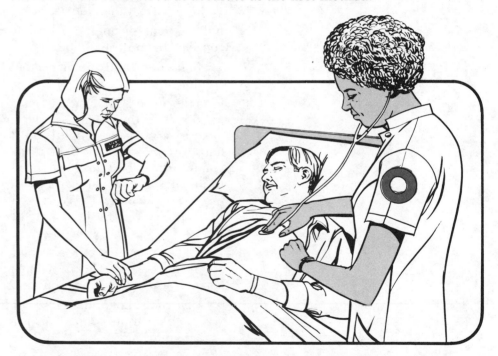

Procedure: Measuring the Apical Pulse

1. Assemble your equipment:
    a) Stethoscope and antiseptic swabs
    b) Watch with a second hand
    c) Temp. board, TPR book, or form used in your institution. Please Note: In many institutions this reading is reported directly to the head nurse or team leader rather than writing it on the form used.
    d) Pencil or pen and note paper
2. Wash your hands.
3. Identify the patient by checking the identification bracelet.
4. Ask visitors to step out of the room.

(continued next page)

Procedure continued

5. Explain to the patient that you are going to take his apical pulse.
6. Pull the curtain around the bed for privacy.
7. Clean the earplugs of the stethoscope with antiseptic solution. Put the earplugs in your ears. Warm the bell or diaphram of the stethoscope by holding it tightly for a few seconds.
8. Uncover the left side of the patient's chest. Avoid overexposing the patient.
9. Locate the apex of the patient's heart by placing the bell or diaphragm of the stethoscope under the patient's left breast. Listen for the heart sounds.
10. Count the heart sounds for a full minute.
11. Write the full minute count on the note paper.
12. Cover the patient and make him comfortable.
13. Clean the earplugs of the stethoscope. Return the equipment to its proper place.
14. Wash your hands.
15. Report to your head nurse or team leader:
    - That you have taken the patient's apical pulse.
    - What the apical pulse rate was.
    - Your observations of anything unusual.

Procedure: Measuring the Apical Pulse Deficit

1. Assemble your equipment:
   a) Stethoscope and antiseptic swabs
   b) Watch with a second hand
   c) TPR book, temp. board, or form used in your institution. Please Note: In many institutions this reading is reported directly to the head nurse or team leader, rather than writing it on the form
   d) Note paper, pen or pencil
2. Wash your hands.
3. Identify the patient by checking the identification bracelet.
4. Ask visitors to step out of the room.
5. Explain to the patient that you are going to take his pulse.
6. Pull the curtain around the bed for privacy.
7. There are two methods of taking the apical pulse deficit:
   - *Method A:* Two nursing assistants do this procedure together at the same time. One counts the radial pulse. The other counts the apical pulse for one full minute. The difference between the two pulses is known as the apical pulse deficit. This method is used for maximum accuracy.
   - *Method B:* The nursing assistant first takes the apical pulse, then the radial pulse. The difference between the two pulses is known as the apical pulse deficit. However, since the readings are not taken at the same time, it is not considered as accurate as the first method.
8. Count the apical pulse and the radial pulse for a full minute, and record both figures.
9. Record the figure for the pulse deficit.
10. Make the patient comfortable.
11. Clean the equipment and return it to its proper place.

(continued next page)

12. Wash your hands.
13. Report to your head nurse or team leader:
    - That you have taken the patient's apical pulse deficit.
    - The apical pulse rate.
    - The radial pulse rate.
    - The pulse deficit.
    - Your observations of anything unusual.

SECTION 4: MEASURING RESPIRATIONS

OBJECTIVES: WHAT YOU WILL LEARN

When you have completed this section, you will be able to:

- Count a patient's respirations accurately
- Determine if the patient's breathing is labored or noisy

**KEY IDEAS:
MEASURING
RESPIRATIONS**

The human body must have a steady supply of air. The body needs the oxygen in the air in order to change food into heat and energy. When you breathe in, air is drawn into the lungs. In the lungs, oxygen is taken out of the air. The oxygen is absorbed into the blood. The blood then carries the oxygen to the body cells. In the body cells the oxygen is used to produce energy for the body (oxidized).

Respiration is the process of inhaling and exhaling. One respiration includes breathing in once and breathing out once. When a person breathes in, his chest gets larger (expands). When he breathes out, his chest gets smaller (contracts). When you count respirations, the patient should be lying on his back. You watch his chest rise and fall as he breathes. Or you feel his chest rise

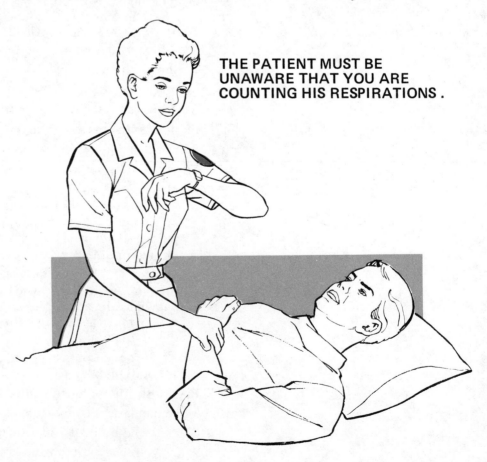

THE PATIENT MUST BE
UNAWARE THAT YOU ARE
COUNTING HIS RESPIRATIONS.

and fall with your hand. Either way, you should count respirations without the patient knowing it. If he thinks his breathing is being counted, he will not breathe naturally. What you want to count is his natural breathing. Besides counting respirations, you will be noticing whether the patient seems to breathe easily or seems to be working hard to get his breath. When a person is working hard to get his breath, it is called **labored respiration**. You must also notice whether his breathing is **noisy**.

Normally adults breathe at a rate of from 16 to 20 times a minute. Children breathe more rapidly. The elderly breathe more slowly. Exercise, digestion, emotional stress, disease conditions, some drugs, stimulants, heat, and cold all can affect the number of times per minute that a person breathes.

Abnormal Respiration

While you are counting the patient's respirations, it is important to observe and make note of anything about his breathing that appears to be abnormal. Different types of abnormal respiration that you should be familiar with are:

a) *Stertorous respiration*—The patient makes abnormal noises like snoring sounds when he is breathing.

b) *Abdominal respiration*—Breathing in which the patient is using mostly his abdominal muscles.

c) *Shallow respiration*—Breathing with only the upper part of the lungs.

d) *Irregular respiration*—The depth of breathing changes and the rate of the rise and fall of the chest is not steady.

e) *Cheyne-Stokes respiration*—One kind of irregular breathing. At first the breathing is slow and shallow; then the respiration becomes faster and deeper until it reaches a kind of peak. The respiration then slows down and becomes shallow again. The breathing may then stop completely for 10 seconds, and begin the pattern again. This type of respiration may be caused by certain cerebral (brain), cardiac (heart), or pulmonary (chest) diseases or conditions.

Procedure: Measuring Respirations

1. Assemble your equipment:
   a) Watch with a second hand
   b) TPR book, temp. board, or form used in your institution
   c) Pen or pencil
2. Wash your hands.
3. Identify the patient by checking the identification bracelet.
4. Ask visitors to step out of the room.
5. Hold the patient's wrist just as if you were taking his pulse. This way he will not know you are watching his breathing. Count the patient's respirations, without his knowing it, immediately after counting his pulse rate.
6. If the patient is a child who has been crying or is restless, wait until he is quiet before counting respirations. If a child is asleep, count his respirations before he wakes up. Always count a child's pulse and respirations before you measure his temperature. (Most children get upset when you measure their temperature.)
7. One rise and one fall of the patient's chest counts as one respiration.
8. If you cannot clearly see the chest rise and fall, fold the patient's arms across his chest. Then you can feel his breathing as you hold his wrist.

(continued next page)

9. Check the position of the second hand on the watch. Count "one" when you see the patient's chest rising as he breathes in. The next time his chest rises, count "two." Keep doing this for a full minute. Report the number of respirations you count.

10. You may be permitted to count for 30 seconds. Count the respirations for one-half minute and then multiply the number you counted by two. For example, if you count 8 respirations in 30 seconds (a half-minute), your number for a full minute is 16.

11. If the patient's breathing rhythm is irregular, always count for a full minute. Observe the depth of the breathing while counting the respirations.

12. Write down the number you counted immediately on the temp. board, in the TPR book, or on the form used by your institution. Be sure you are in the proper column, opposite the correct patient's name.

13. Note whether the respirations were noisy or labored.

14. Make the patient comfortable.

15. Wash your hands.

16. Report to your head nurse or team leader:
    - Whether the respirations were noisy or labored.
    - Whether the respirations were regular.
    - The time they were measured.
    - If the respirations were less than 14 or more than 28 a minute.
    - Your observations of anything unusual.

SECTION 5: MEASURING BLOOD PRESSURE

OBJECTIVES: WHAT YOU WILL LEARN

When you have completed this section, you will be able to:

- Explain systolic pressure
- Explain diastolic pressure
- Demonstrate the use of aneroid and mercury types of blood pressure equipment accurately and efficiently
- Measure a patient's blood pressure accurately

**KEY IDEAS:
BLOOD PRESSURE**

Blood pressure is the force of the blood pushing against the walls of the blood vessels. When you take a patient's blood pressure, you are measuring this force of the blood flowing through the arteries.

There is always a certain amount of pressure in the arteries. This is because the heart, by pumping, is constantly forcing blood to circulate. The blood goes first into the arteries. It then circulates through the whole body. The amount of pressure in the arteries depends on two things:

- The rate of heartbeat.
- How easily the blood flows through the blood vessels.

The heart contracts as it pumps the blood into the arteries. When the heart is contracting, the pressure is highest. This pressure is called the SYSTOLIC PRESSURE. As the heart relaxes between each contraction, the pressure goes down. When the heart is most relaxed, the pressure is lowest. This pressure is called the DIASTOLIC PRESSURE. When you take a patient's blood pressure, you are measuring these two rates—the systolic pressure and the diastolic pressure.

In young healthy adults, the normal blood pressure range is between 100 and 140 millimeters (mm) mercury (Hg) systolic pressure. It is between 60 and 90 millimeters (mm) mercury (Hg) diastolic pressure. The way these figures are written is:

$$120/80 \text{ or } \underline{120} = \text{Systolic}$$
$$80 = \text{Diastolic}$$

When a patient's blood pressure is higher than the normal range for his age and condition, it is referred to as high blood pressure or **hypertension**. When a patient's blood pressure is lower than the normal range for his age or condition, it is referred to as low blood pressure or **hypotension**

Instruments for Measuring Blood Pressure

When you take a patient's blood pressure, you will be using an instrument called a SPHYGMOMANOMETER. Sphygmomanometer is a combination of three Greek words:

- Sphygmo, meaning pulse
- Mano, meaning pressure
- Meter, meaning measure

This instrument, however, is usually called simply the blood pressure cuff. The four main parts of this instrument are: manometer, valve, cuff, and bulb.

Two kinds of instruments are used for taking blood pressure. One is called the **mercury type**. The other is called the **aneroid** (dial) **type**. Both kinds have an inflatable cloth-covered rubber bag, or cuff. The cuff is wrapped around the patient's arm. Both kinds also have a rubber bulb for pumping air into the cuff. The procedure for measuring blood pressure is the same, except for measuring the reading. When you use the mercury type, you will be watching the level of a column of mercury on a measuring scale. When you use the dial (aneroid) type, you will be watching a pointer on a dial.

ANEROID SPHYGMOMANOMETER

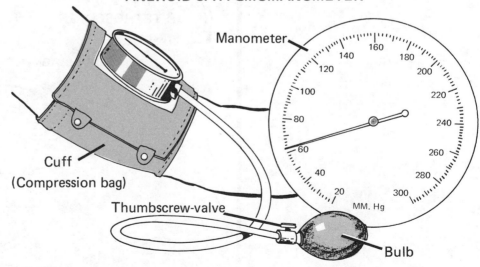

When you measure a patient's blood pressure, you will be doing two things at the same time. You will be listening to the brachial pulse as it sounds in the brachial artery in the patient's arm. You also will be watching an indicator (either a column of mercury or a dial) in order to take a reading.

You will be using a **stethoscope** to listen to the brachial pulse. The stethoscope is an instrument that makes it possible to listen to various sounds in the patient's body, such as the heartbeat or breathing sounds in the chest. The

MERCURY SPHYGMOMANOMETER

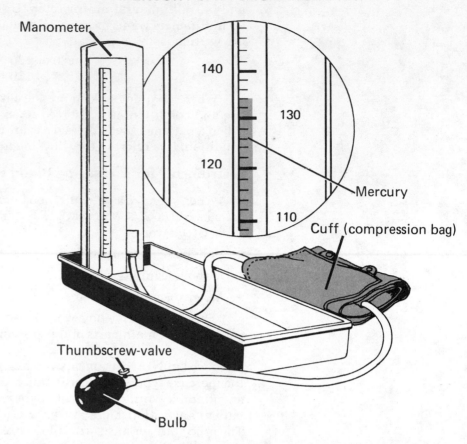

Manometer

140

130

120

Mercury

110

Cuff (compression bag)

Thumbscrew-valve

Bulb

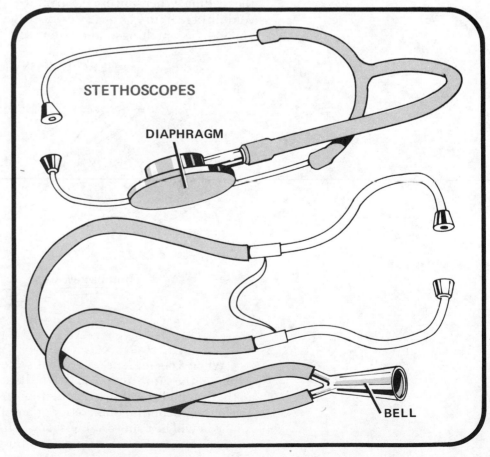

STETHOSCOPES

DIAPHRAGM

BELL

stethoscope is a tube with one end that picks up sound when it is placed against a part of the body. This end is either bell-shaped and is called a **bell**, or it is round and flat and is called a **diaphragm**. The other end of the tube splits into two parts. These parts have tips on the ends and fit into the listener's ears.

In many institutions, the blood pressure equipment hangs on the wall over the bed. A smaller-sized cuff must be used for children or a larger size for obese (overweight) patients. Do not take a blood pressure on an arm that has an IV (intravenous) setup in it.

Procedure: Measuring Blood Pressure

1. Assemble your equipment:
   a) Sphygmomanometer (blood pressure cuff)
   b) Stethoscope
   c) Antiseptic pad
   d) B.P. board, blood pressure book, or form used in your institution
   e) Pen or pencil
2. Wash your hands.
3. Identify the patient by checking the identification bracelet.
4. Ask visitors to step out of the room.
5. Tell the patient that you are going to measure his blood pressure.
6. Wipe the earplugs of the stethoscope with the antiseptic pads.
7. Have the patient resting quietly. He should be either lying down or sitting in a chair.
8. If you are using the mercury apparatus, the measuring scale should be level with your eyes.
9. The patient's arm should be bare up to the shoulder, or the patient's sleeve should be well above the elbow.
10. The patient's arm from the elbow down should be resting fully extended on the bed. Or it might be resting on the arm of the chair, or your hip, well supported, with the palm upward.
11. Unroll the cuff and loosen the valve on the bulb. Then squeeze the compression bag to deflate it completely.
12. Wrap the cuff around the patient's arm above the elbow snugly and smoothly. But do not wrap it so tightly that the patient is uncomfortable from the pressure.
13. Leave the area clear where you will place the bell or diaphragm of the stethoscope.
14. Be sure the manometer is in position so you can read the numbers easily.
15. Put the earplugs of the stethoscope into your ears.
16. With your fingertips, find the patient's brachial pulse at the inner side of the arm above the elbow (brachial artery). This is where you will place the diaphragm or bell of the stethoscope. The diaphragm should be held firmly against the patient's skin, but it should not touch the cuff of the apparatus.
17. Tighten the thumbscrew of the valve to close it. Turn it clockwise. Be careful not to turn it too tightly. If you do, you will have trouble opening it.
18. Hold the stethoscope in place. Inflate the cuff until the dial points to 170.
19. Open the valve counter-clockwise. This allows the air to escape. Let

(continued next page)

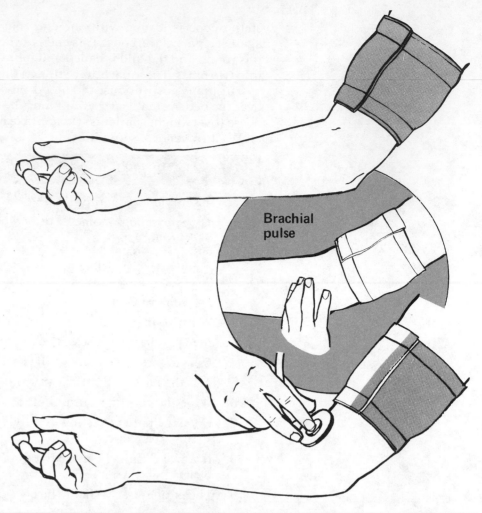

Brachial
pulse

Procedure continued

it out slowly until the sound of the pulse comes back. A few seconds
must go by without sounds. If you do hear pulse sounds immediately, you must stop the procedure. Then completely deflate the cuff.
Wait a few seconds. Then inflate the cuff to a much higher calibration, above 200. Again, loosen the thumbscrew to let the air out.
Listen for a repeated pulse sound. At the same time, watch the indicator.

20. Note the calibration that the pointer passes as you hear the first
    sound. This point indicates the systolic pressure (or the top num-
    ber).

21. Continue releasing the air from the cuff. When the sounds change to
    a softer and faster thud or disappear, note the calibration. This is
    the diastolic pressure (or bottom number).

22. Deflate the cuff completely. Remove it from the patient's arm.

23. Record your reading on the B.P. board, B.P. book, or form used in
    your institution.

24. After using the blood pressure cuff, roll it up over the manometer
    and replace it in the case.

25. Wipe the earplugs of the stethoscope again with an antiseptic swab.
    Put the stethoscope back in its proper place.

26. Make the patient comfortable.

27. Wash your hands.

28. Report to your head nurse or team leader:

(continued next page)

- That you have measured the patient's blood pressure.
- The time that you measured the blood pressure.
- Your observations of anything unusual.

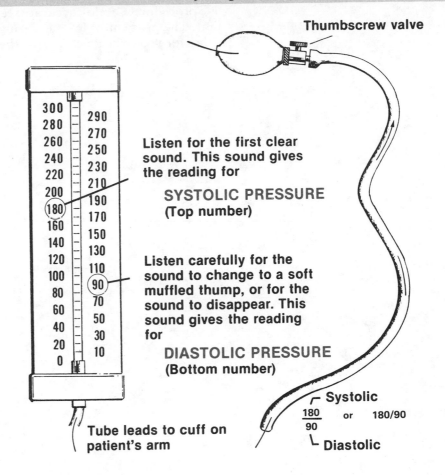

Thumbscrew valve

Listen for the first clear sound. This sound gives the reading for

SYSTOLIC PRESSURE
(Top number)

Listen carefully for the sound to change to a soft muffled thump, or for the sound to disappear. This sound gives the reading for

DIASTOLIC PRESSURE
(Bottom number)

Tube leads to cuff on patient's arm

Systolic

$\frac{180}{90}$ or 180/90

Diastolic

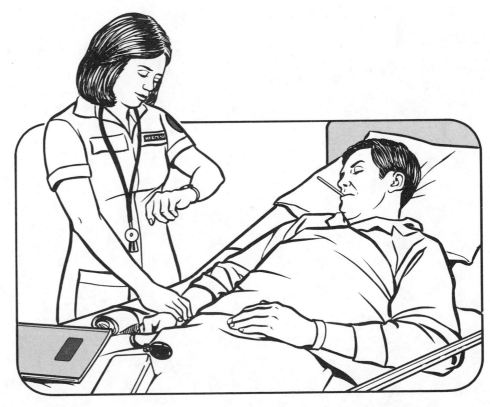

WHAT YOU HAVE LEARNED

The vital signs are temperature, pulse, respiration, and blood pressure. Temperature, pulse, and respiration (TPR) are measured at the same time, as one procedure. Careful, accurate reecording of this information is very important. The procedures for measuring the vital signs must be practiced many times for you to be able to carry them out skillfully and accurately.

13 PATIENT ADMISSION, TRANSFER, AND DISCHARGE

1. Admitting the Patient
2. Transferring the Patient
3. Discharging the Patient

SECTION 1: ADMITTING THE PATIENT

OBJECTIVES: WHAT YOU WILL LEARN

When you have completed this section, you will be able to:

- Admit a patient to the nursing unit by following the correct procedure.
- Welcome the patient and his visitors in a pleasant and courteous manner.
- Observe the patient carefully and record all the information needed.
- Make the patient feel comfortable and help him to adjust to the institutional environment.

**KEY IDEAS:
ADMITTING THE
PATIENT**

A patient coming into a health care institution is occasionally frightened and uncomfortable. He may or may not be seriously ill or in pain. This is a time when you, as a member of the nursing team, are very important to the patient. Being pleasant and courteous will make the patient's arrival easier for him. A nice welcome will create a favorable first impression.

Introduce yourself. Learn the patient's name and use it often. Remember that the way you speak and behave will have a lot to do with the patient's impression of the institution. Smile, be friendly. Do not appear to be rushed or busy with other things. Do your work quietly and efficiently.

Procedure: Admitting the Patient

1. Assemble your equipment on the bedside table:
   a) Admission checklist, if used in your institution
   b) Urine specimen container and laboratory requisition slip
   c) Institution gown or pajamas
   d) Clothing list
   e) Envelope for valuables
   f) Portable scale
   g) Blood pressure cuff and stethoscope
   h) Admission pack
   i) Thermometer
   j) Bedpan and/or urinal, emesis basin, and wash basin
2. Wash your hands.
3. Fanfold the bed covers down to open the bed.
4. Place the hospital gown or pajamas at the foot of the bed.
5. Put the bedpan, urinal, emesis basin, wash basin, and admission pack in their proper place in the bedside table.

(continued next page)

6. When the patient comes up to the floor, introduce yourself to the patient and to his visitors. Smile, be friendly. Call the patient by his name. Shake hands and tell the patient your name and job title.

7. Escort the patient to his room. Introduce him to his roommates, if he has any.

8. Ask the visitors to leave the room while you finish admitting the patient.

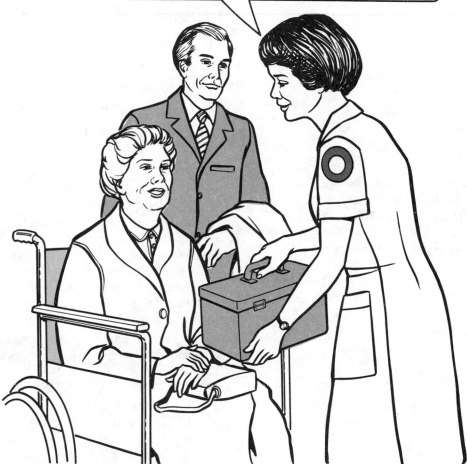

How do you do, Mrs. Jones? I am Mary Hill, your nursing assistant.
How nice to meet you and Mr. Jones.

9. Close the door in a private room. Or draw the curtain around the bed for privacy.

10. Ask the patient to change into the hospital gown or his own pajamas. If necessary, help the patient get undressed and into the gown.

11. Help the patient to get into the bed. (If your head nurse or team leader says the patient may sit in a chair, follow her orders.)

12. Raise the side rails on the bed, if necessary.

13. Complete the admission checklist that follows this admitting procedure. Cover each detail of the admission procedure and checklist. Be

(continued next page)

sure to fill out the list accurately and completely. Write carefully so your writing can be read easily.

14. Make the patient comfortable. Fix the lights the way he wants them. Be sure the top sheets and blankets are arranged properly.

15. Have the patient put his toilet articles and small belongings into or on top of the bedside table. If the patient is unable to do this, do it for him.

16. Ask the head nurse or team leader if the patient is allowed to have drinking water. If he is allowed, fill the water pitcher.

17. To familiarize the patient with his new surroundings, show him where the signal cord is. Attach the signal cord to the bed where the patient can reach it easily. Test the signal cord, explaining how the intercom system works. Permit the patient to work the signal cord light. Show him how to operate the remote-control TV, if there is one.

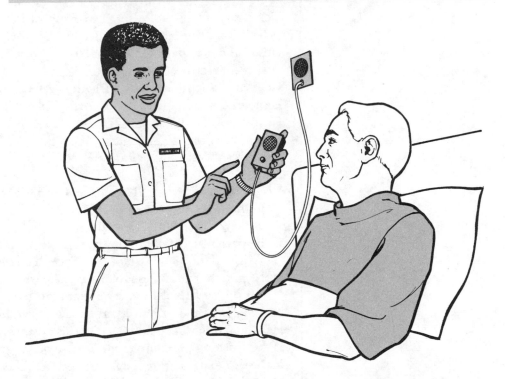

18. Explain the health care institution's policy on radios, television, newspapers, and mail. Tell the patient when his meals will be served. Help the patient to fill out the dietary slip for the next meal.

19. If the patient is allowed to have the head of his bed elevated and the knee gatch adjusted as high or low as is comfortable, adjust these to a position of comfort. If the bed is self-adjustable, explain how the bed works and show the patient how to adjust it.

20. Report to your head nurse or team leader:
    • That you have completed the admission.
    • That the patient is in bed or sitting in a chair.
    • That you have completed the admission checklist.
    • That the side rails are in the up or down position.
    • Your observations of anything unusual.

A SAMPLE ADMISSION CHECKLIST
(Fill in every statement and check every appropriate item)

Patient's name _____ Room number_____

Time of admission _____a.m./p.m.   Date of admission _____

Unit ready to receive patient? Yes☐No☐ Equipment ready? Yes☐No☐

Admitted by stretcher_____ wheelchair_____ walking_____

Check identification bracelet? Yes☐No☐ Bed tag in place? Yes☐No☐

Did the patient need help to get undressed? Yes☐No☐

Is the patient in bed at this time? Yes☐No☐ Time_____a.m./p.m.

Side rails up? Yes☐No☐

Bruises, marks, rashes, or broken skin noted? Yes☐No☐
   If yes, describe _____

Weight_____ Height_____ Scale used? Yes☐No☐

Temperature_____ Pulse_____ Respirations_____ BloodPressure_____

Admission urine specimen collected? Yes☐No☐ Sent to lab? Yes☐No☐

Unusual behavior noted? Yes☐No☐ Unusual appearance noted? Yes☐No☐
   If yes, describe _____

Does the patient have any difficulty with the English language? Yes☐No☐

Is the patient allergic to food? Yes☐No☐ Allergic to drugs? Yes☐ No☐

Reason for admission _____

Complaints _____

Dentures? Yes☐No☐ Partial? Yes☐No☐ Full? Yes☐No☐ Denture cup?
   Yes☐No☐

Vision problems? Yes☐No☐ Does the patient wear glasses? Yes☐No☐

Valuables: Money? Yes☐No☐ Describe _____
   Jewelry? Yes☐ No☐ Describe _____

Is the patient hard of hearing? Yes☐No☐ Hearing aid? Yes☐No☐
   Artificial limb? Yes☐No☐ Brace? Yes☐No☐

Is the patient calm? Yes☐No☐ Is the patient very anxious? Yes☐No☐
   Angry? Yes☐No☐ Is the patient agitated or very excited? Yes☐No☐

Has the patient ever had X rays taken in this hospital before? Yes☐No☐

Has the patient been admitted to this hospital before? Yes☐No☐

Is the clothing list completed? Yes☐No☐ Signed by_____

Is the signal cord attached to the bed? Yes☐No☐

Have drugs brought into the hospital by the patient been given to the charge
   nurse? Yes☐No☐

Name of the nurse drugs were given to _____

Was the patient told not to eat or drink anything until the doctor's visit?
   Yes☐No☐

Admitted by _____

Procedure: Weighing and Measuring the Height of a Patient Who is Able to Stand

1. Assemble your equipment:
    a) Portable balance scale
    b) Paper towel

(continued next page)

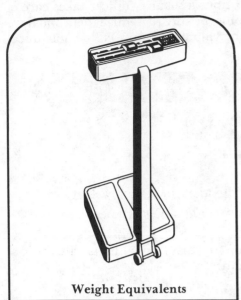

Weight Equivalents

Kilograms (kg)	Ounces (oz)	Pounds (lb)
	4	¼
	8	½
	12	¾
.50	16	1
22.68		50
45.36		100

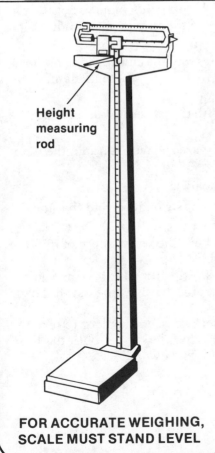

Height measuring rod

FOR ACCURATE WEIGHING, SCALE MUST STAND LEVEL

    c) Note paper

    d) Pen or pencil

2. Wash your hands.

3. Identify the patient by checking the identification bracelet.

4. Ask visitors to step out of the room.

5. Tell the patient that you are going to weigh him.

6. Pull the curtain around the bed for privacy.

7. Balance the scale. To do this, make sure the scale is standing level. Both weights (poises) must point to zero (0). Turn the balance screw until the pointer of the balance beam stays steadily in the middle of the balance area. The scale is now balanced.

8. Place a paper towel on the stand of the scale to protect the patient's feet.

9. Have the patient remove his robe and slippers. Assist him if necessary.

10. Help the patient to stand with both feet firmly on the scale.

11. Ask the patient to place both hands at his side.

12. Adjust the weights (poises) until the balance pointer is again in the middle of the balance area.

13. Note the patient's weight by adding together the numbers on both the large balance and the small balance. Write it down on the note paper.

14. Raise the measuring rod above the patient's head.

15. Have the patient turn so that his back is against the measuring rod. Be sure he is standing very straight, with his heels touching the measuring bar.

16. Bring the measuring rod down so that it rests on the patient's head.

17. Note the patient's height. Write it down on the note paper.

18. Raise the measuring rod. Help the patient to step off the scale.

19. Assist the patient back into bed or help him to put on his robe and slippers.

20. Make the patient as comfortable as possible.

21. Wipe the entire scale with disinfectant solution.

22. Put the scale back where it belongs.

23. Wash your hands.

24. Report to your head nurse or team leader:

- That you have weighed and measured the height of the patient.
- Remind her if the patient has dressings (bandages) or braces, as this must be considered for the correct weight.
- The patient's weight and height.
- Your observations of anything unusual.

PLEASE NOTE: Some institutions have special scales with bars on them to assist the patient in standing straight and to keep the patient from falling. There is a type of bed scale that is used for the complete bedrest patient. Follow your institution's procedures for these different types of scales. If the patient is unable to stand, you will not be required to weigh or measure him.

You may be responsible for taking care of the patient's jewelry, money, or other valuables at the time of admission. In some institutions the admitting office takes care of them, in some institutions a security officer takes care of them. If the family takes the valuables home, be sure to itemize them and have a family member sign that he is taking the valuables home. Follow the procedure used in your institution.

Procedure: Caring for the Patient's Valuables

1. Assemble your equipment on the bedside table:
   a) Valuables envelope
   b) Pen or pencil
2. Wash your hands.
3. Identify the patient by checking the identification bracelet.
4. Ask visitors to step out of the room, unless they are needed as witnesses.
5. Tell the patient that you are going to assist him with his valuables by making an accurate list of them.
6. Pull the curtain around the bed for privacy.
7. Itemize the valuables on the admission checklist or on the appropriate form.
8. When listing the valuables be careful in describing each item. It is not the job of a nursing assistant to decide how much any article is worth. A good description might be: "gold-colored metal earrings," rather than "gold earrings"; a "silver-colored ring with a clear stone," rather than "diamond white gold ring"; a "fur coat," rather than a "mink coat." Never touch the patient's money. Let the patient count it in your presence. Record the amount on the admission checklist.
9. Ask the patient to place his valuables into the envelope that is clearly marked with his name, room number, doctor's name, and identification number.
10. Close the envelope while you are with the patient. Make sure he sees you do this.
11. Have the patient or relative (if they are the witness) sign the itemized list of valuables.
12. Report to the head nurse or team leader:
    - That you have itemized the patient's valuables and that the list is signed.
    - Give the valuables envelope to her. She will dispose of it in the proper way for your institution by:
    a) Having the security officer pick it up and take it to the vault.
    b) Having a relative take it home, after he signs the list that he is doing so.
    c) Having a bonded admission clerk come to the floor to take the valuables envelope to the safe. This clerk gives both the head nurse and the patient a receipt for the valuables.
    - Your observations of anything unusual.

SECTION 2: TRANSFERRING THE PATIENT

OBJECTIVES: WHAT YOU WILL LEARN

When you have completed this section, you will be able to:

- Transfer a patient to another unit within the institution, following the correct procedure.
- Help the patient to stay calm and feel comfortable.

During his stay, a patient may be transferred from one unit to another. This may be done for several reasons:

- He may have asked for a private room, but none was available when he was admitted.
- He may ask to be transferred from a private room to a semi-private room.
- He may be moved to another unit because of a change in his medical condition.

The patient may become alarmed if a doctor orders his transfer. In this case, try to calm the patient. Explain that the change is being made only for his benefit. Before you help in transferring the patient, be sure his new unit is ready to receive him.

**KEY IDEAS:
TRANSFERRING THE
PATIENT**

Procedure: Transferring the Patient

1. Assemble your equipment, according to the needs of the patient:
   a) Wheelchair
   b) Stretcher or the patient's bed
   c) Cart
2. Check to be sure the new unit is ready to receive the patient.
3. Wash your hands.
4. Identify the patient by checking the identification bracelet.
5. Ask visitors to leave the room.
6. Tell the patient you are going to transfer him to his new room.
7. Collect the patient's personal belongings and equipment that is to be moved with him.
8. Transport the patient to the new unit:
   a) The patient can be moved in his own bed from one room to another. Personal belongings can be placed on the bed and moved with the patient. Or, if he has many personal articles, you may use a cart to move them.
   b) You may have to transport the patient by stretcher or wheelchair to his new room. Here you will help the patient from the stretcher or wheelchair into his new bed. In these cases, put the patient's belongings and equipment on a cart. Move them after the patient is settled and safe in the new unit.
9. Follow all safety precautions when wheeling the patient to his new unit. (Some institutions have a transportation service that does this for you.)
10. Give the patient both physical and emotional support. For example, he may need to be reassured that his family and visitors will be given his new room number.
11. Introduce the patient to his new roommate, if there is one.
12. Make the patient comfortable in his new room.

(continued next page)

Procedure continued

13. Introduce him to the nursing staff who will be taking care of him now.

14. Arrange the unit. Help the patient to put away his personal items or possessions. Place the signal cord within the patient's reach.

15. Report to the head nurse or team leader in the new nursing unit. Tell her that the patient is now in the new unit. Describe how the patient reacted to the transfer.

16. Return to your own floor. Strip the bed and take the equipment that was not transferred to the dirty utility room, or follow the procedure used in your institution.

17. Wash your hands.

18. Report to your head nurse or team leader:
    - That the patient has been transferred to the new unit.
    - The time of the transfer.
    - The patient's reaction to the transfer.
    - Your observations of anything unusual.

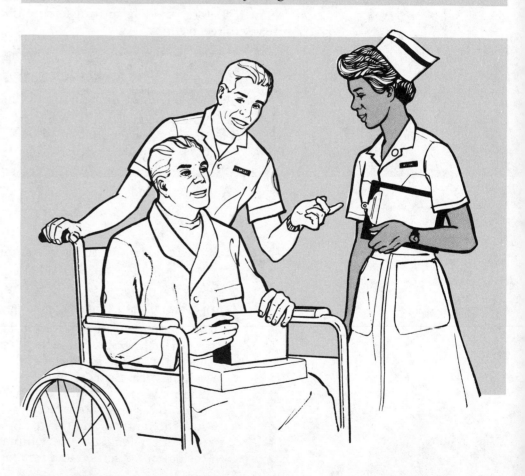

- **Be sure the new unit is ready to receive the patient**
- **Help the patient remain calm**
- **Speak to him in a way that shows you care about him as a person**

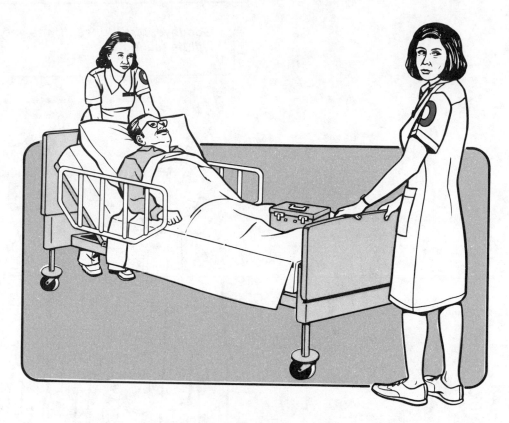

SECTION 3: DISCHARGING THE PATIENT

OBJECTIVES: WHAT YOU WILL LEARN

When you have completed this section, you will be able to:

- Discharge a patient from the health care institution, following the correct procedure.
- Keep the patient from becoming too tired before he is discharged.
- Assist the patient graciously and safely as he leaves the health care institution.

**KEY IDEAS:
DISCHARGING THE
PATIENT**

The patient being discharged is often still weak and may tire easily. Your task at this time is a pleasant one. The patient is usually happy to know he can go home. Written permission from a doctor is required for the patient to be discharged. Your head nurse or team leader will tell you when the doctor has ordered that the patient is to be discharged. If the patient wants to leave and you have not been told that the discharge order has been written by the physician, report this to your head nurse or team leader immediately. Every patient must be taken in a wheelchair to the business office, cashier, or discharge desk (in certain instances a member of the patient's family may do this for him) before he leaves the facility.

Patients are sometimes discharged from one health care institution to another, for example, from a hospital to a nursing home. These patients may leave the facility in an ambulance. Your head nurse or team leader will give you special instructions for the care of these patients.

Normally, there is a certain hour when most patients are discharged. This is so their rooms can be cleaned and made ready for new patients who are often admitted early in the afternoon.

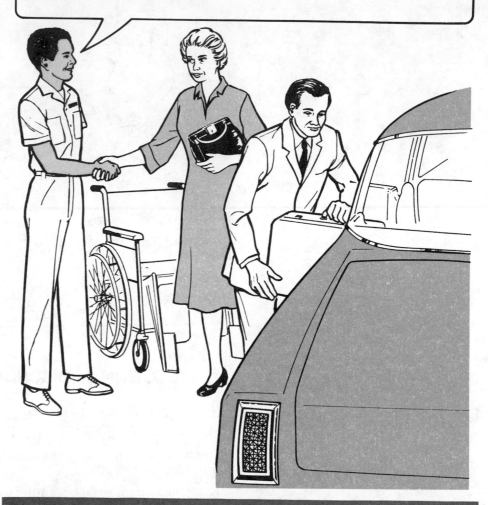

Goodbye, Mrs. Jones. It was very nice meeting you. I hope you will be feeling better.

Procedure: Discharging the Patient

1. Assemble your equipment according to the needs of the patient:
   a) Wheelchair
   b) Stretcher
   c) Discharge slip, if used in your institution
   d) Cart
2. Wash your hands.
3. Identify the patient by checking his identification bracelet.
4. Collect all of the patient's personal possessions for him. Help him to pack everything that belongs to him.
5. Be sure all valuables and medications are returned to the patient by the head nurse or team leader.
6. Help the patient get dressed, if necessary.
7. Check that the patient has the written instructions given to him by the head nurse or team leader, such as:
   a) Doctor's orders to follow at home
   b) Prescriptions
   c) Follow-up schedule of appointments with the doctor or clinic

(continued next page)

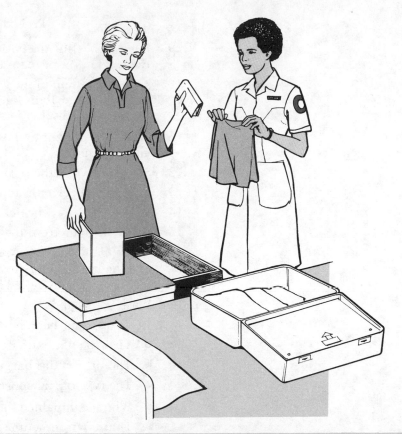

Procedure continued

Please Note: *Many institutions have a special discharge planning nurse* who is notified when the patient is ready to leave. She then sees the patient to check on all of his instructions.

8. Bring the wheelchair to the patient's bedside. Help the patient into it. Remember, all patients being discharged must leave the institution in a wheelchair.

(continued next page)

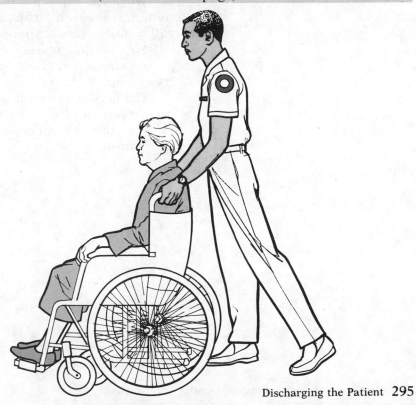

9. Before wheeling the patient off the floor, get the discharge slip from the head nurse or team leader.

10. Take the patient in the wheelchair to the discharge desk, cashier, or business office, if his family has not already done this for him. Give the clerk the discharge slip. Get a release form in return.

11. Wheel the patient to the front door. Help him out of the wheelchair and into his car.

12. Say goodbye to the patient. Wish him well, if appropriate.

13. Take the wheelchair and release form back to the floor.

14. Wipe the entire wheelchair with an antiseptic solution.

15. Strip the linen from the bed. Place it in the dirty linen hamper.

16. Notify environmental service that the discharge has taken place and the unit is ready to be cleaned. (In many institutions environmental service is called housekeeping department.)

17. Wash your hands.

18. Report to your head nurse or team leader:
    - That the patient has been discharged.
    - The time of discharge.
    - The type of transportation used for the discharge.
    - Who accompanied the patient—husband, wife, daughter, friend.
    - That environmental service has been notified that the unit is ready to be cleaned.
    - Give her the release form from the business office, cashier, or discharge desk.
    - Your observations of anything unusual.

WHAT YOU HAVE LEARNED

When you admit a new patient to your nursing unit, you will make him comfortable, ease his fears, and help him adjust to his new surroundings. You will be taking care of your patient's personal possessions and valuables.

You, the nursing assistant, will be helping to transfer a patient from one patient area or unit to another. Most important is relieving the patient of anxiety and making him comfortable in the new unit.

The nursing assistant will have the usually pleasant task of helping the patient get ready for discharge from the health care institution. You will make sure that they take all of their possessions with them and that the discharge goes smoothly.

14 BODY POSITIONS, TUBES, AND TUBING

1. Your Role in the Physical Examination
2. Draping and Positioning the Patient
3. Catheters, Tubes, and Tubing

SECTION 1: YOUR ROLE IN THE PHYSICAL EXAMINATION

OBJECTIVES: WHAT YOU WILL LEARN

When you have completed this section, you will be able to:

- Assemble the equipment necessary for a routine physical examination.
- Prepare the patient for the examination.

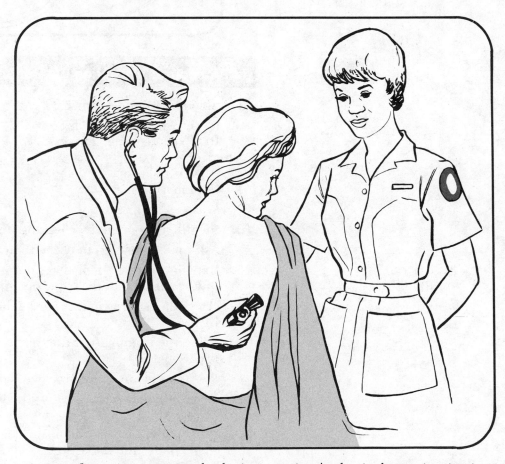

**KEY IDEAS:
THE PHYSICAL
EXAMINATION**

One of your important tasks during a patient's physical examination is to make them as relaxed, comfortable, and reassured as you can. Another important task is to prepare the patient and assemble the equipment for the examination. During the examination, you may help the doctor in several ways.

In preparing for an examination you will be getting the patient ready, putting his unit in order, and collecting the equipment needed for the examination.

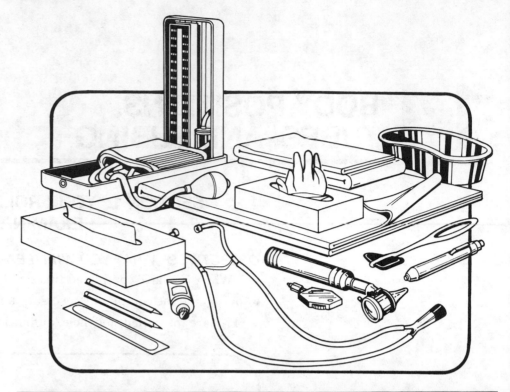

Procedure: Preparing the Patient for a Physical Examination

1. Assemble your equipment:
   a) Examination cart or box
   b) Extra lighting, if necessary
   c) Towel
   d) Bath blanket
   e) Emesis basin
2. Wash your hands.
3. Identify the patient by checking the identification bracelet.
4. Ask visitors to step out of the room.
5. Explain to the patient that you are going to get him ready for a physical examination by the doctor (using the name of the doctor).
6. Check the lighting in the room. If necessary, arrange for additional lighting.
7. Bring the examination cart or box into the unit and put it in its proper place.
8. Pull the curtain around the bed for privacy.
9. If the patient is wearing a hospital gown, untie the gown at the back and neck.
10. If the patient is wearing his or her own nightclothes, have the patient change into a hospital gown to make it easier to remove the gown quickly during the examination.
11. Offer the bedpan or urinal to the patient before the examination. There are several reasons for this:
    a) The patient will be more comfortable if his urinary bladder is empty.

(continued next page)

b) Examination of the abdomen and pelvic regions will be easier for the doctor.

c) You can collect a specimen and be ready for the doctor's request.

12. Cover the patient with a bath blanket or large sheet. Remove the top sheet and bedspread from the bed without exposing the patient.

13. The top sheet, blanket, or bedspread can be used during the examination for draping the patient, if nothing else is available. Draping a patient keeps him from being unnecessarily exposed during the examination. The sheet, blanket, or bedspread may be called the drape.

14. Make the patient comfortable.

15. Wash your hands.

16. Report to your head nurse or team leader:

• That you have prepared the patient for the physical examination.

• Your observations of anything unusual.

Rules to Follow: During the Physician's Examination

a) Wash your hands before and after assisting with the examination.

b) When you hand a tongue depressor to the doctor, first tear the paper disposable covering halfway down. Never touch the tongue depressor with your fingers. As the doctor takes it, pull the paper covering completely off. This way the doctor can take it by one end and put the clean end into the patient's mouth. When the doctor is finished with the tongue depressor, hold out an emesis basin so the doctor can drop it into the basin. The tongue depressor is discarded after the examination.

c) When the doctor asks for a flashlight, turn it on before you hand it to him.

d) The doctor may ask you to shine the flashlight into the patient's mouth. Follow his instructions.

e) When the doctor is ready to examine the patient's body, he will ask you to remove the patient's gown. Have a towel ready to cover the part of the patient's body the doctor is not examining.

f) When the doctor is ready to examine the patient's abdomen, fold the drape down to the patient's hips. Place a gown or towel across the chest.

g) When the doctor has finished this part of the examination, pull the drape back over the patient's chest.

h) When the doctor examines the patient's legs and feet, expose both legs so the doctor can compare them. He may use a percussion hammer to test the patient's reflexes.

i) Sometimes the doctor will ask the patient to stand up while he is examining the patient's feet and body alignment. Place a paper towel on the floor for the patient to stand on. Be sure the patient is properly draped.

j) When the examination is finished, make the patient comfortable. Re-make the top of the bed.

k) Remove all of the equipment. Discard the disposable equipment. Put everything else back in its proper place. Replace used equipment on the examination cart or box, so it is complete and ready to be used for another examination. Follow the procedure used in your institution for the re-stocking of the examination table or box.

EXAMINATION OF PATIENT'S ABDOMEN

- Place towel or gown over patient's chest
- Fold bedding down to patient's hips

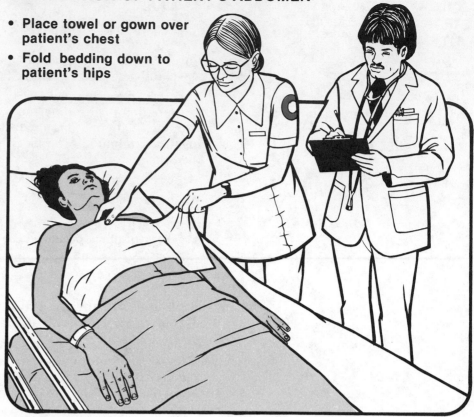

EXAMINATION OF PATIENT'S LEGS

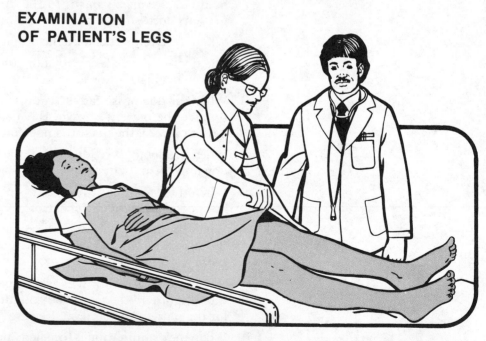

SECTION 2: DRAPING AND POSITIONING THE PATIENT

OBJECTIVES: WHAT YOU WILL LEARN

When you have completed this section, you will be able to:

- Describe the positions used for physical examinations.
- Help the patient into these positions.
- Arrange the patient's drape.

A patient will be standing or lying in different positions for certain kinds of examinations. Learn the name of these positions so you can follow your instructions accurately when positioning the patient.

DORSAL RECUMBENT POSITION

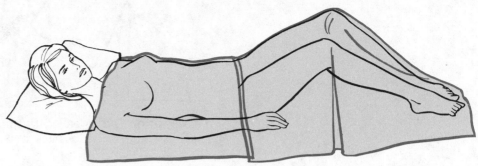

The position is similar to the horizontal recumbent position, except that the patient's legs are parted, the knees are bent, and the soles of the feet are flat on the bed. Drape the female patient by putting a sheet, folded once, across her chest. Put a second sheet crosswise over her legs loosely, so that the perineal region (the area of the body between the thighs) can be exposed for examination.

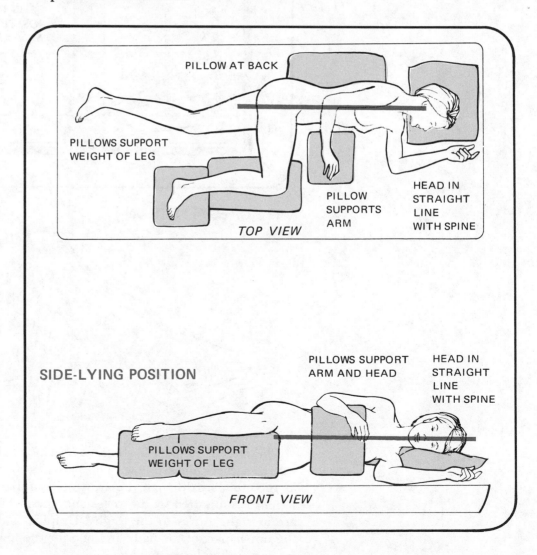

PILLOW AT BACK

PILLOWS SUPPORT
WEIGHT OF LEG

PILLOW
SUPPORTS
ARM

HEAD IN
STRAIGHT
LINE
WITH SPINE

TOP VIEW

SIDE-LYING POSITION

PILLOWS SUPPORT
ARM AND HEAD

HEAD IN
STRAIGHT
LINE
WITH SPINE

PILLOWS SUPPORT
WEIGHT OF LEG

FRONT VIEW

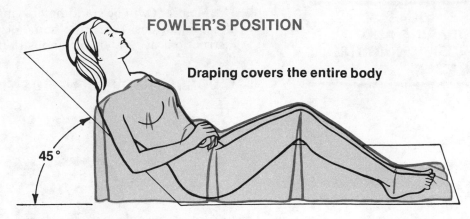

FOWLER'S POSITION

Draping covers the entire body

45°

This position is also called the high Fowler's position. The patient is partly sitting, with the back rest of the bed at a 45° angle. The knees are slightly bent.

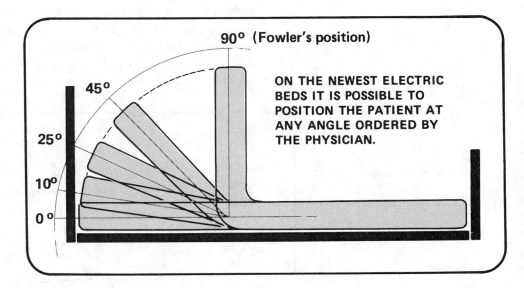

90° (Fowler's position)

45°

25°

10°

0°

ON THE NEWEST ELECTRIC BEDS IT IS POSSIBLE TO POSITION THE PATIENT AT ANY ANGLE ORDERED BY THE PHYSICIAN.

KNEE-CHEST POSITION

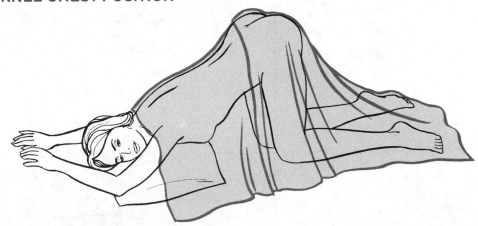

The patient rests on her knees and chest. The head is turned to one side with the cheek on a pillow. The patient's arms are extended slightly, bent at the elbows. Although the arms help support the patient, the main body weight is supported by the knees and chest. The knees are bent so that they are at right angles to the thighs. Draping is done with two sheets, one for the upper part of the body and one for the lower part. This position is used for examining the rectum and vagina.

TRENDELENBURG POSITION
Draping covers the entire body

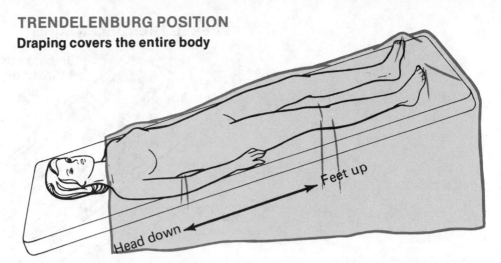

The position is used for surgery on the pelvic organs. The patient's head is low; her body is on an incline, carefully supported to prevent her from slipping out of position or being injured.

DORSAL LITHOTOMY POSITION

- **Drape a folded sheet across the patient's chest**
- **Place a second sheet over the patient's legs**

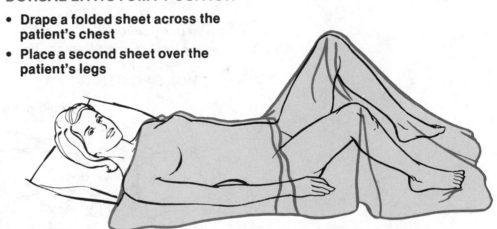

This is the same as the dorsal recumbent position, except that the patient's legs are well separated and the knees are bent more. This position is used often for examination of the bladder, vagina, rectum, and perineum. Sometimes with this position the patient's feet are placed in stirrups if an examination table is being used.

HORIZONTAL RECUMBENT POSITION (SUPINE POSITION)
Draping covers the entire body

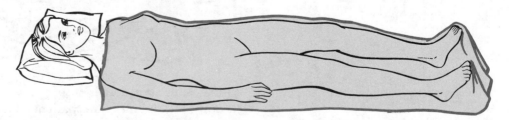

The patient lies on her back with her legs together and extended, or with her knees bent slightly to relax the muscles of the abdomen. A pillow is placed under the patient's head. The drape is spread loosely over the patient's body.

REVERSE TRENDELENBURG

Draping covers the entire body

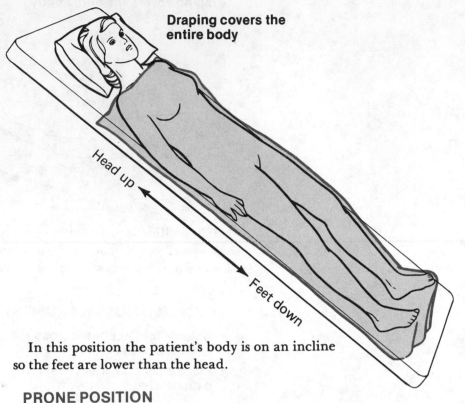

Head up

Feet down

In this position the patient's body is on an incline so the feet are lower than the head.

PRONE POSITION

Draping covers the entire body

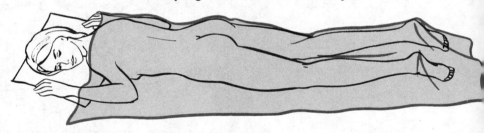

The patient lies on her abdomen with her arms at her sides, or bent at the elbows. Her head is turned to the side.

LEFT SIMS' POSITION
Draping covers the entire body

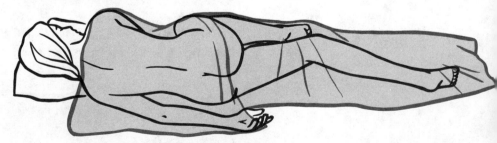

The Sims' position is also called the "semiprone position." The patient lies on her left side. The patient's cheek is resting on a small pillow that is placed under the head. The right knee is bent against the patient's abdomen. The left knee is also bent, but not so much. The left arm is placed behind the body; the right arm rests in a way that is comfortable for the patient. This position is used for rectal examinations and enemas.

LEFT LATERAL POSITION
- Drape top of body with a folded sheet
- Drape lower part of body with a second sheet

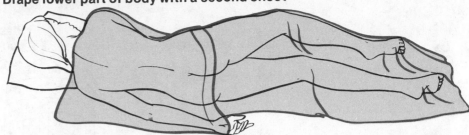

The patient lies on her left side. The hips are closer to the edge of the bed than the shoulders. The knees are bent, one more than the other.

SECTION 3: CATHETERS, TUBES, AND TUBING

OBJECTIVES: WHAT YOU WILL LEARN

When you have completed this section, you will be able to:

- Change the patient's gown with an intravenous (IV) tube running into his body.
- Check the intravenous bottle, drip chamber, tubing, and the patient's arm, so that you can promptly report anything unusual to your head nurse or team leader.
- Describe two methods of giving oxygen to patients.
- Care for patients with nasogastric tubes or indwelling catheter tubing.

KEY IDEAS: INTRAVENOUS (IV) EQUIPMENT

Intravenous tubing is used often in the hospital to put fluids into the patient's body. The tube is connected to a bottle or plastic container. The container holds a fluid that could be a solution of salt or sugar, or perhaps the fluid may contain a prescribed medication or blood.

The other end of the tube is connected to a needle. The needle is inserted by the doctor or the nurse into the patient's vein. The purpose is to give fluids, nourishment, or medications to the patient. It may be used to change the balance of certain chemicals in the patient's body. The solution flows from the bottle into the patient's vein and is circulated through the body.

The amount of fluid that can flow into the patient's body is controlled by a clamp on the tube. This clamp allows only a certain amount of number of drops per minute to flow from the bottle. You, the nursing assistant, should never touch this clamp. Only a doctor or a nurse may change or regulate the amount of flow of a solution. You may have to move the patient in bed or change his position without interrupting the flow of the solution.

Procedure: Changing the Patient's Gown with an IV (Intravenous)

1. Assemble your equipment: Clean hospital gown.
2. Wash your hands.
3. Identify the patient by checking the identification bracelet.
4. Ask the visitors to step out of the room.
5. Tell the patient that you are going to change his gown.

(continued next page)

INTRAVENOUS (IV) EQUIPMENT

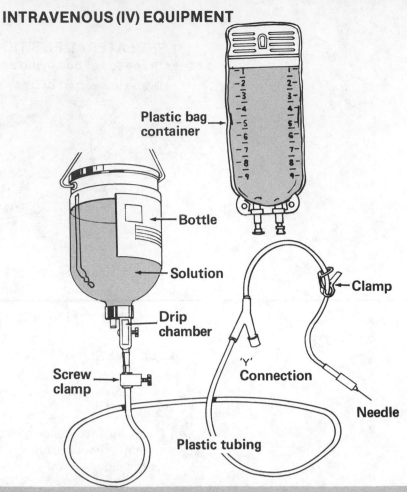

Plastic bag container

Bottle

Solution

Drip chamber

Screw clamp

Clamp

'Y' Connection

Needle

Plastic tubing

Procedure continued

6. Pull the curtain around the bed for privacy.

7. To remove the patient's soiled gown:

   a) Untie the gown.
   b) Remove the arm without the IV from the sleeve.
   c) Remove the gown from the arm with the IV carefully, considering the tube and the container of fluid as part of the arm. Move the sleeve down the arm, over the tubing, and up to the bottle or container.
   d) Remove the container or bottle from the hook, being careful not to lower the bottle below the area on the patient's arm where the needle is inserted.
   e) Slip the gown over the bottle and return the bottle or container to its hook.
   f) Place the soiled gown on a chair.

8. To put the clean gown on the patient, consider the bottle or container and tube as part of the patient's arm.

   a) Lift the bottle from the hook carefully. Do not put the bottle or container below the area on the patient's arm where the needle has been inserted.
   d) Then slip the sleeve of the gown over the bottle or container quickly.
   c) Replace the bottle on the hook.
   d) Slip the gown down the tube and then over the patient's arm.
   e) Then slip the gown over the other arm without the IV.
   f) Tie the back straps for the patient's comfort.

9. Make the patient comfortable.

(continued next page)

10. If the head nurse or team leader has instructed you to keep the patient's arm straight, encourage the patient to do so. He may cut off the flow of solution if he bends his wrist or elbow.

11. Make sure the patient is not lying on top of the IV tubing. Watch for and straighten out any kinks that may form in the tubing. This may happen when the patient changes his position. Pressure or kinks might stop the flow of the solution.

12. Wash your hands.

13. Report to your head nurse or team leader:

    - That you have changed the patient's gown without disturbing the IV.

    - If you cannot see drops of solution passing from the bottle into the tubing, but there is still solution in the bottle.

    - If the plastic drip chamber is filled completely with the solution.

    - If you see blood in the tubing at the needle end.

    - If all the solution has run out of the bottle or that the bottle is almost empty.

    - If the needle has been removed from the patient's arm and whether this occurred deliberately or accidentally.

    - If the tubing has been disconnected and the bed is being saturated while the patient is bleeding freely from the connection.

    - If the patient complains of pain or tenderness at the site (place) where the needle is inserted.

    - If you notice a lumpy, raised, or inflamed (red) area on the patient's skin near the place where the needle is inserted. This might mean that the solution is not running into the vein but, instead, is running into the tissue nearby. This is called infiltration of an IV solution.

    - Your observations of anything else unusual.

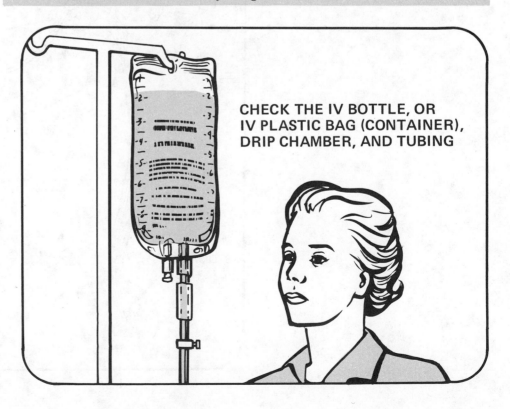

CHECK THE IV BOTTLE, OR IV PLASTIC BAG (CONTAINER), DRIP CHAMBER, AND TUBING

A **nasogastric tube** (also called a levine tube) is inserted through one of the patient's nostrils (naso). Then it is passed down the back of the patient's throat and through the esophagus until the end reaches the patient's stomach (gastric). These tubes may be used for nasogastric, or tube feedings. In such feedings, fluids or liquified (blenderized) foods are given to a patient through the tube at regular times. Nasogastric feeding is also called "**gavage.**"

Nasogastric tubes may also be used to drain fluids by suction from the patient's stomach. Also, sometimes a doctor wants a specimen of the contents of the stomach to be tested. Then the nasogastric tube is used to withdraw the specimen. This is called "**lavage.**" It refers to the washing out of the stomach through a nasogastric tube.

When a nasogastric tube is being used to drain substances out of the stomach or to collect a specimen, the patient is given nothing by mouth (NPO). The food would only be drawn back out through the tube.

Rules to Follow: Caring for the Patient with a Nasogastric Tube

- Never pull on the tube when moving the patient or changing his position.

- Keep the tube clean and free from mucus deposits at the entrance to the nostril.

- Remember to refasten the connecting tubing to the patient's clean gown after you have finished bathing him. This eases the strain on the tube and prevents accidental withdrawal.

- If the patient begins to gag or vomit while the tube is in place, report this immediately to the head nurse or team leader.

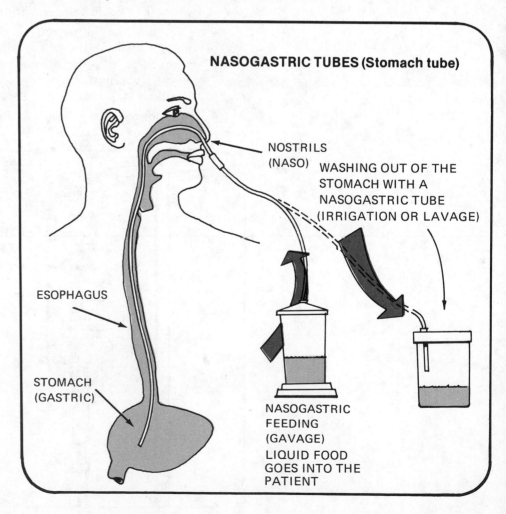

NASOGASTRIC TUBES (Stomach tube)

NOSTRILS
(NASO)

WASHING OUT OF THE
STOMACH WITH A
NASOGASTRIC TUBE
(IRRIGATION OR LAVAGE)

ESOPHAGUS

STOMACH
(GASTRIC)

NASOGASTRIC
FEEDING
(GAVAGE)

LIQUID FOOD
GOES INTO THE
PATIENT

Suction

Fluids are removed from the patient's body through tubes by gravity or **suction**. When fluids are removed by gravity, the collecting container is placed near the patient at a level that is lower than his body. The fluid drips into the container. Suction is also used to remove thick secretions that cannot be drawn out easily by gravity. Sometimes in an emergency situation, suction is used. This may happen when a patient cannot breathe because his respiratory passages are blocked by mucous secretions. Nursing assistants never suction a patient. This procedure is always done by a head nurse, team leader, licensed practical nurse, or a registered nurse.

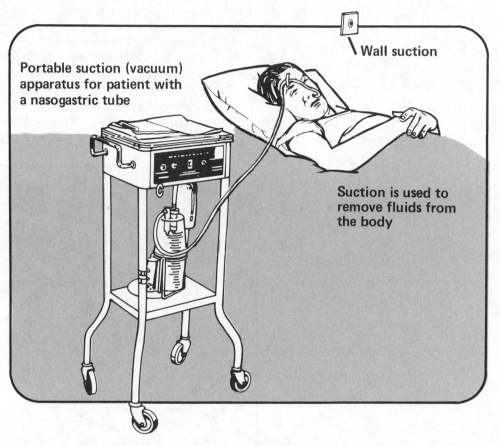

Wall suction

Portable suction (vacuum) apparatus for patient with a nasogastric tube

Suction is used to remove fluids from the body

Rules to Follow: Suction (Vacuum Drainage)

- Report immediately to the head nurse or team leader if you see what appears to be leakage in the tube and suction system.
- Never open the collecting containers to empty the drainage without instructions from your head nurse or team leader.
- Never raise the drainage bottle.
- Never disconnect the tubing.
- Never remove the clamp that is kept at the bedside of a patient who has closed-chest drainage.
- Report to the head nurse or team leader if the level of fluid in the container stops rising. The tubing may be blocked or drainage may be complete.
- The drainage collected through the tubes is measured at regular intervals. The color and kind of material being drained may have to be noted. You may be asked to take these measurements and record them on the output side of the intake and output sheet.
- If a specimen of the drainage is needed, collect the amount specified by the head nurse or team leader.
- If there is a rapid increase in the amount of material being drained, or any change in the material itself, report this to the head nurse or team leader.

Urinary Catheters

The **urinary catheter** is the most common kind of catheter used for taking fluids out of the body. This catheter is made of plastic and inserted through the patient's urethra into his bladder. This catheter also may be used when a patient is unable to void (urinate) naturally. Or it may be used to measure the amount of urine left in the bladder after a patient has voided naturally.

Sometimes a urinary catheter is used for only one withdrawal of urine. Sometimes, however, it is kept in place in the bladder for a number of days or even weeks. In health care institutions only a doctor or a nurse can insert or withdraw a catheter.

Sometimes the bladder-drainage catheter is used to help keep an incontinent patient dry. An **incontinent** patient is one who cannot control his urine or feces. The catheter is specially made so that it will stay in place within the bladder. It really is two tubes, one inside the other. The inside tube is connected at one end to a kind of balloon. After the catheter has been inserted, the balloon is filled with water or air so the catheter will not slip out through the urethra. This is called an **indwelling catheter.** Urine drains out of the bladder

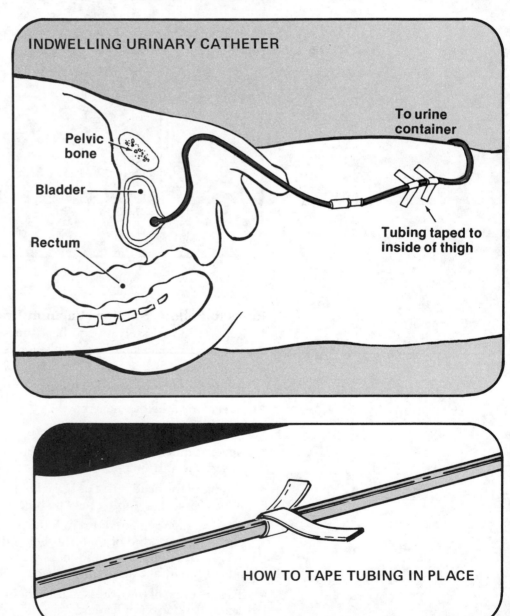

INDWELLING URINARY CATHETER

Pelvic bone

Bladder

Rectum

To urine container

Tubing taped to inside of thigh

HOW TO TAPE TUBING IN PLACE

through the outer tube. The urine collects in a container. The container is attached to the bed frame lower than the patient's urinary bladder. This is always a closed system, which means it is never opened except when emptying the urine collecting bag.

Rules to Follow: Indwelling Urinary Catheter

- Check from time to time to make sure the level of urine has increased. If the level stays the same, report this to your head nurse or team leader.

- If the patient says he feels that his bladder is full, or that he needs to urinate, report this to your head nurse or team leader.

- If the patient is allowed to get out of bed for short periods, the bag goes with the patient. It must be held lower than the patient's urinary bladder at all times, to prevent the urine in the tubing and bag from draining back into the urinary bladder.

- Check to make sure there are no kinks in the catheter and tubing.

- Be sure the patient is not lying on the catheter or the tubing. This would stop the flow of urine.

PLASTIC URINE CONTAINER HUNG ON BED FRAME

Tubing from patient
- **Check tubing for kinks**
- **Be sure patient is not lying on tubing**

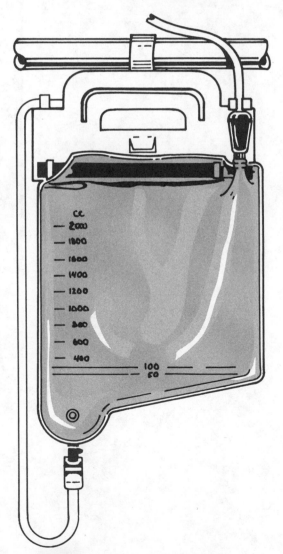

Check level in container for
- **Increase in level**
- **If level remains the same or increases rapidly, report to your head nurse or team leader**

Drain for emptying the container

- The catheter should be taped at all times to the patient's inner thigh. This keeps it from being pulled on or being pulled out of the bladder.
- All patients with urinary drainage through a catheter are on output. You must keep a careful record of urinary output.
- Catheter care should be done as ordered for these patients. (See Chapter 11—Special Treatments, for this procedure.)
- Report to the head nurse or team leader any complaints the patient may have of burning, tenderness, or pain in the urethral area.

Oxygen Therapy

Oxygen therapy can be administered to the patient by physician's order by:

- Tent
- Mask
- Catheter
- Cannula

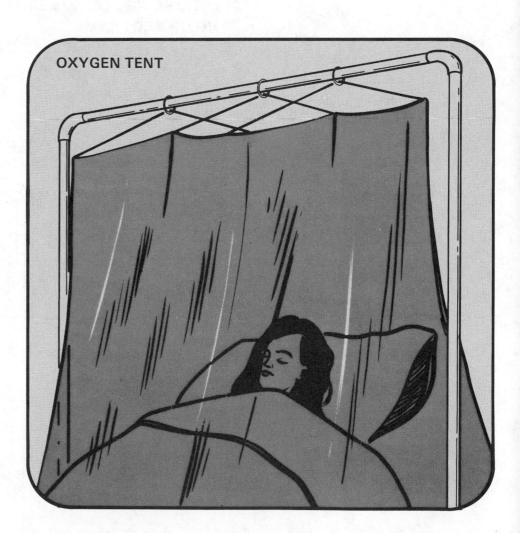

OXYGEN TENT

NASAL CATHETER

This catheter is a piece of tubing that is longer than a cannula. It is inserted through the patient's nostril into the back of his mouth. The nasal catheter is a more effective way to give oxygen to the patient than the nasal cannula. The nasal catheter is used when the patient must have additional oxygen at all times. It is more effective than an oxygen tent or an oxygen mask and is less likely to frighten the patient. The nasal catheter is fastened to the patient's forehead or cheek with a piece of adhesive tape that holds it steady.

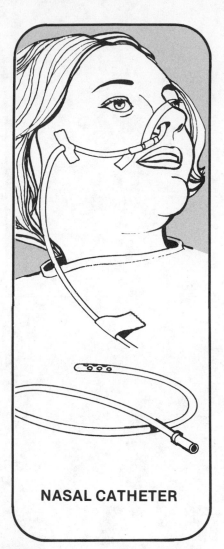

NASAL CATHETER

NASAL CANNULAS

Nasal cannulas, or tubes, are used to give oxygen to a patient. The cannulas are inserted into the patient's nostrils. They are used when the patient needs extra oxygen, not when equipment must provide a patient's total supply of oxygen. The cannula, which is made of plastic, is a half-circle length of tubing with two openings in the center. It fits about one-half inch into the patient's nostrils. Nasal cannulas are held in place by an elastic band around the patient's head and are connected to the source of oxygen by a length of plastic tubing.

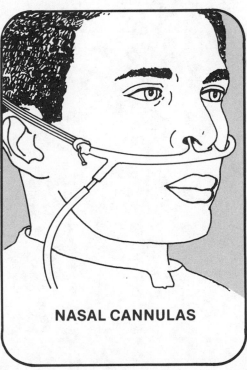

NASAL CANNULAS

OXYGEN FACE MASK

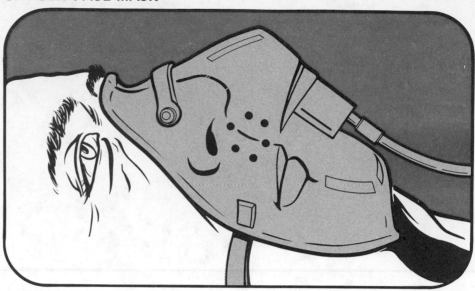

WHAT YOU HAVE LEARNED

As a nursing assistant you will be asked to prepare the patient for a physical examination by the physician. Your role in assisting the doctor includes positioning and draping the patient.

Part of your job description will be observing and checking to make sure that intravenous tubes and other tubes and catheters attached to the patient's body are functioning properly.

All of the tubes and catheters used in modern hospitals today are disposable. This means that these tubes and catheters are discarded in the proper container after one use.

15 WARM AND COLD APPLICATIONS

OBJECTIVES: WHAT YOU WILL LEARN

When you have completed this chapter, you will be able to:

- Explain the principles of warm and cold applications.
- Explain the reasons warm and cold applications are used.
- Explain the difference between moist and dry applications.
- Apply warm and cold applications safely and correctly.
- Apply moist and dry applications safely and correctly.
- Explain what generalized and localized applications mean.

KEY IDEAS: REASONS FOR WARM AND COLD APPLICATIONS

Heat may be applied to an area of the body to speed up the healing process. This is done in the following way: Heat dilates (expands) the blood vessels in the body. This causes more blood to circulate to the injured tissues nearby. Increased circulation can provide the body tissues with more food and oxygen. These are needed for the repair (healing) of body tissue. Warm tub baths, sometimes with medication in the water, are often prescribed for this reason. A **sitz bath** is another example. In this procedure warm water is applied to the patient's perineal or rectal area to speed healing after childbirth or surgery.

Heat may also be applied to an area of the body to ease the pain caused by inflammation and congestion. When the blood vessels become dilated, the increased supply of blood may absorb and carry away the fluids that are causing the inflammation and pain. For example, people with certain bone and joint conditions often get relief from pain and can increase the movement of their body parts because of exercises in warm water.

Cold applications cause the blood vessels to contract (narrow). This contraction may help to prevent or reduce swelling. The cold application helps in the case of a sprained ankle or the beginnings of a black eye. The contraction slows down the flow of blood, therefore it reduces the amount of body fluids that are carried into the injured area. This also prevents or reduces the pain that usually goes along with the swelling. Cold applications may be applied to control bleeding. When cold is applied, the blood flow becomes slower and less blood is able to seep out through a cut or other wound. For example, when a patient has had a tonsillectomy, an ice collar or ice pack may be applied to the neck region.

Cold may be applied to a patient's entire body. This is usually done to lower a patient's body temperature when he has a fever. Special equipment is used to help lower the body temperature including:

- An oxygen tent with a temperature regulator.
- Special thermal blanket and hypothermia machine.
- Alcohol sponge baths.

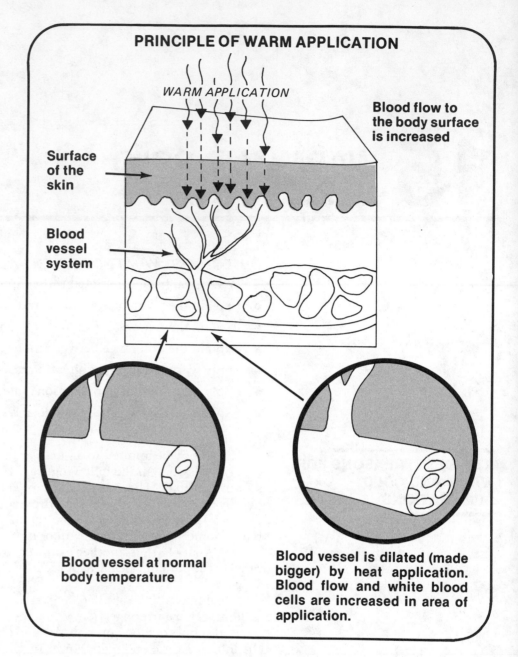

PRINCIPLE OF WARM APPLICATION

WARM APPLICATION

Blood flow to the body surface is increased

Surface of the skin

Blood vessel system

Blood vessel at normal body temperature

Blood vessel is dilated (made bigger) by heat application. Blood flow and white blood cells are increased in area of application.

Temperatures of Applications

For a **warm application**, always use a bath thermometer first to test the temperature of the water. Temperatures for different kinds of heat applications are:

- Warm soak 100°F (37.8°C)

- Warm compress 115°F (46.1°C)

- Warm water bottles 120°F (48.9°C)

- Tub bath 105°F (40.5°C)

For **cold applications**, always use cubed ice with the water. Crushed ice melts too fast. Also it may stick to the cloth and be too cold for the patient's skin. Keep the application cold by adding ice as necessary. Never cover the cold application with linen or any other material after it has been applied to the patient's body. If you cover it, heat will be trapped beneath the cover. Then the application will become warm and will have to be changed sooner than usual.

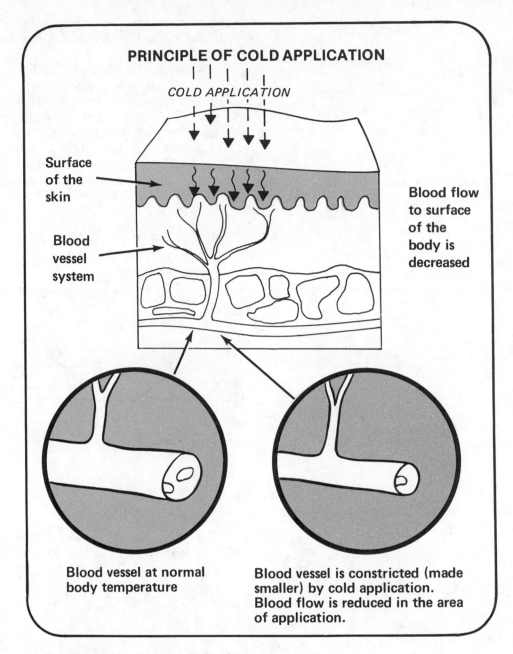

PRINCIPLE OF COLD APPLICATION

COLD APPLICATION

Surface of the skin

Blood vessel system

Blood flow to surface of the body is decreased

Blood vessel at normal body temperature

Blood vessel is constricted (made smaller) by cold application. Blood flow is reduced in the area of application.

Localized and Generalized Applications

Be sure you know exactly where on the patient's body the warmth or cold is to be applied. A **generalized application** is one in which a warm or cold application is applied to a patient's whole body. A **localized application** is one that is applied to a specific part or area of a patient's body.

Moist and Dry Applications

There are several types of both moist and dry applications:

Moist	Dry
Soak—warm or cold	Ice cap and ice collar
Compress—warm or cold	Warm water bottle
Tub	Heat lamp
Alcohol sponge bath	Aquamatic K pad
Sitz bath	Thermal blankets
Cool wet packs	Electric heat cradle
Commercial unit warm pack	Commercial unit cold pack

All applications are either moist or dry. A **moist application** is one in which water touches the skin. A **dry application** is one in which no water touches the skin.

Compresses and soaks are both moist applications. They can be either warm or cold. A compress is a localized application. A soak can be either localized or generalized. In applying a compress, a cloth is dipped into water, wrung out, and applied to the skin. To apply a soak, you immerse the body or body part completely in the water. Warm water bottles, ice caps, and aquamatic K pads are considered dry applications because they have a dry surface. Water is used only inside the equipment and never touches the skin. Dry applications are sometimes used to keep moist applications at the correct temperature.

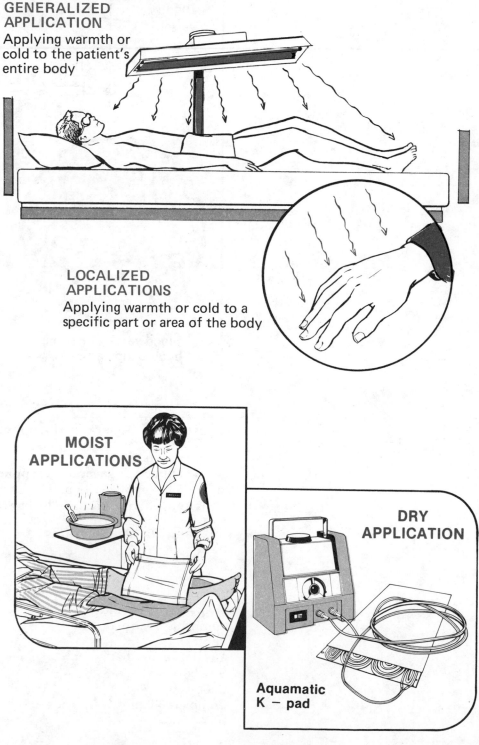

GENERALIZED APPLICATION
Applying warmth or cold to the patient's entire body

LOCALIZED APPLICATIONS
Applying warmth or cold to a specific part or area of the body

MOIST APPLICATIONS

DRY APPLICATION

Aquamatic K – pad

Length of Applications

Follow the instructions given to you by the head nurse or team leader for the exact time to begin the application. Also follow her instructions about how long the application is to stay in place.

In some institutions an ice cap is applied for 10 minutes, removed for 10 minutes, and then reapplied. Following orthopedic surgery, however, ice caps are often ordered continuously on the cast.

Do not put an ice cap or warm water bottle on an area of the body for more than 2 hours at a time. After 2 hours, remove the cap or bottle for one half hour before continuing the application. Soaks and compresses may be kept on the body part for a certain period of time (continuous). Or they may be used for 20 minutes and then taken off for 20 minutes (intermittent).

Checking the Application

Check the application often to keep it at the right temperature throughout the treatment. Suggested times for checking the temperatures of different kinds of applications are:

- Soaks and intermittent compresses: Every 5 minutes
- Heat lamps: Every 5 minutes
- Continuous compresses: Every 30 minutes
- Warm water bottles and ice bags: Every hour

Keeping the Patient Safe

Avoid accidents. Be sure the patient is not in a position where he might fall. Be careful not to spill any water. Be sure electrical equipment does not come in contact with water. Be sure your hands are dry before touching electrical equipment. Be sure the bed is properly protected. Put the side rails in the upright position during the treatment.

Check the patient's skin under warm applications. Watch for too much redness. Look for a darker discoloration that might mean the patient is being burned. Listen when the patient complains. If you think a patient is being burned, remove the heat application immediately and report to your head nurse or team leader at once!

CHECK THE SKIN UNDER THE APPLICATION FOR

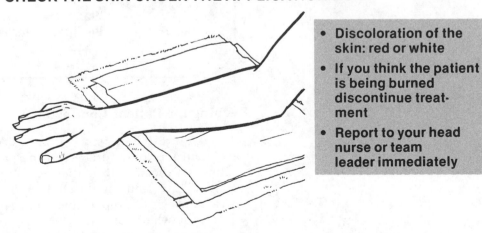

- **Discoloration of the skin: red or white**
- **If you think the patient is being burned discontinue treatment**
- **Report to your head nurse or team leader immediately**

Check the patient's skin where cold is being applied. If the area appears to be blanched, very pale, white, or bluish, tell the head nurse or team leader at once! Watch for changes in the color of parts of the patient's body. For example, if the patient's lips, fingernails, and eyelids look blue or turn a dark color, this is **cyanosis**, which usually is a sign of shock. Stop the treatment immediately and report to your head nurse or team leader.

Always apply the ice cap and warm water bottle with its metal or plastic stopper away from the patient's body. The stopper should never touch the patient's skin. It will be much warmer or colder than the application. It could burn the patient. Remember, ice can also burn the patient's skin. You may be working with an unconscious patient. If so, you may be directed to protect him from a burn by putting a blanket between his skin and the warm water bottle or ice cap.

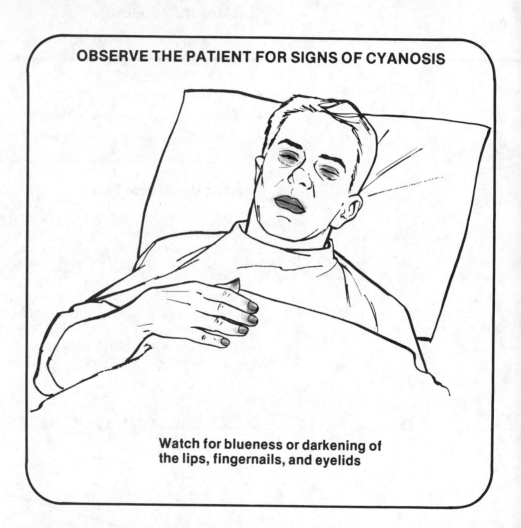

OBSERVE THE PATIENT FOR SIGNS OF CYANOSIS

Watch for blueness or darkening of the lips, fingernails, and eyelids

Keeping the Patient Comfortable

Make sure the patient is in a position that is comfortable for him and convenient for your work. Keep the patient covered and warm during the treatment. Otherwise the patient might become chilled and uncomfortable. If a patient shivers during the cold application, stop the treatment. Cover him with a blanket. Then report this at once to your head nurse or team leader. She will tell you what else to do.

Never put the warm water bottle or ice bag on top of the painful area. The weight probably will increase the pain. Never fill a warm water bottle or ice bag more than half full. It gets too heavy.

Always dry the bottle or bag. Also check it for leaks by turning it upside down. Always place it in a flannel cover. Never let the patient lie on the warm water bottle or ice bag.

When you have finished with an application of moist heat or cold, dry the patient's skin thoroughly and gently, using patting motions. Do not rub the patient's skin to dry it.

Procedure: Applying the Warm Compress (Moist Heat Application)

1. Assemble your equipment:
   a) Disposable bed protector
   b) Basin
   c) Pitcher of water at 115°F (46.1°C)
   d) Washcloth, towel, or gauze pads (compress)
   e) Bath thermometer
   f) Large sheet of plastic
   g) Bath towel
   h) Bath blanket

2. Wash your hands.

3. Identify the patient by checking the identification bracelet.

4. Ask visitors to step out of the room.

5. Tell the patient you are going to apply a warm compress.

6. Pull the curtain around the bed for privacy.

7. Help the patient into a comfortable, safe position. Have the body area exposed that is to be given a warm compress.

8. Place a disposable bed protector under the body area that is to be given the warm compress.

9. Fill the pitcher with warm water. Check the temperature of the water with a bath thermometer (115°F—46.1°C). Then pour the water into the basin.

10. Dip the compress into the water and wring it out thoroughly.

11. Apply the compress gently to the proper area.

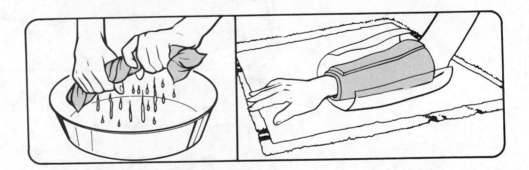

12. Cover the entire compress with a plastic sheet. This keeps the compress warm. Be sure the plastic does not touch the patient's skin. Then wrap the entire area with a large towel.

13. If the patient is cold or chilly, cover him with a blanket.

14. Change the compress and remoisten it, as necessary, to keep it warm. Sometimes a patient is able to apply the compress himself. If your head nurse or team leader gives permission for this, position and assist the patient as necessary.

(continued next page)

15. Check the skin under the application every 5 minutes. If the skin appears red, remove the compress. Cover the area with a towel or blanket. Report this to your head nurse or team leader.

16. A warm compress is usually applied for 15 to 20 minutes. However, follow the instructions given to you by your head nurse or team leader as to how long the warm compress is to be applied.

17. After the treatment is completed, remove the compress and gently pat the area dry with a towel.

18. Make the patient comfortable.

19. Clean standard equipment and put it in its proper place. Discard disposable equipment.

20. Wash your hands.

21. Report to your head nurse or team leader:
    • The time the warm compress was started.
    • How long the compress was in place.
    • The area of application.
    • Your observations of anything unusual.

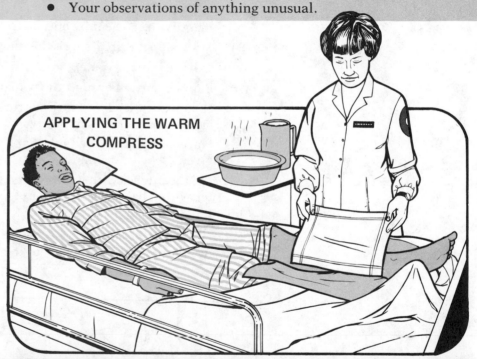

APPLYING THE WARM COMPRESS

Procedure: Applying the Cold Compress (Moist Cold Application)

1. Assemble your equipment:
   a) Disposable bed protector
   b) Basin
   c) Washcloth, towel, or gauze pads (compress)
   d) Bath towel
   e) Bath blanket
   f) Pitcher of cold water (ice cubes, if ordered by the head nurse or team leader)

2. Wash your hands.

3. Identify the patient by checking the identification bracelet.

4. Ask visitors to step out of the room.

5. Tell the patient that you are going to apply a cold compress.

6. Pull the curtain around the bed for privacy.

(continued next page)

7. Help the patient into a comfortable, safe position. Have the area exposed that is to receive the cold compress.

8. Place a disposable bed protector under the body area that is to be given the cold compress.

9. Put cold water in the basin (ice cubes, only if ordered).

10. Dip the compress into the water and wring it out thoroughly.

11. Apply the cold compress to the proper area of the patient's body as quickly as possible. If you are slow, the compress will absorb heat from your hands and the air.

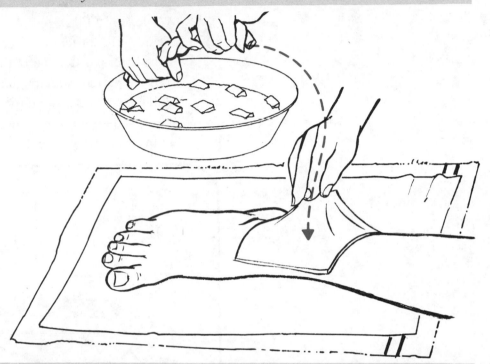

12. If the patient is cold or chilly, cover him with a blanket. Do not cover the compress or the area being treated.

13. Change the compress and remoisten it, as necessary, to keep it cold. Sometimes a patient is able to apply the compress himself. If your head nurse or team leader gives permission for this, position and assist the patient as necessary.

14. Check the patient's skin under the application every 5 minutes. If the skin appears to be blanched or white, remove the compress. Cover the area with a towel or blanket. Report this to your head nurse or team leader.

15. A cold compress is usually applied for 15 to 20 minutes. However, follow the instructions of your head nurse or team leader as to how long the cold compress is to be applied.

16. When the treatment is finished, remove the compress and gently pat the area dry with a towel.

17. Make the patient comfortable.

18. Clean your standard equipment and put it in its proper place. Discard disposable equipment.

19. Wash your hands.

20. Report to your head nurse or team leader:

   • The time the cold compress was started.

   • How long it remained in place.

   • The area of application.

   • Your observations of anything unusual.

Procedure: Applying the Cold Soak
(Moist Cold Application)

1. Assemble your equipment:
   a) Basin, foot tub, or arm basin
   b) Pitcher of cold water (ice cubes only if ordered by head nurse or team leader)
   c) Disposable bed protectors
   d) Bath towel
   e) Bath blanket
2. Wash your hands.
3. Identify the patient by checking the identification bracelet.
4. Ask visitors to step out of the room.
5. Tell the patient you are going to apply a cold soak.
6. Pull the curtain around the bed for privacy.
7. Help the patient into a safe, comfortable position.
8. Fill the pitcher with cold water. Then fill the basin half full.

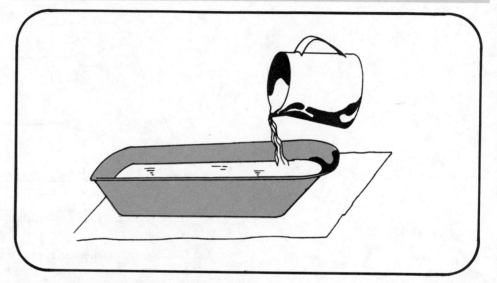

9. Place a disposable bed protector under the body area that is to receive the cold soak.
10. Place the basin in a position so the patient's arm, leg, foot, or hand can be dipped into the basin easily.
11. Place the patient's arm or leg into the water gradually.

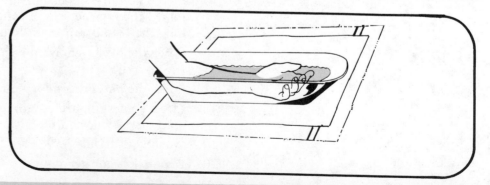

12. When you have to change the water, take the patient's arm or leg out of the basin. Wrap it with a bath towel or bath blanket to keep it warm.

(continued next page)

13. If the patient says he feels weak or cold, stop the treatment. Cover the patient with extra blankets and report this to your head nurse or team leader.

14. Check the skin every 5 minutes. If the skin is blanched or white, stop the treatment. Report to your head nurse or team leader.

15. When the treatment is finished, dry the patient's arm or leg by gently patting with a towel.

16. Make the patient comfortable.

17. Clean standard equipment and put it in its proper place. Discard disposable equipment.

18. Wash your hands.

19 Report to your head nurse or team leader:
   - The time the cold soak was started.
   - The length of treatment.
   - The area of application.
   - Your observations of anything unusual.

Procedure: Applying the Warm Soak (Moist Warm Application)

1. Assemble your equipment:
   a) Basin, foot tub, or arm basin
   b) Pitcher of water at 100°F (37.8°C)
   c) Bath thermometer
   d) Disposable bed protectors
   e) Bath towel
   f) Bath blanket

2. Wash your hands.

3. Identify the patient by checking the identification bracelet.

4. Ask visitors to step out of the room.

5. Tell the patient that you are going to apply a warm soak.

6. Pull the curtain around the bed for privacy.

7. Help the patient into a safe, comfortable position. Have the area to be treated exposed.

8. Fill the pitcher with warm water at 100°F (37.8°C). Check the temperature with a bath thermometer.

9. Pour the water from the pitcher into the basin. Fill the basin one half full.

10. Place a disposable bed protector under the body area that is to receive the soak.

11. Place the basin in a position so the patient's arm, leg, or foot can be placed in it easily.

12. Place the arm or leg into the water gradually.

13. Check the temperature of the water every 5 minutes. When you need to change the water, take the patient's arm, foot, or leg out of the basin. Wrap it with a bath blanket or bath towel to keep it warm.

14. If the patient says he feels weak or cold, stop the treatment. Cover the patient with extra blankets and report this to your head nurse or team leader.

15. Check the skin every 5 minutes. If the skin is red, stop the treatment. Report this to your head nurse or team leader.

(continued next page)

16. When the treatment is finished, dry the patient's arm or leg by patting gently with a towel.
17. Make the patient comfortable.
18. Clean standard equipment and put it in its proper place. Discard disposable equipment.
19. Wash your hands.
20. Report to your head nurse or team leader:
    - The time the warm soak was started.
    - The length of treatment.
    - The area of application.
    - Your observations of anything unusual.

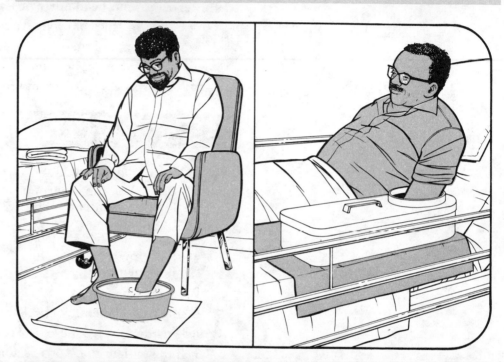

Procedure: Applying the Warm Water Bottle (Dry Heat Application)

1. Assemble your equipment:
   a) Warm water bottle (may be disposable)
   b) Pitcher of water at 120°F (48.9°C)
   c) Bath thermometer
   d) Flannel cover (whatever type of cover used in your institution)
2. Wash your hands.
3. Identify the patient by checking the identification bracelet.
4. Ask visitors to step out of the room.
5. Tell the patient that you are going to apply a warm water bottle.
6. Pull the curtain around the bed for privacy.
7. Fill the pitcher with water at 120°F (48.9°C). Check the temperature of the water with a bath thermometer.
8. Fill the warm water bottle half full of water.
9. Two methods of squeezing the air out of the bottle are:
   METHOD A:
   Place the bag on the edge of a counter. Have the part of the bag containing the water hanging down. Place the part of the bag with-

(continued next page)

out the water lying on the counter top. Put your hand on top of the bag at the edge of the counter. Move your hand slowly toward the opening of the bag, pressing out the air. With the other hand, close the bag.

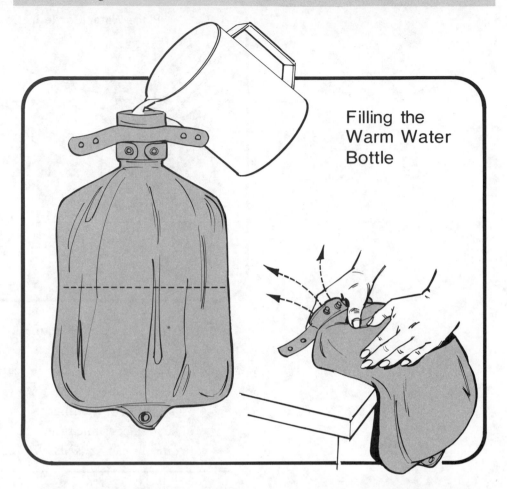

Filling the Warm Water Bottle

METHOD B:

Place the warm water bottle in a horizontal position on a flat surface. Hold the neck of the warm water bottle upright until you can see water in the neck of the bottle. (The water squeezes out the air.)

10. Fasten the top tightly.

11. Dry the warm water bottle. Check for leaks by turning it upside down.

12. Place the warm water bottle in a flannel cover (or type of cover used in your institution).

13. Apply it gently to the proper body area.

14. Never place the warm water bottle on top of a painful area. The weight will increase the pain. Place it on the side.

15. Check the warm water bottle every hour to be sure the temperature is correct. Change the water in the bottle, when necessary, to continue the treatment at the same temperature.

16. Check the skin under the warm water bottle every hour. If the skin is red, remove the warm water bottle and report to your head nurse or team leader.

17. Clean standard equipment and put it in its proper place. Discard disposable equipment.

(continued next page)

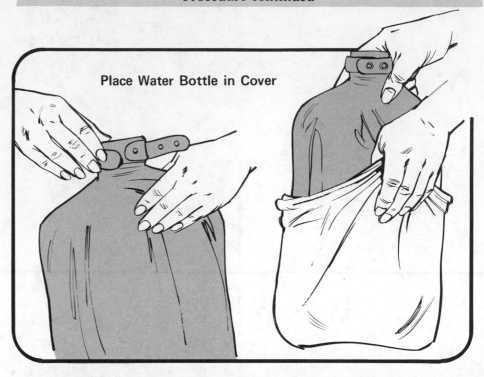

Place Water Bottle in Cover

18. Make the patient comfortable.
19. Wash your hands.
20. Report to your head nurse or team leader:
    - The time the warm water bottle was applied.
    - The length of treatment.
    - The area of application.
    - Your observations of anything unusual.

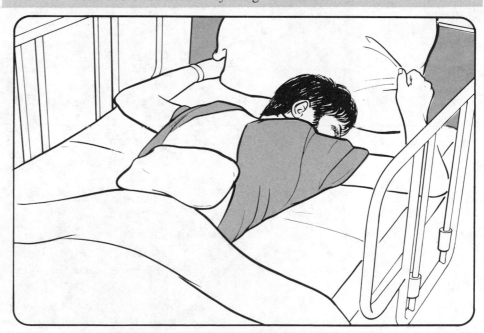

WARM WATER BOTTLE INSIDE COVER

Procedure: Applying the Ice Bag, Ice Cap, or Ice Collar (Dry Cold Application)

1. Assemble your equipment:
   a) Ice bag, ice cap, or ice collar (may be disposable)
   b) Flannel cover (whatever type of cover used in your institution)
   c) Ice cubes in a clean container
   d) Bath blanket
2. Wash your hands.
3. Identify the patient by checking the identification bracelet.
4. Ask visitors to step out of the room.
5. Tell the patient that you are going to apply the ice bag, ice cap, or ice collar.
6. Pull the curtain around the bed for privacy.
7. Pour cold water over the ice cubes to melt the sharp edges.
8. Fill the ice collar, ice bag, or ice cap one-half full of ice.
9. Squeeze the sides of the ice bag to force the air out of it.
10. Fasten the stopper tightly.
11. Dry the outside of the ice bag with a paper towel.
12. Invert the ice bag to test for leaking.

(continued next page)

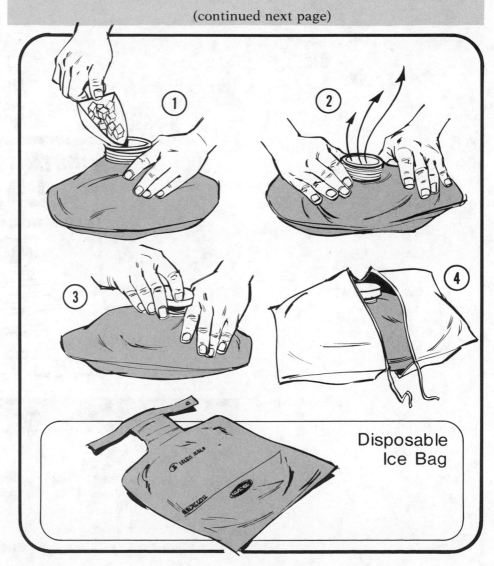

Disposable Ice Bag

13. Place the ice bag into the flannel cover (or type of cover used in your institution).

14. Apply the ice bag to the proper area of the patient's body.

15. If the patient is cold or chilly, cover him with a blanket. Do not cover the ice bag or the area being treated.

16. Do not leave the ice bag on an area of the body for more than 2 hours at a time. Follow the instructions from your head nurse or team leader. After one hour replace the ice in the bag. This will keep it cold enough for proper application. After 2 hours, remove the ice bag for a half hour before continuing the cold application.

17. Check the skin under the application every 10 minutes. If the skin appears to be blanched or white, remove the ice bag. Cover the area with a towel and report to your head nurse or team leader.

18. Clean standard equipment and put it in its proper place. Discard disposable equipment.

19. Make the patient comfortable.

20. Wash your hands.

21. Report to your head nurse or team leader:
    - The time the ice bag was applied.
    - The length of treatment.
    - The area of application.
    - Your observations of anything unusual.

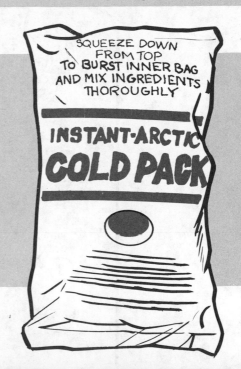

Procedure: Applying the Commercial Unit Cold Pack (Dry Cold Application)

1. Assemble your equipment:
   a) Commercial unit single-use cold pack
   b) Flannel cover (whatever type of cover used in your institution)
   c) Bath blanket

2. Wash your hands.

3. Identify the patient by checking the identification bracelet.

(continued next page)

4. Ask visitors to step out of the room.

5. Tell the patient that you are going to apply a cold pack.

6. Pull the curtain around the bed for privacy.

7. Place the flannel cover on the cold pack (or whatever type of cover used by your institution).

8. Hit the cold pack with your hand. A single blow to the surface activates the unit.

9. Apply the pack to the proper area of the patient's body.

10. Check the skin under the application every 10 minutes. If the skin appears blanched or white, remove the pack and cover the area with a blanket. Report this to your head nurse or team leader.

11. If the treatment is continuous, replace it as necessary with a new cold pack.

12. Discard disposable equipment.

13. Make the patient comfortable.

14. Wash your hands.

15. Report to your head nurse or team leader:

    - The time the cold pack was applied.
    - The length of treatment.
    - The area of application.
    - Your observations of anything unusual.

Procedure: Applying the Commercial Unit Heat Pack - (Moist Warm Application)

1. Assemble your equipment:
   a) Commercial unit single-use warm pack that has been warmed in the heating lamp unit
   b) Disposable bed protectors
   c) Large sheet of plastic

2. Wash your hands.

3. Identify the patient by checking the identification bracelet.

4. Ask visitors to step out of the room.

5. Tell the patient that you are going to apply a warm pack.

6. Pull the curtain around the bed for privacy.

7. Place the bed protector under the body part that is to receive the warm pack.

8. Tear the foil covering from the warm pack.

9. Place the moist warm pack on the proper body area.

10. Cover the pack with the sheet of plastic. This will keep the pack warm.

11. Check the skin under the application every 10 minutes. If the skin appears red, remove the pack and cover the area with a blanket. Report this to your head nurse or team leader.

12. If the treatment is continuous, replace it as necessary with a new warm pack.

13. When the treatment is finished, discard disposable equipment.

14. Make the patient comfortable.

15. Wash your hands.

(continued next page)

Procedure continued

16. Report to your head nurse or team leader:
    - The time the warm pack was applied.
    - The length of treatment.
    - The area of application.
    - Your observations of anything unusual.

Procedure: Applying a Heat Lamp (Dry Warm Application)

1. Assemble your equipment:
   a) Heat lamp
   b) Bath blanket
   c) Bath towel
   d) Tape measure
2. Wash your hands.
3. Identify the patient by checking the identification bracelet.
4. Ask visitors to step out of the room.
5. Tell the patient that you are going to apply a heat lamp.
6. Pull the curtain around the bed for privacy.
7. Expose only the body area that is to receive the heat. Drape the patient so that heat is directed to the proper area of the skin. Cover the rest of the patient's body with the bath blanket or towel.

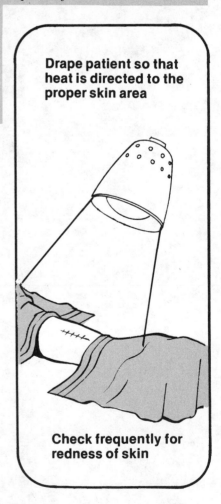

Drape patient so that heat is directed to the proper skin area

Check frequently for redness of skin

(continued next page)

8. The part of the patient's body that is being treated should be at least 18 inches away from the heat lamp. Use a tape measure to check the distance. Drape the patient so that the heat is directed to the proper skin area.

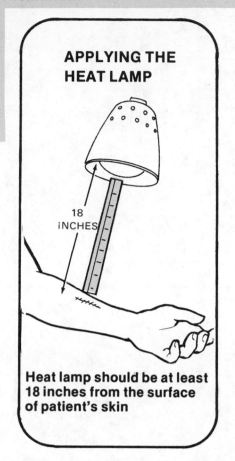

APPLYING THE HEAT LAMP

18 INCHES

Heat lamp should be at least 18 inches from the surface of patient's skin

9. Check the skin after 5 minutes. If the patient's skin becomes red, stop the treatment and report to your head nurse or team leader.

10. There is a danger of fire when a heat lamp is being used. Therefore, keep all linen away from the lamp.

11. Leave the heat lamp on the patient from 5 to no more than 10 minutes, unless you have other instructions from your head nurse or team leader.

12. After the treatment, remove the lamp.

13. Make the patient comfortable.

14. Wipe the lamp with disinfectant solution and put it back in its proper place.

15. Wash your hands.

16. Report to your head nurse or team leader:
    ● The time the heat was applied.
    ● The length of treatment.
    ● The area of application.
    ● Your observations of anything unusual.

**KEY IDEAS:
PERINEAL HEAT LAMP**

When you are using the heat lamp as a perineal, or "peri" lamp, help the patient into the lithotomy position. Place her feet on the mattress. Bend the knees and separate them. Place the lamp 18 inches away from the perineum. Remove the peripad to expose the perineal area. Remove the patient's pillow. Instruct the patient to keep her head flat, exposing more of the perineum. Watch for excessive heat. The light should be on from 5 to 10 minutes. When the treatment is finished, remove the lamp. Put a new peripad in place and make the patient comfortable.

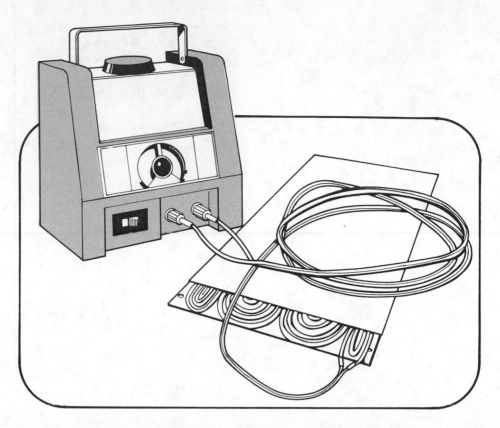

Procedure: Applying the Aquamatic K-Pad (Dry Heat Application)

1. Assemble your equipment:

   a) Aquamatic K-pad and control unit. (The temperature is pre-set by CSR (central supply room). The container is filled with distilled water by CSR.)

   b) Cover for pad (pillowcase or flannel cover)

2. Wash your hands.

3. Identify the patient by checking the identification bracelet.

4. Ask visitors to step out of the room.

5. Explain to the patient that you are going to apply the K-pad.

6. Pull the curtain around the bed for privacy.

7. Inspect the K-pad for leaks and to make sure the cord and plug are in good condition.

8. Plug the cord into an electrical outlet.

9. Place the pad in the cover. DO NOT USE ANY PINS!

10. Place the container on the bedside table. Arrange the tubing at the level of the pad. Do not allow the tubing to hang below the level of the bed.

11. Gently apply the pad in its cover to the proper body area.

12. Check the skin under the pad every hour.

13. When the treatment is finished, return the equipment to its proper place.

14. Make the patient comfortable.

(continued next page)

15. Wash your hands.
16. Report to your head nurse or team leader:
    - The time the K-pad was applied.
    - The length of treatment.
    - The area of application.
    - Your observations of anything unusual.

DISPOSABLE SITZ BATH KIT

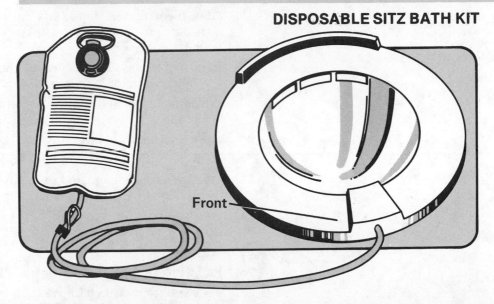

Front

Procedure: Using the Disposable Sitz Bath (Moist Warm Application)

1. Assemble your equipment:
   a) Disposable sitz bath kit containing:
      - Plastic bowl with a large brim
      - Water bag
      - Tubing and stopcock (clamp)
   b) Plastic laundry bag
   c) Bath thermometer
   d) Bath towels
   e) Pitcher of water at 105°F (40.5°C)
2. Wash your hands.
3. Identify the patient by checking the identification bracelet.
4. Ask visitors to step out of the room.
5. Tell the patient that you are going to give him a sitz bath.
6. Pull the curtain around the bed for privacy.
7. Help the patient to put on his slippers and robe.
8. Help the patient into the bathroom.
9. Raise the toilet seat.
10. Check the temperature of the water with the bath thermometer. It should be 105°F (40.5°C).
11. Put the plastic bowl into the toilet bowl. Be sure that the opening for overflow is toward the front of the toilet.
12. Pour the water into the bowl, filling it half full.
13. Close the stopcock on the tubing. Fill the water bag with water (105°F, 40.5°C) from the pitcher. Close the bag.

(continued next page)

14. Hang the container for water 12 inches higher than the bowl.

15. Help the patient remove his robe and pajamas and sit down into the sitz bath. Be sure the patient can reach the signal cord.

16. Place the tubing inside the bowl with the opening of the tube under the water level. The tube fits into a little groove in the front of the basin.

17. Open the stopcock and adjust the flow if necessary.

18. Have the patient sit in the sitz bath with water running in for from 10 to 20 minutes. Follow the instructions of your head nurse or team leader.

19. If the patient says he feels weak or faint, stop the treatment. Turn on the signal light for help in getting the patient out of the bathroom.

20. When the treatment is finished, remove the tubing. Help the patient out of the sitz bath.

21. Pat the patient's body gently with a towel to dry.

22. Help the patient back into bed. Make him comfortable.

23. Clean your equipment and return it to its proper place. If it is not to be used again, discard the disposable equipment.

24. Put the dirty towels in the plastic laundry bag. Bring the bag to the dirty linen hamper in the dirty utility room.

25. Wash your hands.

26. Report to your head nurse or team leader:
    - The time the sitz bath was started.
    - The length of time the patient was in the sitz bath.
    - Your observations of anything unusual.

Procedure: Using the Portable Chair-Type or Built-In Sitz Bath (Moist Warm Application)

1. Assemble your equipment:
   a) Portable chair or built-in sitz bath
   b) Disinfectant cleanser
   c) Bath towels
   d) Bath blanket
   e) Bath thermometer
   f) Plastic laundry bag

2. Wash your hands.

3. Identify the patient by checking the identification bracelet.

4. Ask visitors to step out of the room.

5. Tell the patient that you are going to give him a sitz bath.

6. Pull the curtain around the bed for privacy.

7. Bring the portable chair-type sitz bath into the patient's room. Or help the patient (using a wheelchair if necessary) to the bathroom with the built-in chair-type sitz bath.

8. Clean the sitz bath with disinfectant cleanser.

9. Rinse it well.

10. Fill it half full with water at 105°F (40.5°C).

11. Place a towel on the seat and on the front edge of the sitz bath.

12. Help the patient to undress, except for his gown and slippers.

13. Help the patient to sit down in the tub. Hold his gown up so it does not get wet.

(continued next page)

14. Cover the patient's shoulders with a bath blanket if he complains of being cold.

15. Continue the treatment for 10 to 20 minutes, unless you have other instructions from your head nurse or team leader.

16. Check the patient every 5 minutes.

17. If the patient says he feels weak or faint, stop the treatment. Put the signal light on for help in getting the patient out of the tub. Let the water out of the tub.

18. When the treatment is finished, help the patient out of the tub.

19. Pat his body gently with a towel to dry.

20. Help the patient back to bed. Make him comfortable.

21. Clean the sitz tub with disinfectant cleanser.

22. Put the portable chair-type tub back in its proper place.

23. Place the used towels in the plastic laundry bag. Bring the bag to the dirty linen hamper in the dirty utility room.

24. Wash your hands.

25. Report to your head nurse or team leader:
   - The time the sitz bath was started.
   - The length of time the patient was in the sitz bath.
   - Your observations of anything unusual.

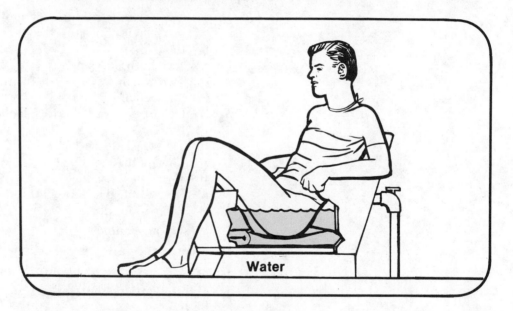

Water

KEY IDEAS: THE ALCOHOL SPONGE BATH

You have had the experience of perspiring on a warm summer day. You often feel cooler as the moisture evaporates from your skin. As perspiration evaporates into the air, it carries some heat with it. This cools the body. An alcohol sponge bath cools a patient's body in the same way. Alcohol is applied to the patient's body because it will evaporate from the skin much faster than water. The purpose of the alcohol sponge bath is to lower the patient's body temperature.

Rules to Follow: Giving the Alcohol Sponge Bath
- Alcohol sponge baths are never given without the doctor's orders.
- You will place ice bags on certain areas of the patient's body. Often the areas are the armpits or the groin (the area where the thighs meet the trunk of the body). These are places where many blood vessels are close to the surface of the body.

- You will put warm water bottles around the patient's feet. This prevents the patient from becoming chilled. The feet are the area of the body farthest from the heart, therefore they have the poorest circulation.

- Never apply alcohol to the patient's face.

- You may add ice cubes to the cooling solution. This is done only if you are given this instruction by your head nurse or team leader.

- If the patient becomes chilled and starts to shiver, stop the treatment. Call the head nurse or team leader. If the patient's shivering cannot be controlled, the alcohol sponge bath will do no good. This is because the shivering causes increased cell and muscle activity. This produces more heat and causes the body temperature to rise.

- Alcohol sponge baths are not given to children. This treatment is too severe for a child.

Two other methods to lower the body temperature are sometimes used for generalized cold applications. These are thermal blankets and oxygen tents. Such applications also lower the patient's body temperature. A cool-mist air tent is sometimes used if an infant or child has a high fever. The coolness and increased humidity from the fine mist help to reduce the fever.

Procedure: Giving the Alcohol Sponge Bath (Moist Cold Application)

1. Assemble your equipment:
   a) Alcohol 70% (rubbing alcohol)—cool water (one cup of alcohol mixed with one cup of cool water)
   b) Basin
   c) Two bath blankets
   d) Two warm water bottles with covers
   e) Six ice bags with covers
   f) Ice cubes, if ordered for alcohol-water solution
   g) Bath towels
   h) Two washcloths
   i) Thermometer
   j) Two small towels
   k) Disposable bed protectors
   l) Plastic laundry bag

2. Wash your hands.

3. Identify the patient by checking the identification bracelet.

4. Ask visitors to step out of the room.

5. Tell the patient that you are going to give him an alcohol sponge bath.

6. Pull the curtain around the bed for privacy.

7. Take the patient's temperature, pulse, respiration, and blood pressure.

8. Record the information in the proper place.

9. Put the bath blanket on top of the bedspread and top sheet.

10. Tuck the blanket under the patient's shoulders. Without exposing the patient, remove the top sheet and bedspread from under the blanket the patient is holding in place.

11. Remove the patient's gown without uncovering him.

12. Place the disposable bed protectors and bath blanket under the patient by turning him from side to side.

(continued next page)

13. Help the patient to move close to the side of the bed where you will be working.

14. Place a small dry towel between the patient's legs to cover the genital area.

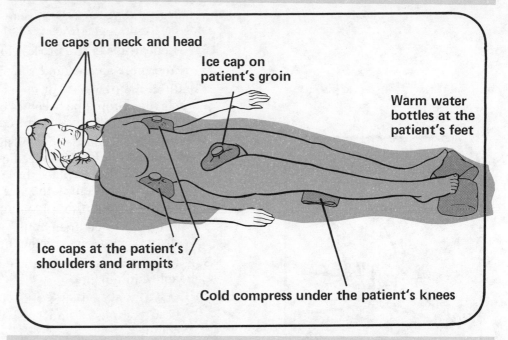

Ice caps on neck and head

Ice cap on patient's groin

Warm water bottles at the patient's feet

Ice caps at the patient's shoulders and armpits

Cold compress under the patient's knees

15. Fill the ice bags with ice cubes. Cover them with flannel covers. Place one on each side of the patient's neck, one in each armpit, one on the groin, and one on top of the patient's head.

16. Wet one small towel with cold water and place it under both knees.

17. Fill both warm water bottles. Place one at the bottom of each of the patient's feet.

18. Mix the solution as instructed, or put one cup of alcohol with one cup of cool water into the basin.

19. Put both washcloths into the water-alcohol solution.

20. Alternate the washcloths throughout this procedure.

21. Place a bath towel under the arm farthest away from you.

22. Make a mitt with a washcloth. Dip it into the solution. The washcloths should not be wrung out. They should be dripping wet.

23. Sponge the entire arm and underarm with long, even strokes. Do not dry the area. Place the arm under the blanket wet. Then remove the towel.

24. Repeat the step on the arm closer to you.

25. Fold the bath blanket down to the patient's waist. Place a towel across the blanket to keep it dry.

26. Sponge the front of the patient's neck and chest to the waistline. Do not dry, but cover with a towel.

27. Fold the bath blanket to the groin. Place a second towel across the groin area.

28. Sponge the entire abdomen with the alcohol solution. Then cover the abdomen and chest with the blanket. Remove both towels as you cover him with the blanket.

29. Expose the leg farthest from you. Place a towel under the leg. Sponge the entire leg with the alchohol solution. Do not dry, but cover the leg with the blanket and remove the towel.

(continued next page)

30. Repeat the process on the leg closest to you.

31. Turn the patient on his side. Spread a towel over the mattress near his back. Sponge the back of his neck, his back, and his buttocks with long, even strokes.

32. Do not dry. Turn the patient on his back. Cover him with the blanket. Remove the towel.

33. Repeat this entire process for 20 minutes.

34. Add more alcohol and water as needed.

35. Stop the treatment if the patient complains of being cold or if he shivers. Stop if he becomes cyanotic or if you observe anything unusual. Report this to your head nurse or team leader.

36. When the treatment is finished, remove the bath blankets. Change the sheets if they have become damp. Remove all ice bags and warm water bottles. Replace the gown, the top sheet, and the bedspread. Cover the patient with extra blankets if you are instructed to do so by the head nurse or team leader.

37. Place all soiled linen in the plastic laundry bag. Take the bag to the dirty linen hamper in the dirty utility room.

38. Clean your equipment and put it in its proper place. Discard disposable equipment.

39. Measure the patient's vital signs 10 minutes after the treatment has been completed and one-half hour after the treatment has been completed.

40. Record in the proper place.

41. Make the patient comfortable.

42. Wash your hands.

43. Report to your head nurse or team leader:
    - The time the alcohol sponge bath was started.
    - How long it was given.
    - The patient's vital signs before the treatment, 10 minutes, and one-half hour after the treatment has been completed.
    - Your observations of anything unusual.

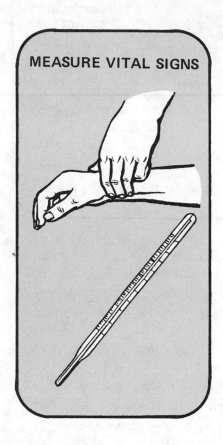

MEASURE VITAL SIGNS

WHAT YOU HAVE LEARNED

You have studied the principles and purposes of warm and cold and dry and moist applications. You have been given the procedures for applying warm and cold compresses; warm and cold soaks; warm water bottles; ice bags, caps, and collars; heat lamps; the aquamatic K-pad; the commercial unit cold pack; the portable chair-type and built-in sitz bath; and alcohol sponge baths. Keep alert and observe the patient carefully during the time you are giving both warm and cold and dry and moist applications.

16 PREOPERATIVE AND POSTOPERATIVE NURSING CARE

1. Preoperative Nursing Care
2. Postoperative Nursing Care
3. Binders and Elastic Bandages

SECTION 1: PREOPERATIVE NURSING CARE

OBJECTIVES: WHAT YOU WILL LEARN

When you have completed this section, you will be able to:

- Complete a preoperative checklist accurately.
- Shave a patient in preparation for surgery.
- Help the preoperative patient feel calm and relaxed.
- Get the patient's unit ready for his return from the operating or recovery room.

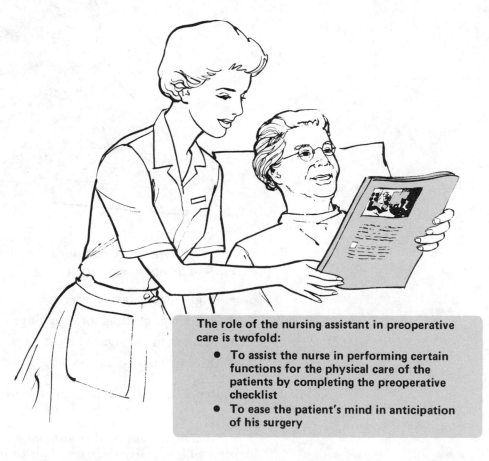

The role of the nursing assistant in preoperative care is twofold:

- **To assist the nurse in performing certain functions for the physical care of the patients by completing the preoperative checklist**
- **To ease the patient's mind in anticipation of his surgery**

**KEY IDEAS:
PREOPERATIVE CARE**

Two very important words are used often in this chapter. They are: preoperative and postoperative.

- The word **operative** means an operation or surgery.
- **Pre** means before.
- **Post** means after.
- **Preoperative** means before surgery.
- **Postoperative** means after surgery.

Almost every patient who enters a hospital for surgery will be a little nervous and upset. Part of your job as a nursing assistant is to make the patient feel as calm and relaxed as possible.

Some things that might upset the preoperative patient are:

- Concern for one's family.
- Being away from work; financial fears.
- A possible disability because of the operation.
- The possibility of death or serious complications.
- Fear of the unknown.

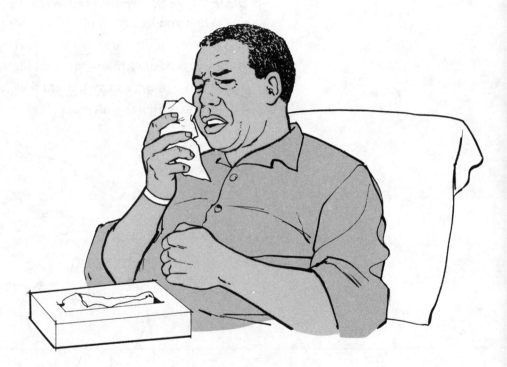

To prevent chest complications following surgery, watch for these symptoms in preoperative patients:

- Signs of respiratory infection
- Sneezing, sniffling, or coughing
- Complaints or signs of chest pains
- Elevated temperature

Report any of these immediately to your head nurse or team leader.

Good physical and emotional preoperative care can help to reduce anxiety and fears. Give the patient all your attention. Make him feel that you care about him and how the operation comes out. Listen and show interest in what the patient says. Many frightened people relieve their tension by talking a lot and by asking lots of questions. Others do not say anything. You can give support to your patient just by being there when he needs assistance, by staying calm if he seems upset, and by being tactful. Alert the head nurse or team leader if the patient appears abnormally upset or fearful.

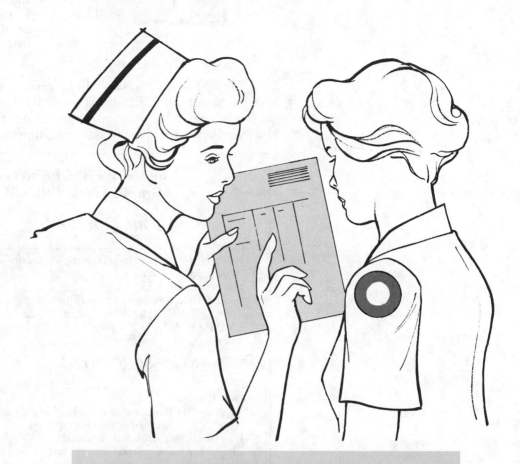

YOUR HEAD NURSE OR TEAM LEADER WILL GIVE YOU THE PREOPERATIVE CHECKLIST AND INSTRUCT YOU AS TO:

- What each patient has been told about his operation.
- What you are to tell the patient to prepare him for his surgery and postoperative care.
- How to handle and answer the patient's questions.
- What care to give the patient the evening before surgery.
- What care to give the patient the morning of surgery.
- What she wants you to complete from the patient's answers on the checklist.

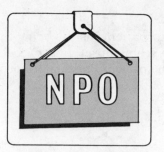

You may be asked to take away the patient's water pitcher and glass at midnight and to post a sign saying *NPO*. NPO is taken from the Latin, *nils per os*, which means "nothing by mouth." The sign is usually put at the head or foot of the bed; follow your head nurses's or team leader's instructions.

In most hospitals, you will be given a preoperative checklist along with your instructions. The checklist shown here is a sample. It is like the one actually used in the hospital. By filling out this checklist, the nursing staff can be sure the patient has been prepared properly for surgery.

SAMPLE PREOPERATIVE CHECKLIST
COMPLETED BY NURSING ASSISTANT

EVENING BEFORE SURGERY

Patient's Name _____

Identify the patient by checking his identification bracelet Yes_____ No_____

Skin prep done by _____ at _____ p.m.

Skin prep checked by _____ at _____ p.m.

Food restrictions, if any, explained to patient . . . . Yes_____ No_____

"NPO AFTER MIDNIGHT" sign put on patient's bed
AND EXPLAINED TO THE PATIENT . . . . Yes_____ No_____

Enema administered by _____ at _____ p.m.

MORNING OF SURGERY

Bath . . . . Yes_____ No_____

Oral hygiene . . . . Yes_____ No_____

False teeth (dentures) & removable bridges removed . . . . Yes_____ No_____

Jewelry and pierced earrings removed . . . . Yes_____ No_____

Hairpiece, wig, hairpins removed . . . . Yes_____ No_____

Lipstick, makeup, and false eyelashes removed . . . . Yes_____ No_____

Sanitary belts removed . . . . Yes_____ No_____

Nail polish removed . . . . Yes_____ No_____

Eyeglasses and contact lenses removed . . . . Yes_____ No_____

Prosthesis (artificial hearing aid, eye, leg, arm, and so forth)
    removed . . . . Yes_____ No_____

All clothing removed except clean hospital gown . . . . Yes_____ No_____

Patient allergic or sensitive to drugs . . . . Yes_____ No_____

Pre-op urine specimen obtained and sent to lab . . . . Yes_____ No_____

Urinary drainage bag emptied . . . . Yes_____ No_____

Side rails in up position . . . . Yes_____ No_____

Temperature _____ Pulse _____ Respiration _____

Blood Pressure _____ Weight _____ lbs. Height _____ ft. _____ in.

Time patient leaves for the operating room _____

Observations _____

Signature and title _____

KEY IDEAS:
SKIN PREPARATION

Before an operation, the patient's skin in the operative area must be free of hair and as clean as possible. Hair on the body is a breeding place for microorganisms. Because hair cannot be sterilized, it must be removed by shaving. The area on the body that is shaved is where the operation is going to be done. When you are shaving a patient before an operation, watch for scratches, pimples, cuts, sores, or rashes on the skin. If you see anything on the skin that looks unusual, be sure to report this to the head nurse or team leader.

In some hospitals, the patient is sent to the operating room suite one hour before he is scheduled for surgery. At that time the nurses in the operating room will prep the patient (shave the skin in preparation for surgery). This is done in those hospitals that have anterooms to the operating rooms. In the anteroom, each patient has his own cubicle, which is merely a curtained-off area. In other hospitals, the staff does the prep the evening before surgery. The operating room staff does another complete prep after the patient is on the operating room table.

The prep is done with a special prep kit. This is obtained from the central supply room for each patient. After it is used, it is discarded in the dirty utility room. Each kit contains a safety razor and a sponge filled with soap. Most hospitals have a special place to dispose of razors in the dirty utility room. It is usually a covered metal container. If your hospital does not supply a disposable prep kit, get the individual items from CSR.

Procedure: Shaving a Patient in Preparation for Surgery

1. Assemble your equipment:
   a) Disposable prep kit containing:
      - Razor and razor blades
      - Sponge filled with soap
      - Tissues
   b) Basin of water at 115°F (46.1°C)
   c) Bath blanket
   d) Towels

DISPOSABLE PREP KIT

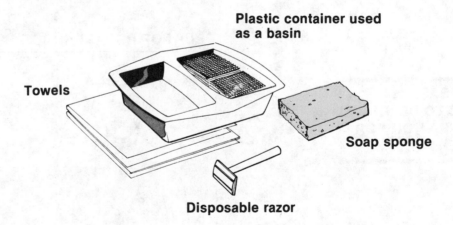

Plastic container used as a basin

Towels

Soap sponge

Disposable razor

2. Wash your hands.
3. Identify the patient by checking his identification bracelet.
4. Ask visitors to step out of the room.
5. Explain to the patient that you are going to shave him.
6. Pull the curtains around the bed for privacy.
7. Raise the bed to its highest horizontal position.
8. Place the bath blanket over the bedspread and top sheet. Ask the patient to hold the blanket in place. Fanfold the top sheets to the foot of the bed. Do this from underneath the blanket without exposing the patient.
9. Adjust the bedside lamp so that the area is well lighted. There should be no shadows where you will be working.

(continued next page)

10. Open the disposable prep kit.

11. Wet the soap sponge in the basin of water. Then soap the area to be shaved. Work up a good lather with the sponge.

12. Check to be sure the razor blade is in the correct position in the razor.

13. Hold the skin taut with a dry tissue. Shave in the direction the hair grows. Rinse the razor often. Keep the razor and the patient's skin wet and soapy throughout the shaving procedure.

14. Clean the patient's umbilicus (navel), if it is in the area to be shaved.

15. Wash the soap off the patient's skin. Dry thoroughly with the towel.

16. Clean your equipment and put it in its proper place. Discard disposable equipment.

17. Cover the patient with the top sheet and bedspread. Ask him to hold them while you take the bath blanket from underneath, without exposing the patient.

18. Make the patient comfortable.

19. Lower the bed to its lowest horizontal position.

20. Wash your hands.

21. Report to your head nurse or team leader:

    • The time at which you shaved the patient.

    • Your observations of anything unusual.

**KEY IDEAS:
AREAS TO BE SHAVED IN
PREPARATION FOR
SURGERY**

PREP FOR BREAST SURGERY

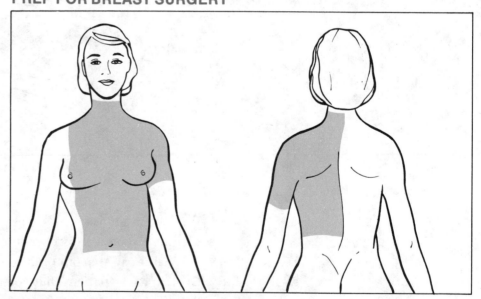

The area not being operated on is called the *unaffected* side. The area where the operation will be done is called the *affected side.* Shave from the nipple line of the unaffected side to the middle of the patient's back on the affected side. On the affected side, shave from the chin down to the umbilicus (navel), the axilla (armpit), and part of the upper arm.

CHEST PREP FOR THORACIC SURGERY

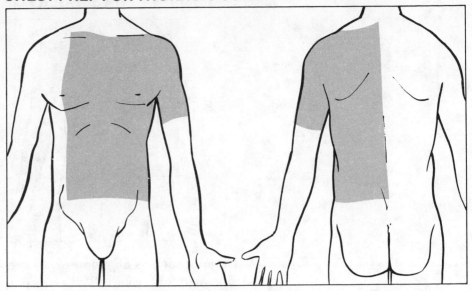

Shave the area extending from the nipple on the unaffected side, across the chest area of the affected side, and across the back, from the top of the shoulders down to the pubic hair.

ABDOMINAL PREP

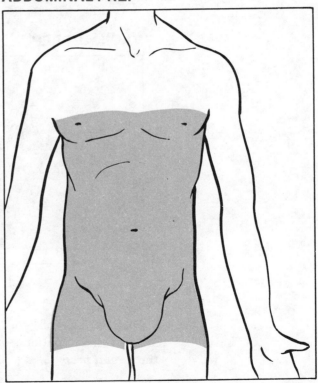

Shave from the nipple line on male patients, and from below the breasts on female patients, down to and including the pubic area. Shave the width of this area to each side of the body.

PREP FOR SURGERY OF EXTREMITY (ARM OR LEG)

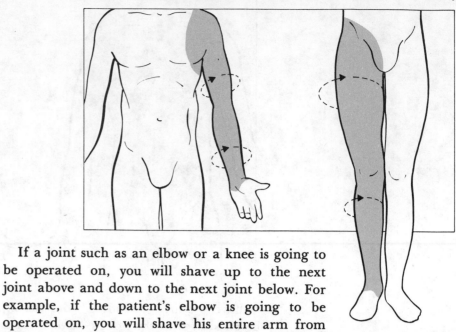

If a joint such as an elbow or a knee is going to be operated on, you will shave up to the next joint above and down to the next joint below. For example, if the patient's elbow is going to be operated on, you will shave his entire arm from the shoulder down to the wrist. If an area between joints is going to be operated on, you will shave the entire area, including the joints above and below. Shave all around an arm or a leg.

VAGINAL PREP

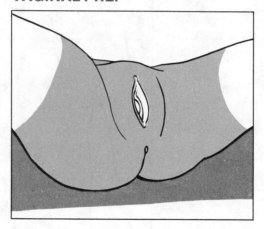

The words *vaginal prep* mean the preparation of the genital area of female patients.

SCROTAL PREP

Preparation of the genital area of male patients is called the *scrotal prep*.

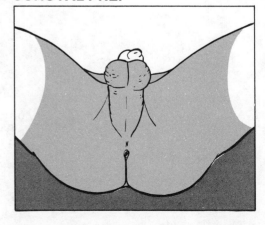

BACK PREP

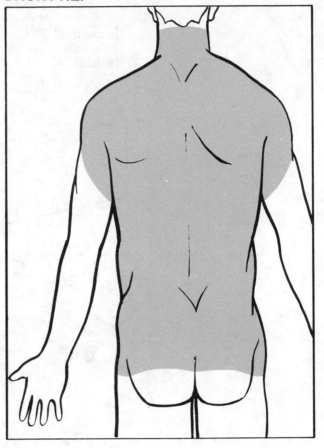

Shave the patient's entire back from the hairline on the neck down to the middle of the buttocks, including the axillary area.

After the patient has been given his preoperative medications by the medication nurse:

- Keep the side rails in the up position.
- Remind the patient that he is not to smoke or eat.

The transportation attendant or the operating room assistant will come to the floor at the proper time to take the patient to the operating room suite. Move the furniture out of the way. Make the room ready for the stretcher to be brought in. Assist with moving the patient from the bed to the stretcher. Tell the patient you will see him in his room after the surgery.

The transportation assistant will then wheel the patient on the stretcher to the head nurse's desk. At this time, the head nurse will give the attendant the patient's chart. She will check the name on the identification bracelet against the name on the chart. The attendant then takes the patient to the operating room.

Preparing the Patient's Unit to Receive the Patient After Surgery

Your next task is to strip the linen from the bed, make the operating room bed, and prepare the unit to receive the patient postoperatively.

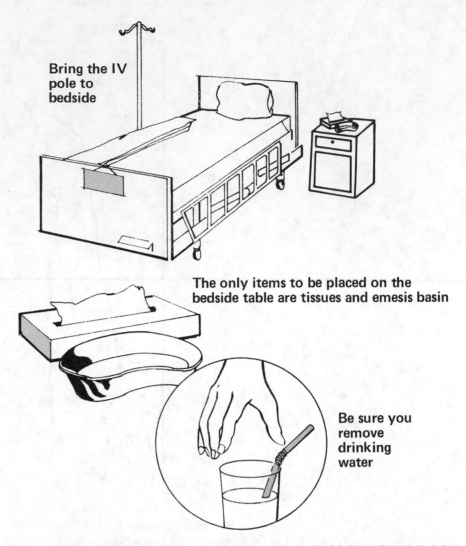

Bring the IV pole to bedside

The only items to be placed on the bedside table are tissues and emesis basin

Be sure you remove drinking water

WHEN TRANSPORTING THE PATIENT TO THE OPERATING ROOM:

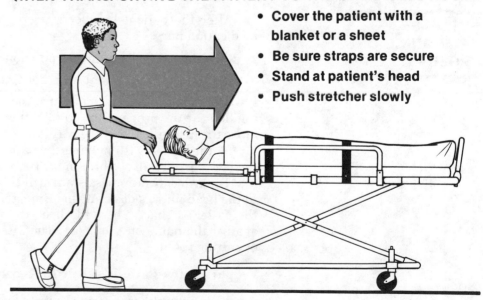

- Cover the patient with a blanket or a sheet
- Be sure straps are secure
- Stand at patient's head
- Push stretcher slowly

SECTION 2: POSTOPERATIVE NURSING CARE

OBJECTIVES: WHAT YOU WILL LEARN

When you have completed this section, you will be able to:

- Observe the patient for signs of postoperative problems.
- Provide a safe environment for the postoperative patient.

**KEY IDEAS:
THE POSTOPERATIVE
PATIENT**

Postoperative care means taking care of a patient right after surgery. Most patients are taken to a surgical recovery room immediately following surgery. They remain in the recovery room until they begin to recover from the effects of anesthesia. When the patient returns to his room, you will begin assisting with postoperative nursing care.

Anesthesia

Before surgery, the patient is given special medications that cause a loss of feeling in all or part of the body. This loss of feeling means the patient feels no pain. When the patient is under the influence of these special medications, called **anesthetics**, he is in a state of anesthesia. Some anesthetics cause the loss of sensation in the whole body. These are called general anesthetics. Some anesthetics cause a numbness or loss of feeling in only a part of the body. These medications are called local anesthetics. A spinal anesthetic causes loss of feeling in a large area of the body, usually from the umbilicus down to and including the legs and feet.

The doctor who administers the anesthetic to the patient in the operating room is known as an **anesthesiologist**. The registered nurse who administers the anesthetic to the patient in the operating room is known as an **anesthetist**.

Chest Complications Following Anesthesia
May Happen for Several Reasons:

- The anesthetic may irritate the patient's respiratory passages (mouth, nose, trachea, lungs) and cause the secretions in these passages to increase. This might raise the chance of an infection in the lungs or other parts of the respiratory system.

- Smoking tends to irritate the whole respiratory system. Smoking may increase the secretion of mucus, which also could raise the chance of an infection.

- After surgery, many patients are so sore they cannot breathe deeply. They cannot cough up the increased amount of mucous material being secreted in the lungs. This could cause a respiratory infection, such as pneumonia.

- A patient might vomit while he is still unconscious after surgery. The vomitus (vomited material) might be aspirated, that is, drawn back into the lungs. This could very quickly cause an infection or even the patient's death. Saliva might also be drawn into the throat and block the air passages, which could cause an infection.

- Unconsciousness and inactivity during anesthesia allow mucus to accumulate in the patient's respiratory passages. If ordered by the physician, the head nurse or team leader will call the inhalation therapy department (Pulmonary Medicine). Staff persons from that department will treat the patient with chest complications.

When the Patient Comes Back from Surgery

The patient will be coming back to his unit on a stretcher. Move the furniture out of the way and make sure the bedside area is clear. The stretcher then can be brought easily and quickly to its place next to the bed.

When the patient is brought back to the unit, you will do the following things:

- Help to move the patient safely from the stretcher to the bed.
- Be sure the patient is covered with blankets to keep him warm.
- Be sure the bedside rails are raised after the patient is in bed.
- Measure the patient's vital signs (T.P.R. & B.P.) as instructed by head nurse or team leader.
- Place signal cord within the patient's reach.

WHEN THE PATIENT AWAKENS FROM THE ANESTHESIA

Call the patient by his first name

This reassures the patient that someone who knows him is present

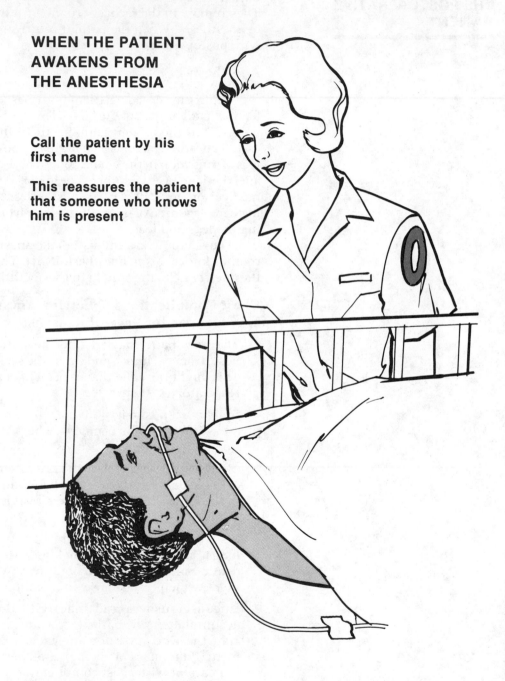

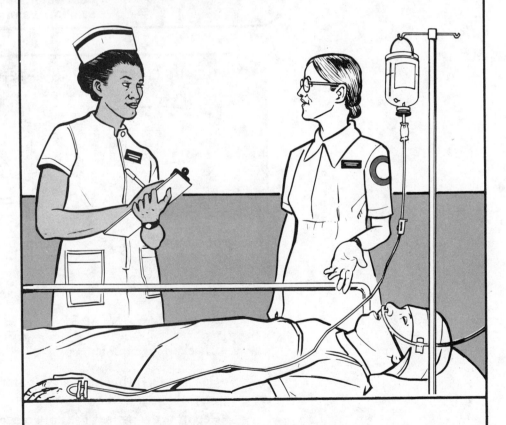

SIGNAL FOR YOUR HEAD NURSE OR TEAM LEADER IMMEDIATELY IF YOU NOTICE ANY OF THESE SYMPTOMS

Observe the patient for

- Rise or fall of blood preassure
- Choking
- Pulse: fast (above 100), slow (below 60) or an irregular pulse beat
- Respirations: rapid (above 30), labored
- Skin, lips, fingernails: very pale or turning blue (CYANOSIS)
- Thirst: patient asks for water often
- Unusual or extreme restlessness
- Moaning or complaining of pain
- Sudden bright red bleeding
- Any other noticeable sudden changes

- A patient may appear to be unconscious, but not really be. . . He may be able to hear you
- Say only those things you would want the patient to hear if he were fully conscious

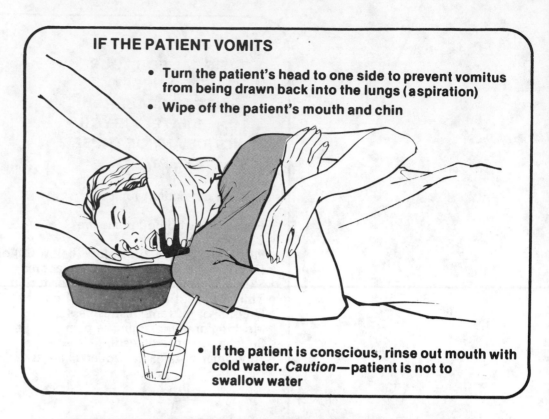

IF THE PATIENT VOMITS

- Turn the patient's head to one side to prevent vomitus from being drawn back into the lungs (aspiration)
- Wipe off the patient's mouth and chin

- If the patient is conscious, rinse out mouth with cold water. *Caution*—patient is not to swallow water

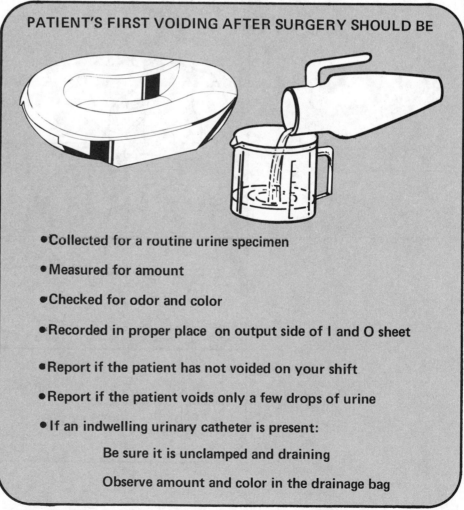

PATIENT'S FIRST VOIDING AFTER SURGERY SHOULD BE

- Collected for a routine urine specimen

- Measured for amount

- Checked for odor and color

- Recorded in proper place on output side of I and O sheet

- Report if the patient has not voided on your shift

- Report if the patient voids only a few drops of urine

- If an indwelling urinary catheter is present:

    Be sure it is unclamped and draining

    Observe amount and color in the drainage bag

WHEN A PATIENT IS RECEIVING IV FLUIDS:

- Check the IV solution or blood transfusion for proper flow of fluid
- Check the skin for swelling, bleeding, or pain around the needle
- Do not adjust the clamps or flow rate
- Signal for your head nurse or team leader immediately if the patient's skin around the needle is swollen or bleeding, or if the fluid is not running properly

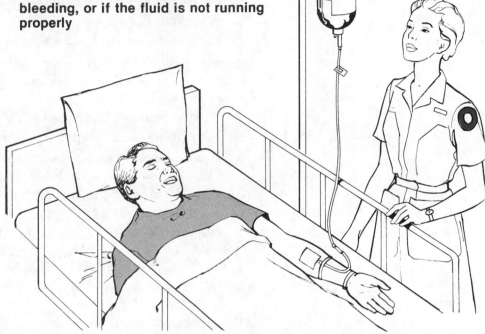

TURNING THE POSTOPERATIVE PATIENT

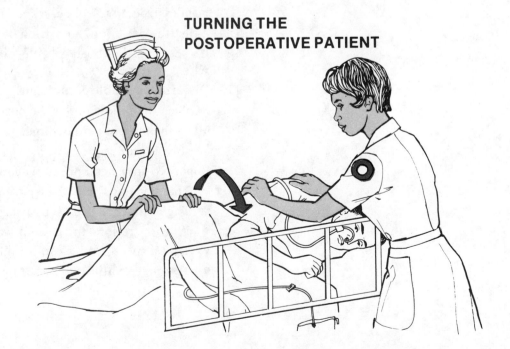

Unless you are instructed not to, you should move a postoperative patient into a new position every 2 hours (q2h). This helps him rest better, protects his skin, promotes healing and helps prevent pneumonia. Each time the patient is moved he should be turned onto his opposite side so he faces the other side of the bed. Move the patient's legs at the same time.

If the patient's gown becomes wet, change it immediately. Change the bed linens whenever they become damp and soiled. Take the blankets off the bed if the patient complains of being too warm. Keep the side rails up at all times.

KEY IDEAS: DEEP-BREATHING EXERCISES

Deep-breathing exercises expand the lungs by increasing lung movement and assist in bringing up lung secretions. These exercises will help in preventing postoperative pneumonia or pneumonitis.

Procedure: Helping the Patient with Deep-Breathing Exercises

1. Assemble your equipment:
   a) Pillow
   b) Specimen container, if a specimen is ordered
   c) Tissues
2. Report to the medication nurse that you are ready to start deep-breathing exercises. If she wishes to give the patient medication to relieve him of any discomfort or pain, she will do so at this time.
3. Wash your hands.
4. Identify the patient by checking the identification bracelet.
5. Ask visitors to step out of the room.
6. Tell the patient that you are going to help him with deep-breathing exercises.
7. Pull the curtain around the bed for privacy.
8. Offer the patient a bedpan or urinal.
9. Dangle the patient's legs over the side of the bed, if allowed. If not, place the patient in as much of a sitting position as possible.
10. Place the pillow on the patient's abdomen for support.
11. Ask him to breathe deeply 10 times.
12. Count the respirations out loud to the patient as he inhales and exhales. If the patient cannot breathe deeply, ask him to cough. Coughing is just another way of breathing deeply.
13. Ask the patient to feel his chest as he breathes to encourage deeper breathing.
14. Tell the patient to cough up all loose secretions into the tissues, if a specimen is not necessary, or into a specimen container, if you have been instructed to collect a specimen.
15. Assist the patient to a position of comfort and safety in bed.
16. If a specimen has been collected, label it, and send to the laboratory with a requisition slip.
17. Discard disposable equipment.
18. Replace the pillow under the patient's head.
19. Make the patient comfortable.
20. Wash your hands.
21. Report to your head nurse or team leader:
    - That you have helped the patient with deep-breathing exercises.
    - The number of breathing exercises.
    - What secretions the patient was able to cough up.
    - That a specimen was collected and sent to the lab.
    - Your observations of anything unusual.

SECTION 3: BINDERS AND ELASTIC BANDAGES

OBJECTIVES: WHAT YOU WILL LEARN

When you have completed this section, you will be able to:

- Apply the five types of binders.
- Apply elastic bandages and anti-embolism elastic stockings.
- Apply triangle sling bandages.

Binders are wide cloth bandages, usually made of cotton. They are used on different parts of a patient's body for several reasons. Binders can be used postoperatively, or after childbirth, or whenever it is desirable to:

- Give support to a weakened body part.
- Hold dressing and bandages in place.
- Put pressure on parts of the body to make the patient more comfortable.

The head nurse or team leader will tell you if a particular patient is to have a binder applied and what kind of binder is to be used. Remember that, unless the binder is put on properly, it can be more uncomfortable for the patient than if it had not been used at all. Binders are obtained from the central supply room (CSR).

Rules to Follow: Binders

- Keep the binder smooth and clean. Otherwise it will be uncomfortable in the same way that crumbs or wrinkles in the patient's bed are uncomfortable. Bedsores (decubitus ulcers) can be caused by wrinkles or wetness of a binder.
- Watch for reddened areas on the patient's skin. Report these to your head nurse or team leader.
- Use the correct type of binder. Be sure it is the correct size.
- There are five different types of binders commonly used:

STRAIGHT ABDOMINAL BINDER

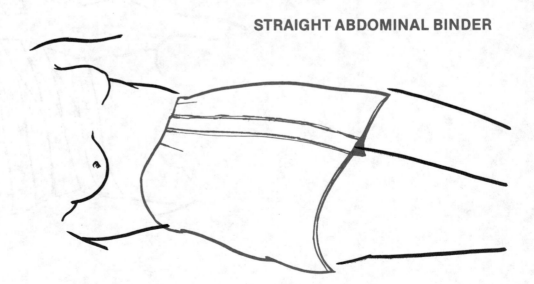

The straight abdominal binder is used for the same purposes as the scultetus binder. It usually is applied from the bottom up (toward the heart), and darts are pinned to the top of the binder to make sure it will fit snugly. The straight abdominal binder may be fastened with velcro.

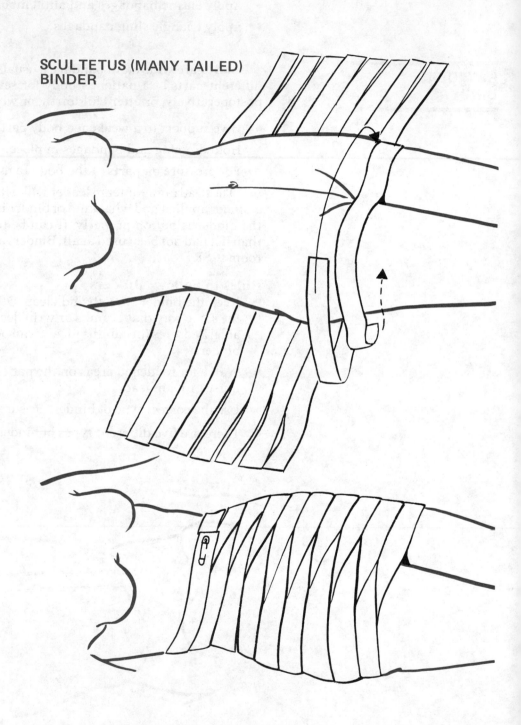

SCULTETUS (MANY TAILED) BINDER

The scultetus binder is called the many-tailed binder because of its shape. It is used to hold dressings in place and to provide pressure and support. It is applied from the bottom up (or toward the heart) and is fastened with one safety pin at the top tail.

BREAST BINDER

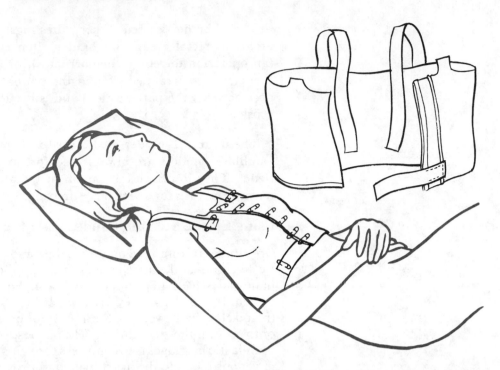

The breast binder sometimes is used with female patients after childbirth or after breast surgery. The binder gives support to the breasts and holds dressings in place. Sometimes the binder is used to compress the breasts when it is necessary to dry up the patient's milk, as with a patient who will not be breast feeding her baby. The binder is first fastened at the shoulders. It then is fastened along the front, working from the middle to the top and bottom. Darts are pinned at the waist to provide room and support for the breasts and also to help make the binder fit better. Ask the patient to support her breasts inward and upward with her hands, outside the binder, as you pin it together.

T BINDER

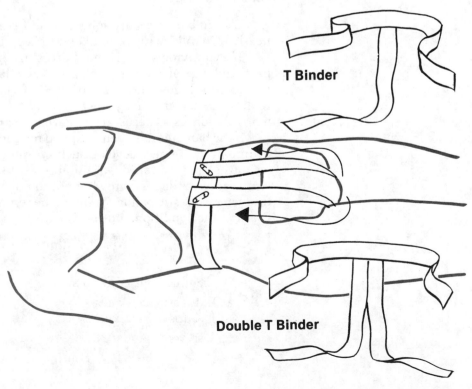

T Binder

Double T Binder

The T binder is used to keep dressings in place on the perineal (genital) area and rectal area. This binder often is used after a hemorrhoidectomy (an operation to remove hemorrhoids), or after the delivery of a baby. The binder is first wrapped around the patient's waist. Part of the binder then goes between the patient's legs and is brought back up to be fastened at the waist.

The double T binder is also used for holding perineal dressings in place. Double T binders are always used for holding these dressings on male patients. They sometimes are used on female patients if rectal surgery is extensive and calls for a very large dressing.

Using Elastic Stockings and Elastic Bandages

Binders are applied mainly to the torso of the patient. Anti-embolism elastic stockings and elastic bandages are applied to the body extremities (arms, hands, legs, feet). In postoperative care, they are most often used on the lower extremities, or legs. They are used either as treatment for thrombophlebitis (blood clots in the veins of the leg), or for phlebitis (inflammation of the veins) or to prevent these conditions. The purpose of anti-embolism elastic stockings and elastic bandages is to compress the veins and therefore improve the return of venous blood to the heart, which improves circulation.

In cases of sprain or strain at the joint, they are used to provide support and comfort.

Applying Anti-Embolism Elastic Stockings

Anti-embolism elastic stockings can be either knee-length or full-length. Be careful to smooth out all the wrinkles. Be sure the stocking is pulled up firmly. Elastic stockings must be removed and reapplied at least once every day and more often if the doctor has so ordered. These stockings come in various sizes. Be sure they are the right size and fit the patient. They should be applied while the patient is lying down (not sitting in a chair) before getting out of bed.

Elastic Bandages

Elastic bandages are long strips of elasticized cotton. They are wound neatly into rolls, with a metal clip to keep the end in place.

They provide support, hold dressings in place, apply pressure to a body part, and improve return circulation. Bandages may be ordered toes to knees, toes to mid-thighs, toes to groin, or heel free, (heel free means heel uncovered). Follow the instructions given to you by the head nurse or team leader. Use as many bandages as necessary to cover the area as ordered.

If the bandage has been wrapped too tightly, the patient's circulation may be impaired. He may develop such symptoms as paleness, coldness, blueness (cyanosis), pain, swelling, or numbness in the extremities. Be very careful to wrap these bandages firmly but not too tightly. Check the patient's condition frequently. Elastic bandages should be removed and re-applied once per shift. Observe the condition and color of the skin every hour (q.h.).

Procedure: Applying Elastic Bandages

1. Assemble your equipment:
   a) Elastic bandages
   b) Clips or safety pins
2. Wash your hands.

(continued next page)

ELASTIC STOCKINGS AND BANDAGES

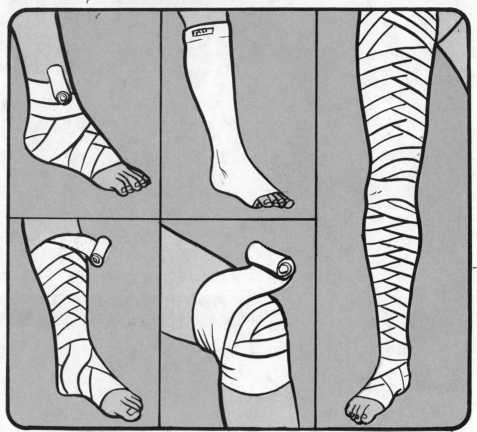

Procedure continued

3. Identify the patient by checking the identification bracelet.

4. Ask visitors to step out of the room.

5. Tell the patient that you are going to wrap his leg or arm (or whatever area is to be wrapped) with an elastic bandage.

6. Pull the curtain around the bed for privacy.

7. Place the patient in a comfortable position that is convenient for you to work. Expose the area to be wrapped.

8. Extend the part of the body to be bandaged. Support the patient's heel or wrist.

9. Stand directly in front of the patient or facing the part to be bandaged.

10. Hold the bandage with the loose end coming off the bottom of the roll.

11. Anchor the bandage by two circular turns around the body part at its smallest point. This usually is the ankle or the wrist.

12. Apply the bandage in the same direction as venous circulation, that is, toward the heart.

13. Roll the bandage smoothly and wrap it firmly but not too tightly.

14. Exert even pressure. Keep the bandage smooth. Be sure no skin areas show between the turns.

15. If possible, leave the toes or fingers exposed for observation of circulatory changes.

(continued next page)

16. Continue wrapping upward with a spiral turn. Each turn should overlap the one before about one-half width of the bandage.

17. After applying the bandage, secure the terminal end by pinning it with a safety pin or by applying bandage clips.

18. If more than one bandage is used, overlap them to prevent the bandages from slipping.

19. To remove the bandage, unwind it gently. Gather it into a loose mass, passing the mass from hand to hand as the bandage is unwound. Then roll the bandage smoothly so it is ready for the next application.

20. Make the patient comfortable.

21. Wash your hands.

22. Report to your head nurse or team leader:

    - That you have applied or removed the elastic bandages.

    - The area of application.

    - Your observations of anything unusual.

Procedure: Applying a Triangle Sling Bandage

1. Assemble your equipment:
   a) Triangle of material, or a square of cloth folded into a triangle, or a commercially packaged triangle bandage
   b) Pin
   c) Small pieces of soft absorbent material

2. Wash your hands.

3. Identify the patient by checking his identification bracelet.

4. Ask all visitors to leave the room.

5. Tell the patient that you are going to apply the sling bandage.

6. Pull the curtains around the bed for privacy.

7. Assist the patient to a comfortable position. If the patient is permitted to sit on the side of the bed (dangle), have him do so.

8. Place small pieces of soft absorbent material wherever two areas of skin touch. This will prevent body parts from rubbing against each other, causing friction. Areas to place these absorbent pieces are the folds of the body where skin touches skin, such as under the breasts, between the arm and the chest, and in the axilla.

9. Place one end of the triangle over the shoulder on the uninjured side with the point of the triangle extending under the injured arm or shoulder.

10. Be gentle. Bring the other end of the triangle over the shoulder on the injured side, allowing enough of the bandage to reach around the back of the neck.

11. The patient's hand must be higher than the elbow and be supported to prevent "wrist drop."

12. To give desired support, adjust the sling to the patient's size.

13. Tie the ends of the bandage at the side of the neck.

14. To avoid a pressure point, use a square knot.

(continued next page)

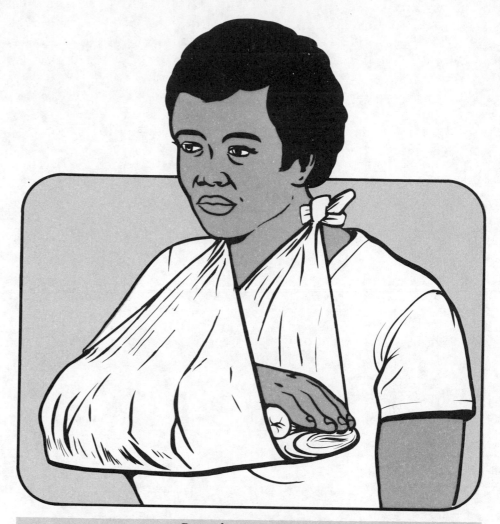

15. Tie a knot or fold the corner of the bandage at the elbow and pin it in place to keep the elbow from moving out of the support.

16. Check this patient every hour (q.h.) for skin color, positioning, circulation, and comfort.

17. Make the patient comfortable.

18. Wash your hands.

19. Report to your head nurse or team leader:

    • That the triangle bandage has been applied.

    • The time it was applied.

    • The patient's comments as to the comfort of the bandage.

    • Your observations of anything unusual.

WHAT YOU HAVE LEARNED

As a nursing assistant, you will be part of both preoperative and postoperative care. Giving good nursing care before and after surgery is very important for the well-being of the patient.

Shaving the operative area in preparation for surgery, filling in all blanks on the preoperative checklist, and following the instructions of your head nurse or team leader are your main duties when working with surgical patients.

17 EXTENDED CARE PATIENTS

1. Care of the Incontinent Patient
2. Care of the Diabetic Patient
3. Care of the Orthopedic Patient
4. Care of the Ostomy Patient
5. Care of the Seizure Patient

SECTION 1: CARE OF THE INCONTINENT PATIENT

OBJECTIVES: WHAT YOU WILL LEARN

When you have completed this section, you will be able to:

- Care for the patient's skin to help prevent bedsores.
- Recognize the signs of a bedsore (decubitus ulcer).
- Care for the incontinent patient.
- Re-toilet train the incontinent patient.

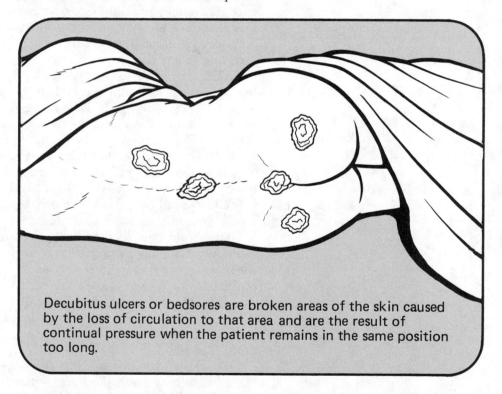

Decubitus ulcers or bedsores are broken areas of the skin caused by the loss of circulation to that area and are the result of continual pressure when the patient remains in the same position too long.

**KEY IDEAS:
DECUBITUS ULCERS**

Decubitus ulcers, called bedsores or pressure sores, are areas where the skin has broken because of prolonged pressure. Injury to the skin comes from pressure on a part of the body where there is loss of circulation (blood flow). Then the tissues are destroyed. If decubitus ulcers are not treated, they quickly get larger, become very painful, and usually become infected.

The direct cause of bedsores is interference with the circulation of blood in a part of the body. The interference usually is caused by pressure over the **bony prominences.** These are places where bones are close to the surface of the body.

The pressure can come from the weight of the body lying in one position for too long or from splints, casts, or bandages. Even wrinkles in the bed linen can be a cause of bedsores.

Bedsores are often made worse by continued pressure, heat, moisture, and lack of cleanliness. Irritating substances on the skin such as perspiration, urine, feces, material from wound discharges, or soap that has been left on the skin after a bath all tend to make bedsores worse.

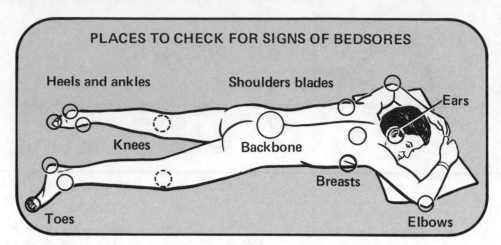

PLACES TO CHECK FOR SIGNS OF BEDSORES

Heels and ankles • Shoulders blades • Ears • Knees • Backbone • Breasts • Toes • Elbows

Preventing bedsores is the responsibility of the entire nursing team. These sores are usually the result of carelessness or a lack of knowledge and skill in caring for the patient. Once even a mild bedsore has formed, it is very hard to cure. Therefore, as a nursing assistant, you have to know how to prevent bedsores and how to recognize them when they do occur. Report the first sign of a bedsore to your head nurse or team leader so that steps can be taken to prevent further damage.

The signs of a bedsore on the skin are heat, redness, tenderness, discomfort, and a feeling of burning. When the skin is broken, a bedsore has formed. Specific treatment for a bedsore is prescribed by a doctor. The wound, however, must be kept clean and the rules of asepsis must be followed. As you have learned, the skin is where the battle for asepsis begins.

Places to check on the body for signs of bedsores are the bony areas. These are, for example, the shoulder blades, elbows, knees, heels, ankles, and backbone. Usually these areas are covered only by a thin layer of skin. They receive a smaller supply of blood than other areas of the body. These are the areas where bedsores are most likely to occur.

Obese patients tend to develop bedsores where body parts rub against each other, causing friction. Places to check on obese patients are the folds of the body where skin touches skin, such as under the breasts, between the folds of the buttocks, and between the thighs.

The doctor may order special equipment to reduce the pressure on the skin. One way is to use an air cushion or a sponge rubber cushion under the base of the spine, sacrum, or lower back. If you use an air cushion, do not fill it more than half full.

There are special devices that can be used to reduce the pressure on the heels, the elbows, and the back of the head, such as sheepskin booties and sheepskin elbow pads. Also used are pillows, pads, air mattresses, alternating pressure mattresses, flotation beds or pads, and commode flotation pads. The roto-rest bed, which constantly turns the patient, is an excellent device to minimize pressure points.

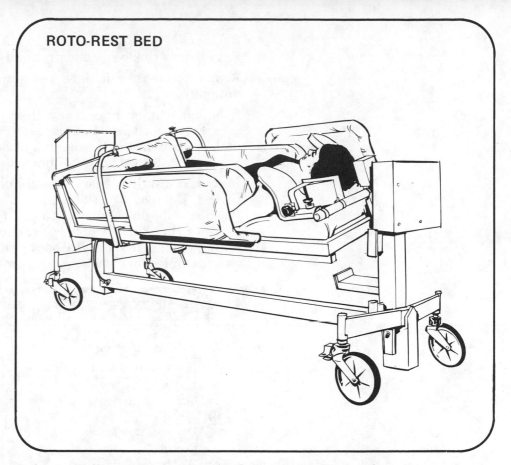

ROTO-REST BED

Rules to Follow: Preventing Bedsores (Decubitus Ulcers)

You, the nursing assistant, can help to prevent bedsores by doing the following:

- Turn the patient often. You should change the patient's position every two (2) hours.

- Be careful when using bedpans because pressure from sitting on the rim and friction when putting the patient on the pan or when taking the patient off can create or worsen bedsores. Never leave the patient on the bedpan longer than necessary. Use care when removing the bedpan to avoid spilling urine on the skin as urine could irritate and cause further damage to the reddened or tender area. Covering the bedpan with pads can reduce some pressure and powdering the rim will minimize friction.

- Keep the patient's body as clean and dry as possible. Change the patient's gown if it is damp. Wash the patient's skin with mild soap to remove urine or feces. Use lotion on the skin to prevent contact with discharged materials from wounds, which can cause irritation.

- If a part of the patient's body shows signs of developing a bedsore, gently rub the area with skin lotion. This should be done every two hours. Rub with a circular motion, away from the affected part of the body, but not directly on the affected area as too much rubbing may break the skin. Rubbing, that is, friction, stimulates the circulation of blood in the affected area.

- Use powder or corn starch where skin surfaces come together and form creases. However, use it sparingly. Examples are under the breasts of women patients, between the buttocks, and in the folds of skin on the abdomen. Corn starch helps keep these areas dry. When bathing the patient be sure to wash the corn starch off completely. This is especially important in caring for obese patients.

- Keep linen wrinkle-free and dry at all times.

- Remove crumbs, hair pins, and any other hard objects from the bed promptly.

- If the patient is incontinent, use a disposable bed protector. This allows the area that is soiled to be cleaned easily and often. These protect the linen the patient has to lie on. Be sure that plastic never touches the patient's skin and change the bed protector immediately when it becomes wet.

- In some institutions a large disposable diaper is used for the incontinent patient. However, the skin underneath must be watched carefully for a reaction to the diaper material and to irritations caused by urine and feces touching the skin. The diaper prevents the urine and bowel movement from spreading to the entire body of the patient. However, it needs to be changed immediately when soiled or wet.

Procedure: Preventing Decubitus Ulcers (Bedsores) in the Incontinent Patient

1. Assemble your equipment:
   a) Basin of water at 115°F (46.1°C)
   b) Soap
   c) Corn starch or powder
   d) Towels
   e) Disposable gloves
   f) Lotion
   g) Washcloths

2. Wash your hands.

3. Identify the patient by checking the identification bracelet.

4. Ask visitors to step out of the room.

5. Tell the patient you are going to wash him.

6. Pull the curtain for privacy.

7. Put on the disposable gloves.

8. Using the toilet tissue, wipe away as much feces as possible, then wash the area that has urine or feces on it very well, removing all waste material from the skin.

9. Rinse with water, changing the water frequently.

10. Dry with a circular motion to stimulate blood circulation.

11. Apply lotion to the buttocks and back, massaging to stimulate blood circulation.

12. Wipe off any excess lotion.

13. Apply corn starch or powder only where skin surfaces touch other skin surfaces (creases).

14. Leave the top sheets loose so air can get to every part of the patient's body.

15. Turn the patient to a different position every two hours.

16. Keep the patient dry at all times by checking the patient every two hours. Re-make the bed as necessary.

17. Make the patient comfortable.

18. Discard disposable equipment.

19. Place dirty soiled linen in the laundry bag, and then place the bag into the dirty linen hamper in the utility room.

(continued next page)

Procedure continued

20. Remove and discard gloves.
21. Wash your hands.
22. Report to your head nurse or team leader:
    - That the patient is incontinent of urine and/or feces.
    - That the patient was washed and his skin is now clean and dry.
    - That the patient's position was changed every two hours, and the time of each position change.
    - Any signs of decubitus ulcers.
    - The color, amount, and consistency of the feces and urine you cleaned.
    - Your observations of anything unusual.

KEY IDEAS: RE-TOILET TRAINING THE INCONTINENT PATIENT

Incontinent patients are those who have lost all or only part of their control over their excretory functions. In some cases of incontinence re-toilet training or rehabilitation may be used to help the patient regain some or all of this lost control. Offering the patient the bedpan or urinal at regularly scheduled intervals helps the patient avoid incontinence.

If prescribed by the physician, a rectal suppository ordered on a regular schedule can help train the patient to empty his rectum while he is on the bedpan. Follow the instructions of your head nurse or team leader for the time and type of suppository to be used. Follow the procedure for the insertion of the suppository (Chapter 11, Section 1).

Procedure: Re-Toilet Training and Rehabilitation of the Incontinent Patient

1. Assemble your equipment:
   a) Urinal, if appropriate
   b) Bedpan or bedside commode
   c) Container of warm water 105°F (40.5°C)
   d) Towel
   e) Suppositories, as ordered by the physician
2. Wash your hands.
3. Identify the patient by checking the identification bracelet.
4. Ask visitors to step out of the room.
5. Tell the patient that you are going to give him a bedpan.
6. Pull the curtain for privacy.
7. To stimulate evacuation of the bowel and bladder, place the patient on a bedpan or on the bedside commode or walk him to the bathroom every two hours.
8. Pour warm water at 105°F (40.5°C) over the genital area into the bedpan to stimulate elimination.
9. Dry the patient with toilet tissue.
10. Remove the bedpan.
11. Help the patient back into bed from the bedside commode or toilet.
12. Wash the patient's hands.
13. Make the patient comfortable.
14. Wash your hands.

(continued next page)

15. Report to the head nurse or team leader:
    - That the patient was placed on the bedpan, commode, or toilet on a regular basis.
    - The time this was done.
    - If the patient urinated or moved his bowels into the bedpan, commode, or toilet.
    - Your observations of anything unusual.

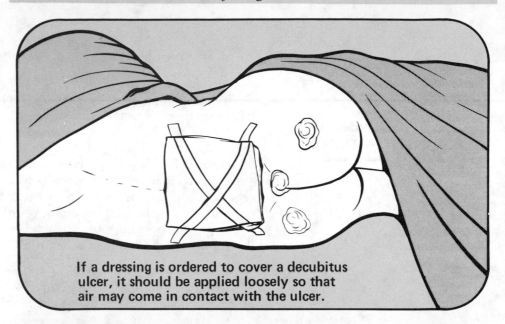

If a dressing is ordered to cover a decubitus ulcer, it should be applied loosely so that air may come in contact with the ulcer.

Procedure: Special Back Care (Back Rub) to Prevent Decubitus Ulcers

1. Assemble your equipment:
   a) Towels
   b) Lotion, standing in a basin of warm water 115°F (46.1°C)
2. Wash your hands.
3. Identify the patient by checking the identification bracelet.
4. Ask visitors to step out of the room.
5. Tell the patient you are going to give him a back rub.
6. Pull the curtain around the bed for privacy.
7. Ask the patient to turn on his side so that his back is toward you, or have him turn on his abdomen. If he is unable to turn, turn him into whichever of these two positions is most comfortable for the patient and yourself.
8. The side rail should be in the up position on the far side of the bed.
9. Lotion should be warmed by placing the container in a basin of warm water 115°F (46.1°C).
10. Open the ties on the gown. Put a towel lengthwise on the mattress close to the patient's back.
11. Pour a small amount of lotion into the palm of your hand.
12. Rub your hands together to warm the lotion using friction.

(continued)

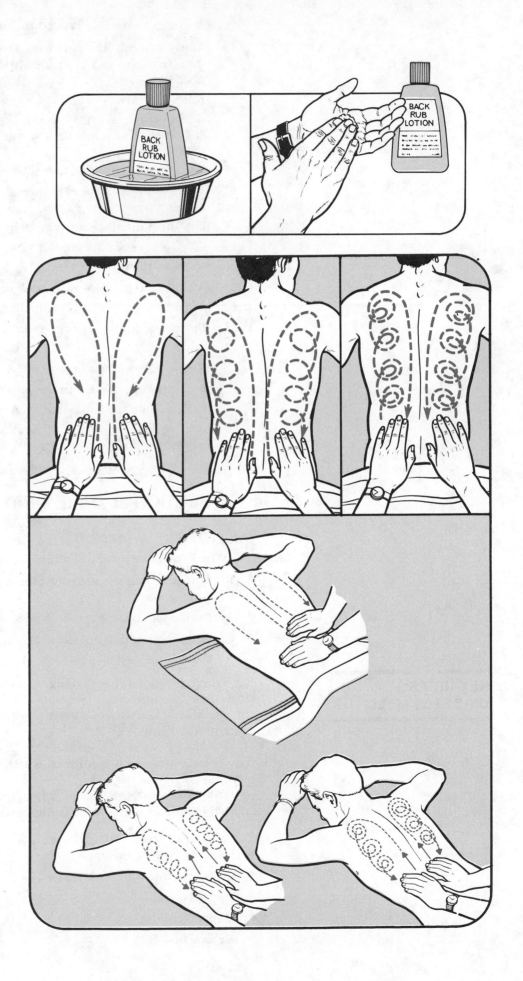

13. Apply lotion to the entire back with the palms of your hands. Use long, firm strokes from the buttocks to the shoulders and back of the neck.

14. Keep your knees slightly bent and your back straight.

15. Exert firm pressure as you stroke upward from the buttocks to the shoulders. Use gentle pressure as you stroke downward from shoulders to buttocks.

16. Use a circular motion on each bony area.

17. This rhythmic rubbing motion should be continued for one and one-half to three minutes.

18. Dry the patient's back by patting gently with a towel.

19. Close and re-tie the gown.

20. Remove the towels.

21. Assist the patient to turn back to a comfortable position.

22. Arrange the top sheets of the bed neatly.

23. Put your equipment back in its proper place.

24. Wash your hands.

25. Report to your head nurse or team leader:
    - That you have given the patient special back care.
    - The time the care was given.
    - The number of times this care was given on your shift. (This is done if the special back care is ordered every two hours.)
    - Your observations of anything unusual.

SECTION 2: CARE OF THE DIABETIC PATIENT

OBJECTIVES: WHAT YOU WILL LEARN

When you have completed this section, you will be able to:

- Recognize the signs and symptoms of diabetes mellitus, insulin shock, and diabetic coma.
- Test urine for sugar, acetone, and ketones.
- Collect a fresh fractional urine specimen.

**KEY IDEAS:
DIABETES MELLITUS**

When the body cannot change starches and sugar into energy and cannot store them because of an imbalance of hormones (insulin), the result is the chronic disease known as **diabetes mellitus**, which is a disturbance of carbohydrate metabolism.

Insulin shock is a condition that occurs in patients with diabetes when they receive too much insulin or when they miss a meal or have too much physical activity.

Diabetic coma may occur when the diabetic patient does not receive enough insulin or when there is increased stress or infection.

Terms Often Used with Diabetes Mellitus:

- FBS—fasting blood sugar
- GTT—glucose tolerance test
- Hypoglycemia
- Hyperglycemia
- Ketone bodies

- Gangrene—necrosis
- S&A test—sugar and acetone test
- Pancreas—Islands of Langerhans—endocrine and exocrine glands
- PPBS—post-prandial blood sugar
- Fresh fractional urine specimen

Signs and Symptoms of Diabetes Mellitus:
- Fatigue, tiredness
- Loss of weight
- Vaginitis—inflammation of the vagina
- Skin erosions—sores heal poorly and slowly
- Hyperglycemia—high blood sugar
- Glycosuria—sugar in the urine
- Polyuria—frequent and large amounts of urine
- Polydipsia—excessive thirst
- Poor vision—eyesight affected

Signs and Symptoms of Insulin Shock (Hypoglycemia/Low Blood Sugar—Insulin Reaction):
- Excessive sweating, perspiration
- Faintness, dizziness, weakness
- Hunger
- Irritability, personality change, nervousness
- Numbness of tongue and lips
- Not able to awaken, coma, unconciousness, stupor
- Headache
- Tremors, trembling
- Blurred or impaired vision
- Upon examination: a) Low blood surgar; b) No sugar in the urine

Signs and Symptoms of Diabetic Coma (Hyperglycemia/High Blood Sugar—Diabetic Acidosis):
- Air hunger, heavy labored breathing, increased respirations
- Loss of appetite
- Nausea and/or vomiting
- Weakness
- Abdominal pains or discomfort
- Generalized aches
- Increased thirst and parched tongue
- Sweet or fruity odor of the breath
- Flushed skin
- Dry skin
- Increased urination
- Soft eyeballs
- Dulled senses
- Upon examination: a) Large amounts of sugar and ketones in the urine; b) High blood sugar

When caring for a diabetic patient, you may be asked to perform certain diagnostic tests on the patient's urine. There are two basic tests: one for sugar (the **Clinitest**) and one for acetone (the **Acetest**). In your work you will collect the **fresh fractional urine specimen**. However, the actual test may be done in a laboratory or by the medication nurse, head nurse, or team leader. In certain situations you may do the tests. The term **fractional urine** is used to mean the specimen collected for both sugar and acetone tests. The results of these tests are needed by the doctor and the medication or primary nurse to determine changes that must be made in the diabetic patient's diet and medications.

These tests are usually done four times a day: one-half hour before breakfast, lunch, supper, and at bedtime.

For each test you will be using either a reagent strip or a reagent tablet. A **reagent** is a substance used in a chemical reaction to determine the presence of another substance. The names for these tablets or strips vary greatly according to geographical area and the pharmaceutical company from which they are purchased. When testing for sugar—doing the Clinitest—you will be using Clinitest tablets, Tes-tape, Clinistix, or Uristix. When testing for acetone—doing the Acetest—you will be using Ketostix, Tes-tape, Acetone Tablets, Uristix, or Labstix.

Some institutions have a small individual disposable kit for these tests, which is ordered from the central supply room or from the pharmacy for each patient. The patient's name should be written on the container. It should be kept in the patient's bathroom or in a designated place in the dirty utility room.

Instructions for these tests are usually posted in every dirty utility room. You also will find instructions for these tests on the package of reagent strips or reagent tablets. All tablets and strips used for these tests are **poisonous**. Always put equipment in a safe place where children cannot reach it. Heat is generated during the Clinitest. Do not touch the bottom of the glass test tube while doing the tests as it will be hot and you could burn yourself.

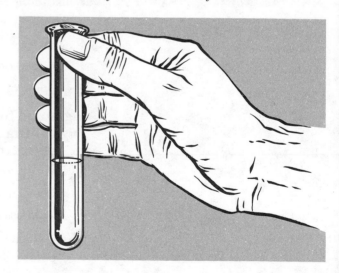

Fresh Specimens

A fresh specimen is needed for each testing. However, since the sugar test and the acetone test are done at the same time, one specimen is needed. The word **fresh** is used to refer to urine that has been accumulated recently in the patient's urinary bladder. To obtain fresh urine, it is necessary to discard the first urine voided because this urine has remained in the urinary bladder for an unknown length of time. One-half hour after discarding the urine, collect a fresh urine specimen for the test. This will be urine recently accumulated in the urinary bladder. The word **fractional** is used to refer to a small portion of the urine voided. Only a very small amount of urine is needed for these tests.

Procedure: Collecting a Fresh Fractional Urine (FR.U.) Specimen

1. Assemble your equipment:
   a) Bedpan and cover, urinal, or specipan
   b) Urine specimen container with cover
   c) Graduate, to measure output if the patient is on intake and output
   d) Label, if necessary. You will write on the label or on the cover of the container depending on the policy of the institution
   e) Disposable gloves (optional)

2. Wash your hands.

3. Identify the patient by checking the identification bracelet.

4. Ask visitors to step out of the room.

5. Tell the patient you need some urine for a urine test.

6. Pull the curtain around the bed for privacy.

7. Ask the patient to urinate into the bedpan, urinal, or specipan one-half hour before the test is to be done, in order to empty the bladder. If the patient is unable to void at this time, report this to your head nurse or team leader and follow her instructions.

8. If the patient is on intake and output, measure the urine and record the amount on the intake and output sheet.

9. Throw away this urine.

10. Prepare a label for the container with the patient's name, copying from the patient's identification bracelet. Record the date and time of collection and the name of the specimen. Place the correct label on the specimen container for the correct patient.

11. Have the patient void again at the correct time for the test so that fresh urine is used for the test.

12. Take the covered bedpan or urinal to the patient's bathroom or to the dirty utility room.

13. If the patient is on intake and output, measure and record the amount on the intake and output sheet.

14. If the urine is to be tested on the patient care unit, test it at this time. If the specimen is to be tested in the laboratory, pour the urine into the urine specimen container and label it. Send or take the specimen with a requisition or laboratory request slip to the lab immediately.

15. Discard the remaining urine. Wash the bedpan or urinal and put it in its proper place.

16. Wash the patient's hands and make him comfortable.

17. Wash your hands.

18. Report to your head nurse or team leader:
   - That the fresh fractional urine specimen has been obtained.
   - The result of the test or that the specimen has been sent to the laboratory or that it is in the proper place for testing.
   - The date and time of collection.
   - Your observations of anything unusual.

The Clinitest and Clinistix test are tests done to determine the amount of **glucose** (sugar) in the patient's urine. **Urine glucose level** refers to the amount of sugar in the urine.

Procedure: The Clinitest

1. Assemble your equipment:
   a) Fresh fractional urine specimen labeled with the patient's name
   b) Clean and dry test tube
   c) Color chart
   d) Medicine dropper
   e) Clinitest reagent tablets
   f) Paper cup of water for rinsing dropper
   g) Paper cup of clean water for test
   h) Paper towel
   i) Disposable gloves (optional)
2. Wash your hands.
3. Place the paper towel on the countertop that will be your working area.
4. Rinse the dropper in the paper cup of water that is used for rinsing only.
5. With the dropper in the upright position, place 5 drops of urine in the center of the test tube.
6. Rinse the dropper.
7. Place 10 drops of clean water in the center of the test tube.
8. Place one Clinitest tablet in the test tube by dropping the tablet into the cover of the bottle and then dropping the tablet into the test tube from the cover. Never touch the tablet with your hands. (If your hands are wet and you touch the tablet, the moisture will activate the reaction and you will be burned.) Then cap the bottle immediately. If the tablets are individually wrapped, open the foil carefully and drop the tablet into the test tube without touching the tablet.

(continued next page)

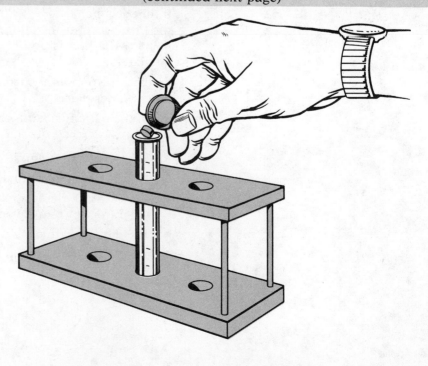

9. Wait 15 seconds after the reaction (boiling) has stopped. Then gently shake the test tube.

10. Compare the test tube contents with the color chart.

11. Match the color of the liquid in the test tube to the nearest matching color on the chart. Be sure to use the color chart that goes with the tablets you have used for the test. If the color is questionable, consult your head nurse or team leader.

12. Read the number inside the matching color box. For example, if the color is bright orange, it will say 2% or 4++++(plus) inside the orange-colored box.

13. Throw away used disposable equipment. Wash the test tube with cold water. Replace it upside down so that any remaining water will drain out. The test tube will then be ready for the next test. Rinse the medicine dropper with cold water. Put it in the rack in the upright position.

14. Wash your hands.

15. Report to your head nurse, team leader, or medication nurse:
   - That you have completed the Clinitest.
   - Your findings (the number from the matching color box) so that she can enter the information on the patient's chart.
   - Your observations of anything unusual.

Procedure: The Clinistix Test

1. Assemble your equipment:
   a) Fresh fractional urine specimen, labeled with the patient's name
   b) Clinistix reagent strips
   c) Disposable gloves (optional)

2. Wash your hands.

3. Dip the reagent strip into the urine in the specimen container.

4. Remove it immediately.

5. Tap the edge of the strip against the side of the urine container to remove excess urine.

6. Hold the strip in a horizontal position to prevent the mixing of the chemical from the adjacent reagent area.

7. Read the results 10 seconds after removing the strip from the urine. Clinistix reagent strips are used for the glucose level and, therefore, should be read at 10 seconds for qualitative results.

8. Read the results from the color chart, matching the color carefully. The color chart is on the bottle label that holds the Clinistix.

9. Discard disposable equipment.

10. Wash your hands.

11. Report to your head nurse, team leader, or medication nurse:
   - That you have completed the Clinistix test.
   - Your findings from the matching color chart, so that she can enter the information on the patient's chart.
   - Your observations of anything unusual.

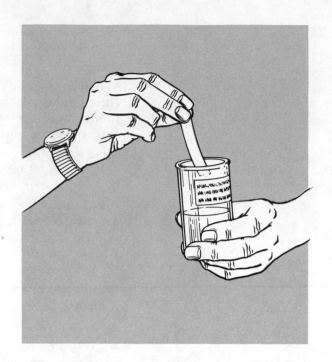

The **Acetest** and **Ketostix** reagent strip test determine the amount of acetone or ketones in the patient's urine. Acetone level refers to the amount of acetone in the urine. Ketone level refers to the amount of ketones in the urine.

Procedure: The Acetest

1. Assemble your equipment:
   a) Fresh fractional urine specimen, labeled with the patient's name
   b) Color chart
   c) Medicine dropper
   d) Acetest reagent tablets
   e) Paper cup of water for rinsing dropper
   f) Paper towel
   g) Disposable gloves (optional)
2. Wash your hands.
3. Place the paper towel on the countertop that will be your working area.
4. Place one Acetest tablet on the paper towel.
5. Never touch the tablet, but drop it into the cover of its container. Then place it on the paper towel from the cover.
6. Rinse the medicine dropper with water from the paper cup.
7. Drop one drop of urine on the tablet. Wait 30 seconds.
8. Compare it to the color chart.
9. Match the tablet color to the closest matching color on the chart.

(continued next page)

10. Read the results from the chart. For example, if the color is dark purple, it will say "Large Quantity."
11. Throw away used disposable equipment.
12. Wash your hands.
13. Report to the head nurse, team leader, or medication nurse:
    - That you have completed the Acetest.
    - Your findings, so that she can enter them on the patient's chart.
    - Your observations of anything unusual.

Procedure: The Ketostix Reagent Strip Test

1. Assemble your equipment:
   a) Fresh fractional urine specimen, labeled with the patient's name
   b) Ketostix reagent strips
   c) Disposable gloves (optional)
2. Wash your hands.
3. Dip the Ketostix strip into the urine in the container.
4. Remove it immediately.
5. Tap the edge of the strip against the side of the urine container to remove excess urine.
6. Hold the strip in a horizontal position to prevent possible mixing of the chemical from the adjacent reagent area.
7. Read the results 15 seconds after removing the strip from the urine. The ketone test is read at 15 seconds.
8. Read the results from the color in good lighting, matching the color carefully. The color chart is on the Ketostix bottle label.
9. Throw away used disposable equipment.
10. Wash your hands.
11. Report to your head nurse, team leader, or medication nurse:
    - That you have completed the Ketostix test.
    - Your findings, so that she can enter them on the patient's chart.
    - Your observations of anything unusual.

SECTION 3: CARE OF THE ORTHOPEDIC PATIENT

OBJECTIVES: WHAT YOU WILL LEARN

When you have completed this section, you will be able to:

- Describe the scope and nature of conditions requiring orthopedic equipment.
- Identify the basic types of orthopedic equipment.
- Demonstrate the required skill to use or assist in the use of common types of equipment.

Orthopedics (also spelled orthopaedics) is the science of the prevention and correction of deformities and the treatment of diseases of the bones, muscles, joints, and fasciae (supporting membranes), either by manipulation, by special apparatus, or by surgery. Orthopedic nursing requires special knowledge and skills in addition to routine patient care. To care for the orthopedic patient, the nursing assistant will need knowledge of body mechanics and specialized procedures peculiar to the treatment of this type of patient. Nursing assistants will need to be familiar with special equipment such as splints, casts, traction devices, and turning frames.

Common Orthopedic Conditions

A. Fractures:
1) Simple
2) Compound

B. Dislocations

C. Sprains

D. Bone Diseases:
1) Osteomyelitis
2) Tuberculosis

E. Joint Diseases:
1) Arthritis
2) Inflammation

F. Injury to the central nervous system may be neurological in nature:
1) Poliomelitis (not seen often)
2) Trauma or accidental injury damaging the spinal cord and resulting in paralysis of some area of the body.
3) Guillain-Barré Syndrome—a disease of the nervous system

Orthopedic Treatment

Orthopedic care offers a double challenge to the nursing assistant.
1) Routine nursing care is difficult to give when a patient is in a cast or traction. It will be necessary to devise ways to carry out some procedures with the least possible disturbance to these orthopedic devices.
2) The patient himself presents a challenge. Because of the long hospitalization, and his fear of deformity, the patient may become unduly depressed or discouraged. Your understanding and encouragement will do much to support the patient's morale. Encourage the patient to do as much for himself as possible. Offer the patient help only when he asks for it and only if he needs it, as he should be self-reliant. It is important that this type of patient does not feel isolated and useless.

Orthopedic Equipment

Modern science constantly is developing new ways and means to help the orthopedic patient. Some of these methods involve the use of special equipment. All devices of orthopedic equipment have a two-fold aim:

1) To provide support for the injured part until it heals.

2) To prevent deformity and weakness in the injured muscles and joints.

Support for the injured part may be provided by bandages, adhesive strapping, splints, or plaster casts applied externally. Support may also be applied directly to a bone by using pins, metal plates, or prosthetic devices, for example, the replacement of a joint. These specialized **prostheses** (artificial aids) are applied in the operating room using specialized surgical procedures. To prevent stiffness or deformity, the patient will be asked to use the affected part within the limits as ordered by the doctor. Frequently, the patient needs the support of a brace, crutches, or a walker.

Skin Care

Besides routine nursing care, the orthopedic patient needs special skin care. Since he is often confined to his bed and, in many cases, is immobile because of a cast or traction, he is particularly susceptible to bedsores. Follow the instructions in Section 1 of this chapter to prevent decubitus ulcers. You should change the patient's position every two hours following the doctor's instructions, give special back care, and change the area of pressure as often as is possible. Providing a smooth, clean, dry bed and keeping the cast clean helps prevent itching skin at the groin and axilla edge of a cast.

Plaster Casts

Patients in plaster casts often suffer feelings of restriction and fatigue. A trapeze, suspended from an over-the-bed frame allows the patient to move himself.

Turning Frames

The **turning frame** is simply a hospital bed designed to provide a variety of positions for the patient whose position in bed can only be changed with great care and under controlled conditions. The main difference between an ordinary bed and the turning frame is that it contains two frames on which the patient can lie, the anterior frame for lying flat on the stomach, and the posterior for lying flat on the back. The extra frame is stored on a rack on the bottom when not in use. The other principle parts are the arm boards, reading board, bedpan rack, traction pulleys and the "T" traction bar.

The turning frame that the patient lies on is at standard bed height. It is flexible enough to accommodate patients of any size. Traction applied to the head and/or feet is maintained while the patient is being turned. Only one safety lock keeps the frames and the patient secure.

The Advantages of the Turning Frame are:
- The patient may be turned with ease.
- Turning does not alter the position or alignment of the patient.
- The patient may be kept in hyperextension at adjustable points and heights.
- Traction may be maintained while turning.
- The danger of bedsores is minimized.
- The bedpan is easily placed under the patient without having the patient move.
- The patient can eat, read, and write in the prone position.
- Bathing is made easy and comfortable for the patient.
- Hyperextension (overextension) is maintained without the use of plaster casts.
- Spacing of the frames is adjustable for thin or heavy patients.
- Bed height is correct for nursing care.
- Neurosurgeons find the turning frame is valuable in the care of spinal cord injuries that result in paralysis and then in incontinence.

- The turning frame is used in the treatment of sacral bedsores and body burns that are extensive.

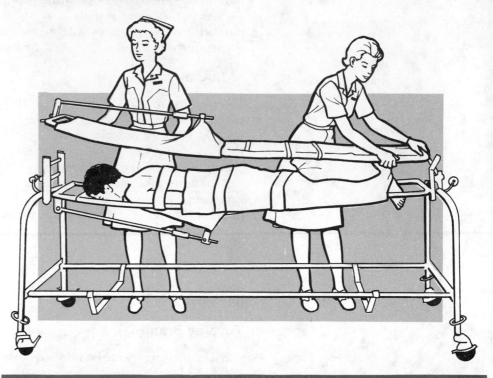

Procedure: Turning the Patient on a Manually Operated Turning Frame

1. Assemble your equipment:
   a) Sheepskin
   b) Second frame
2. Wash your hands.
3. Identify the patient by checking the identification bracelet.
4. Ask visitors to step out of the room.
5. Tell the patient that you are going to turn him on the frame, to his other side (back to stomach or stomach to back).
6. Pull the curtains around the bed for privacy.
7. Remove the patient's gown.
8. Remove the foot support from the posterior frame.
9. Release the stabilizer arms and remove the arm boards.
10. Position the patient's arms and hands along his trunk.
11. Cover the patient's trunk and extremities with the sheepskin, so when he is turned he is positioned on top of the sheepskin.
12. If there is a catheter in place, it must be clamped off for the turning procedure.
13. Inspect the anterior frame cover for tautness (tightness). Remove the top locking nuts and position the anterior frame over the patient and the sheepskin.
14. Adjust the face piece to fit without undue pressure on the chin and forehead. Replace the top locking nuts and screw them tightly.
15. Fasten the three web restraining straps securely around the frame at the level of the patient's shoulders, hands, and knees.

(continued next page)

16. The patient is now ready for turning. Have two other nursing assistants stand in position, trunks bending slightly. They will both be standing on the same side of the patient and will be facing the frame. Correct body mechanics will help prevent back strain and at the same time provide adequate leverage during the turn. Turn the patient.

17. After the patient has been turned, remove the web restraining straps, place the arm boards in position, remove the posterior frame and store the cart assembly bars in the correct place.

18. If a catheter is in place, unclamp it. Adjust the utility board for the patient's use.

19. Adjust the stabilizer arms and secure them for further immobilization.

20. After the turn, make special note that the patient's hands and feet are not in a position to cause foot drop or contractures.

21. The patient should now be lying on the sheepskin. Cover the patient with a small loose sheet.

22. Make the patient comfortable.

23. Wash your hands.

24. Report to your head nurse or team leader:

    - That the patient has been turned.
    - The time the patient was turned.
    - How the patient tolerated the procedure.
    - Your observations of anything unusual.

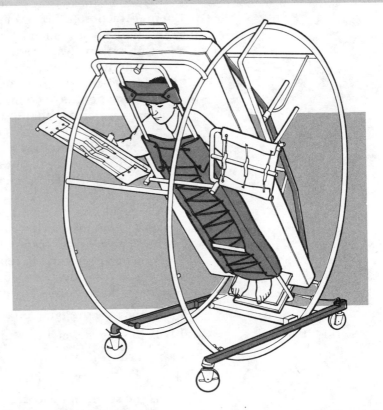

As a nursing assistant, you will have limited contact with the orthopedic device known as a circular double frame electric bed. In this bed the turning is done by an electric motor controlled from a panel similar to that on regular hospital electric beds.

The circular double frame electric bed is used for a patient requiring complete immobilization but for whom it is desirable to maintain a normal posture and position. It can be used for patients who cannot be lifted or moved.

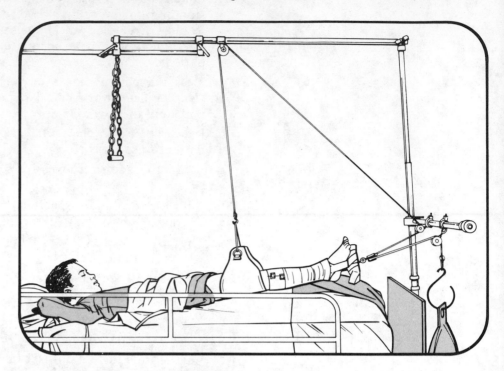

Care of the Patient in Traction

Traction means the exertion of pull by means of weights and pulleys. **Counter traction** (exertion of pull in the opposite direction) must be present to maintain body alignment. Traction is used to promote and maintain alignment of broken (fractured) bones and for other orthopedic conditions and treatment. It may be applied to the skin externally, or to the bone internally through surgery. It is maintained by the use of a special frame on the bed.

If the patient is uncomfortable, tell the head nurse or team leader. Often sand bags are used with traction. These are cloth bags filled with sand to make them heavy. Ask for permission before moving the bags. If the head nurse or team leader tells you they may be moved, follow her instructions. When you have finished, be sure to put the bags back in the same position they were in before, very slowly. Never change the patient's body position without permission from the head nurse or team leader.

A nursing assistant will never set or adjust any of the equipment in use on a patient in traction. This is strictly a function of the physician or registered nurse. The nursing assistant, however, is expected to check continually on the traction apparatus and to report any defect to the head nurse or team leader. The following questions concern points that a nursing assistant should observe as he performs any nursing task involving patients in traction.

a) Is the rope dragging on the bed or floor?

b) Is the bag of weights resting on the floor or against the bed?

c) Is a rope off its pulley?

d) Has the patient slid down in the bed?

e) Is the splint in the correct position?

f) If there is a cast, is it causing pain?

g) Is the skin on the body part where the cast ends blue in color? Is that part cold to the touch?

h) Does the patient complain of pain?

IF THE ANSWER TO ANY OF THESE QUESTIONS IS "YES," REPORT THE SITUATION TO THE HEAD NURSE OR TEAM LEADER IMMEDIATELY, AS THESE ARE ALL CONDITIONS THAT SHOULD NOT EXIST, AND SHOULD RECEIVE PROMPT ATTENTION.

Purposes and Types of Plaster Casts

Plaster casts are, in reality, a form of a bandage. They are used as a support to hold injured bones in alignment while they are healing. Casts are wet when applied, then allowed to dry. The plaster of paris hardens as it dries and the whole cast becomes rigid. Plastic or fiberglass casts perform the same task but are lighter, cleaner, and easier to use and remove.

While a plaster cast is drying, the patient's position must be maintained and the cast left uncovered. Pillows are placed to support the cast so it will not bend or move while still soft.

Observing Patients in Plaster Casts

Casts are confining and can be very uncomfortable. The skin area near the edges of the cast can become irritated and develop pressure bedsores from chafing.

Casts may restrict circulation, but should not. The nursing assistant should observe patients in casts for signs of pain, pallor, bluish color, and coldness to the touch. You should ask the patient for signs of tingling or numbness. These are signs of poor circulation. The nursing assistant should feel the exposed part of the limb to note whether or not it is cold. Any symptom of circulatory impairment should be reported immediately to the head nurse or team leader.

Patients may complain of itching. The feeling of restriction in a cast may affect them emotionally. These effects should be noted and reported to the head nurse or team leader.

Nursing assistants should be sure that casts are not soiled while bedpans and urinals are being used. Keeping the cast clean goes a long way toward avoiding discomfort and other skin irritations.

Unusual odors coming from the cast should be reported to the head nurse or team leader at once. This could be a sign that a decubitus ulcer or infection is forming under the cast.

SECTION 4: CARE OF THE OSTOMY PATIENT

OBJECTIVES: WHAT YOU WILL LEARN

When you have completed this section, you will be able to:

- Define an ostomy.
- Give ostomy care.

**KEY IDEAS:
THE OSTOMY**

The creation of an ostomy is a surgical procedure (operation). A new opening is created in the abdomen for the release of solid wastes (feces) from the body. The opening is called a **stoma**. A stoma is created surgically to change the path of the patient's feces from the rectum. This is done when his colon is diseased or injured. The ostomy is most often performed when it is necessary to remove tumors. Sometimes the surgery is done to permit repair of bowel injuries.

A person with a stoma must wear an **ostomy appliance** to collect fecal matter released through the stoma. This is a collecting bag held over the opening by special types of material like a paste or adhesive and/or a belt.

As a nursing assistant, you will be taking care of the ostomy after the patient has been fitted with an ostomy appliance. This is sometimes referred to as a "old ostomy." A fresh surgical patient with a new ostomy is always cared for by a registered nurse.

Sometimes the patient is able and wants to care for the ostomy himself. In this case, get permission from the head nurse or team leader.

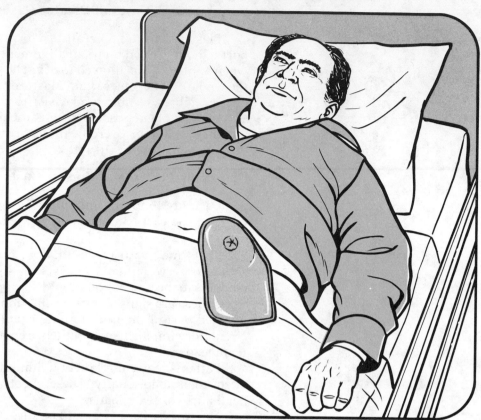

OSTOMY APPLIANCE IN PLACE OVER THE STOMA

Procedure: Caring for an Ostomy

1. Assemble your equipment:
   a) Bedpan
   b) Disposable bed protector
   c) Bath blanket
   d) Large emesis basin
   e) Clean ostomy belt (ostomy appliance), adjustable
   f) Clean stoma bag
   g) Toilet tissue
   h) Basin of water at 115°F (46.1°C)
   i) Soap or cleanser as ordered by head nurse or team leader
   j) Disposable washcloth
   k) Disposable gloves
   l) Towels
   m) Lubricant or skin cream as ordered

2. Wash your hands.

3. Identify the patient by checking the identification bracelet.

4. Ask visitors to step out of the room.

5. Tell the patient that you will take care of and change his ostomy appliance.

(continued next page)

6. Pull the curtain around the bed for privacy.

7. Cover the patient with the bath blanket. Ask the patient to hold the top edge of the blanket. Without exposing him, fanfold the top sheet and bedspread to the foot of the bed under the blanket.

8. Place the disposable bed protector under the patient's hips. This is to keep the bed from getting wet or dirty.

9. Place the bedpan and emesis basin within easy reach.

10. Fill the wash basin half full with water at 115°F (46.1°C). Have soap or cleanser as ordered, disposable washcloth, and bath towels on the bedside table.

11. Remove the soiled plastic stoma bag from the belt.

12. Open the belt. Protect it if it is clean and can be used again. If the belt is dirty, remove it. It will have to be replaced with a clean one.

13. Put the soiled plastic bag into the bedpan. Wipe the area around the ostomy with toilet tissue. This is to remove any loose feces. Place the dirty tissue in the bedpan or emesis basin.

14. Wet and soap the washcloth. Wash the entire ostomy area with a gentle circular motion.

15. Rinse the entire area very well. Be careful not to leave any soap on the skin. (Soap has a drying effect and may irritate the skin.)

16. Dry the area gently with a bath towel.

17. Apply a small amount of lubricant (if ordered) around the area of the ostomy. The lubricant is to prevent irritation to the skin around the ostomy. Wipe off all excess lubricant so the ostomy device will adhere to the skin.

18. Put a clean adjustable belt on the patient. Place a clean stoma bag in place through the loop.

19. Remove the disposable bed protector. Change any damp linen.

20. Replace the top sheet and bedspread and remove the bath blanket.

21. Make the patient comfortable.

22. Remove all used equipment. Dispose of waste material in the large hopper or into the toilet.

23. Discard disposable equipment.

24. Clean the bedpan and put it where it belongs.

25. Empty the wash basin. Wash it thoroughly with soap and water. Rinse and dry it and return it to its proper place.

26. Wash your hands.

27. Report to your head nurse or team leader:
    - That the ostomy was cleaned.
    - The amount of drainage.
    - The consistency of the excretions.
    - The color and appearance of the stoma and ostomy area.
    - Your observations of anything unusual.

Following surgery, the type of discharge from a sigmoid or descending colostomy may be semi-liquid until, through management of diet, the discharge begins to resemble a normal bowel movement.

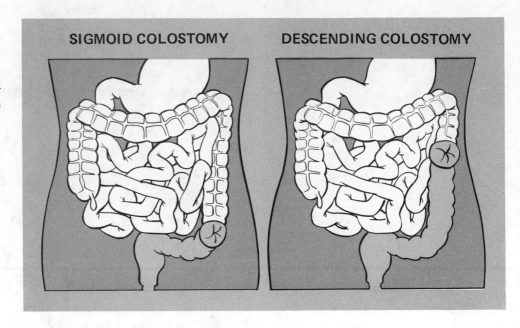

SIGMOID COLOSTOMY   **DESCENDING COLOSTOMY**

Frequently the transverse-single barrel, the transverse-double barrel, and the transverse-loop colostomy are temporary. Common patient problems in these types of ostomies include skin irritation, leakage from the appliance, and odor control.

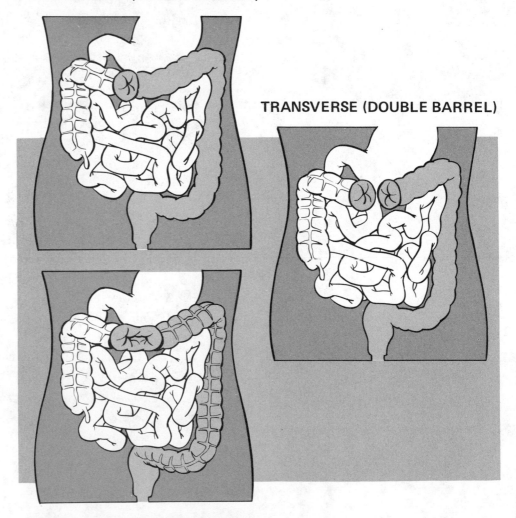

TRANSVERSE (SINGLE BARREL)

TRANSVERSE (DOUBLE BARREL)

TRANSVERSE—LOOP COLOSTOMY

Urinary diversion urostomy is performed for malfunction of the urinary bladder. When the patient has a bilateral cutaneous ureterostomy or an ileal conduit, prevention of leakage and skin protection are of utmost importance.

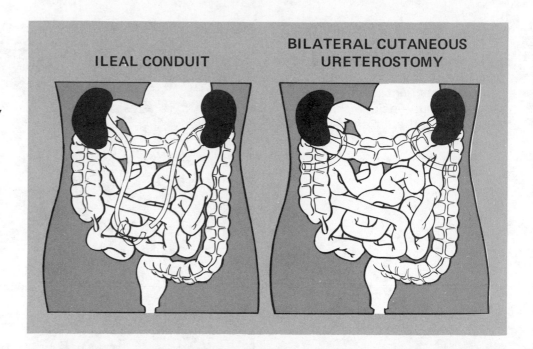

ILEAL CONDUIT

BILATERAL CUTANEOUS URETEROSTOMY

The ascending colostomy is essentially the same as the transverse colostomy; however, it usually is not temporary. Common patient problems in the ascending colostomy include skin irritation, leakage from the appliance, and odor control.

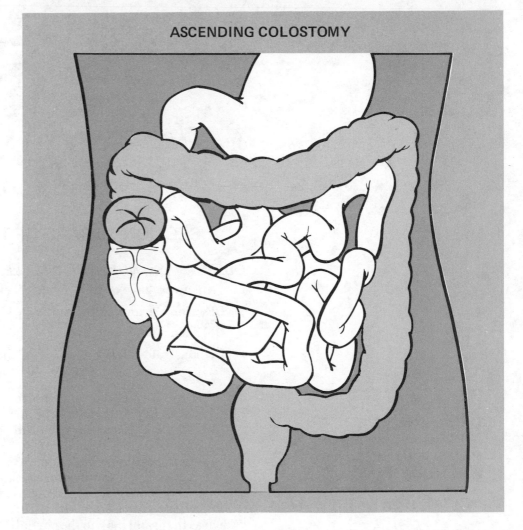

ASCENDING COLOSTOMY

The ileostomy frequently is performed in young adults. Common patient problems in the ileostomy include skin irritation and odor control.

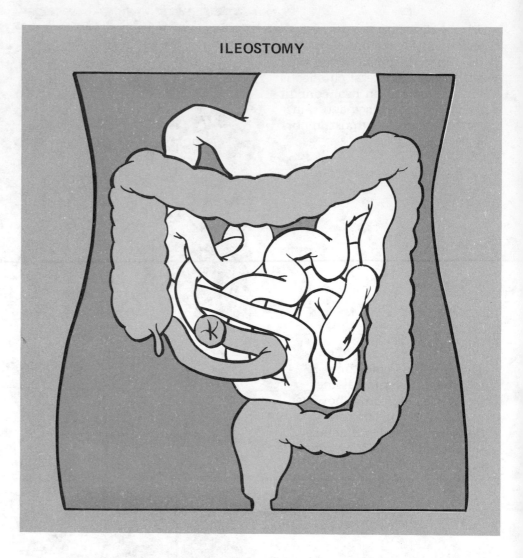

ILEOSTOMY

SECTION 5: CARE OF THE SEIZURE PATIENT

OBJECTIVES: WHAT YOU WILL LEARN

When you have completed this section, you will be able to:

- Describe a grand mal seizure.
- Describe a petit mal seizure.
- Demonstrate safety measures for the patient having a seizure.

**KEY IDEAS:
CREATING A SAFE
ENVIRONMENT FOR A
PATIENT HAVING
A SEIZURE**

A **seizure** is caused by an abnormality within the central nervous system. This abnormality is thought to be an electrical problem in the nerve cells.

Seizures can occur from the time of birth or may be the result of head injury, cancer, or disease.

As a nursing assistant, you may be present when a patient has a seizure. Therefore, it is important for the nursing assistant to know what the warning signals of a seizure are and what to do if one occurs.

There are several types of seizures, ranging from the total body seizure known as the **grand mal**, to the partial small seizure, known as the **petit mal**. In the grand mal seizure, there may be stiffness of the total body followed by a jerking action of the muscles. Sometimes the patient's tongue may be bitten and usually the patient becomes unconscious. In the petit mal seizure, the patient may appear to be daydreaming, his eyes may roll back, and there may be some quivering of the body muscles. The petit mal seizure usually lasts less than 30 seconds. The grand mal seizure may last for several minutes and varies greatly.

The major role of the nursing assistant in caring for a patient having a seizure is to prevent the patient from injuring himself. If you are present at the beginning of a seizure, you may place a padded tongue depressor or tongue blade in the patient's mouth, if this is the policy of your health care institution. Some health care institutions prefer that you simply turn the patient's head to the side. If the patient's jaw is already tight or he has his teeth clenched, *DO NOT TRY TO PRY HIS TEETH APART TO INSERT A TONGUE DEPRESSOR.* Help the patient to lie down. If you are not at his bedside, carefully help him to the floor. Loosen his clothing and move any equipment that he might bump into. Place a pillow or something soft under his head. *TURN HIS HEAD TO THE SIDE TO PROMOTE DRAINAGE OF SALIVA OR VOMITUS. NEVER TRY TO MOVE OR RESTRAIN THE PATIENT.* Stay with him and pull the emergency signal cord for help.

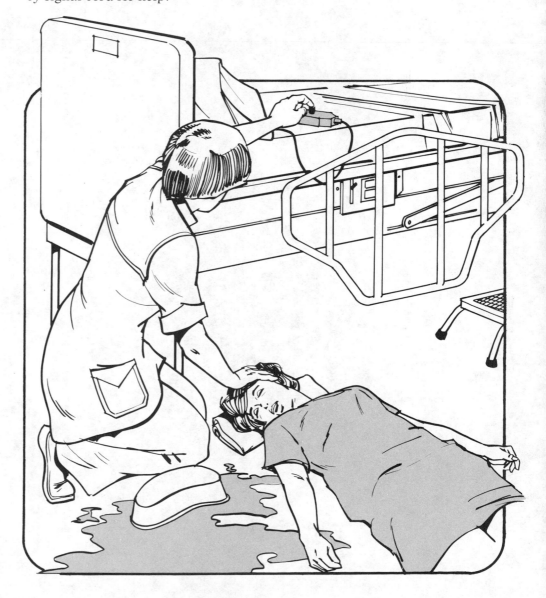

WHAT YOU HAVE LEARNED

The special skills you have learned in this chapter will be a great aid to you in understanding and caring for the long-term patient. Proper care for the prevention of decubitus ulcers is one of the most important things you can do for any extended care patient. Patients with diabetes require special attention and frequent testing of their urine. You will be using highly specialized equipment in the care of patients with orthopedic conditions. It is important that you know how to use them correctly and safely.

Keeping the skin clean around the ostomy is the main physical goal of the nursing care you will deliver to these patients. The information in this chapter has provided you with the background necessary for you to assist the nurse in giving good care to these patients.

18 HOME HEALTH CARE

1. Introduction to Home Health Care
2. Geriatric Care in the Home
3. Newborn and Infant Care in the Home
4. Household Management

SECTION 1: INTRODUCTION TO HOME HEALTH CARE

OBJECTIVES: WHAT YOU WILL LEARN

When you have completed this section you will be able to:

- List the tasks the home health assistant is expected to do.
- Describe potential safety hazards in the home.

**KEY IDEAS:
THE HOME HEALTH
ASSISTANT**

The home health assistant always works under the direct supervision of a registered nurse or physician. With professional supervision, the home health assistant is able to assist the patients with the activities of daily living and maintain a safe, clean, and comfortable environment.

All the nursing skills and principles explained in this book can be applied by the home health assistant. The patient in the home should receive the same high quality nursing care given to patients in health care institutions. This is important whether you are giving a bed bath or measuring the patient's blood pressure. As a home health assistant you will be:

- Communicating with the patient because you will spend more time with the patient than any other health care person.

- Observing, recording, and reporting any changes in the patient's condition as well as keeping records of patient care activities.

- Controlling the spread of microorganisms in the home by using proper handwashing techniques and by sufficient housecleaning to maintain a clean environment for the patient.

- Assisting the patient during the use of special equipment such as a wheelchair, walker, or a commode.

- Making the patient's bed and changing the linens as often as necessary to maintain a clean, dry, and wrinkle-free bed for the patient.

- Maintaining a safe environment for the patient.

- Cleaning any equipment used in the care of the patient.

- Washing the patient's clothing, bed linens, and towels.

- Lifting, moving, and transporting the patient, including assisting with ambulation.

- Assisting with range of motion exercises.

- Assisting with personal care, including oral hygiene, bathing, dressing, shampooing and combing the hair, shaving the beard, and using the bedpan, urinal, bedside commode or bathroom facilities.

- Recording intake and output.

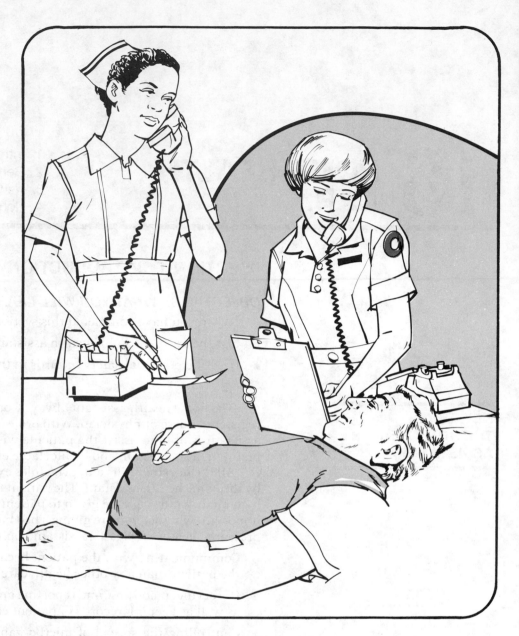

- Preparing and serving the patient's food. This may include grocery shopping, menu planning, cooking, following prescribed therapeutic diets, feeding helpless patients, and offering between-meal nourishments.
- Collecting specimens.
- Observing, measuring, and recording vital signs.
- Assisting during physical examinations by the registered nurse or doctor.
- Applying binders and elastic bandages or stockings.
- Assisting with ostomy care.
- Preventing decubitus ulcers through proper skin care and frequent back rubs.
- Performing basic urine tests for sugar and/or acetone.

In general, you will do these tasks the same way you would do them in any health care institution. It is important to follow the procedures given throughout this book accurately and carefully. Due to lack of equipment or supervision you may have to deviate from standard institutional procedure and improvise. Remember that aseptic technique—handwashing—is part of everything you do.

Helpful Personal Qualities

As a member of the health care team you are expected to maintain a professional attitude in the home. The same qualities that will make you a successful nursing assistant in a health care institution will be necessary if you are to be successful as a home health assistant. The best home health assistants are those who are dependable, trustworthy, considerate, tactful, ethical, courteous, sympathetic, energetic, polite, careful, observant, and sensitive. Communication skills are an essential part of your job. You will be in close contact with the patient, family members, and visitors.

The atmosphere and life-style will be different in every home in which you work. You must respect the rights of the patient and his family to have beliefs and opinions, culture and customs that might be different from your own. People of different backgrounds may eat foods you have never seen or tasted; they may behave differently toward their family members than you would; their religious beliefs may seem unusual to you; and their standards of cleanliness or general life-style may be different than yours. Accept these differences with respect and understanding, without judging or criticizing. Let the patient know it is your pleasure, not just your job, to assist him.

Procedures Home Health Assistants May Not Do

The nursing tasks home health assistants are not permitted to do in the home vary from state to state. In most areas of this country home health assistants may NOT do the following tasks:

- Change sterile dressings.
- Irrigate body cavities (this includes administering enemas and irrigation of ostomies or wounds).
- Gastric lavage or gavage.
- Catheterization.
- Administer medications.
- Apply heat by any method.
- Care for a tracheostomy tube.
- Perform any activity that has not been included in your assignment by your supervisor.

The reason the home health assistant may not perform the above tasks is that they have not been trained in these areas and do not have the knowledge or background necessary.

Safety in the Home

Because of age or illness, patients are prone to having accidents in the home and are often unable to take care of themselves in case of an emergency. You, as the home health assistant, will be responsible for the patient's safety while you are present in the home. You can create a safe environment for your patient and yourself by eliminating, preventing, or correcting conditions that could cause accidents. By avoiding risks you can prevent accidents. Safety in the home includes proper infection control, electrical and fire safety, and accident prevention.

Safety Hazards. As you go about your work, be alert and look for **hazards** like frayed electrical wires or loose rugs. Make a note of these things and bring them to the attention of the family member responsible and to your supervisor. Some of the most common safety hazards in the home are:

- Damaged electrical wiring on both large and small appliances.
- Faulty stairs.

- Poisoning (highest incidence in children due to medication and cleaning solutions).

- Flammable cleaning rags, mops and brooms. (These should be cleaned after each use and stored in a well-ventilated place.)

- Sharp objects such as knives, razors, and lawn tools.

- Kitchen accidents such as fires and burns. (These are often caused by grease left on a burner or by spilling hot foods.)

- Helpless patients or partially ambulatory patients falling down. (Many fractured bones occur this way.)

- Slipping on a wet floor. (Spills hould be wiped up immediately.)

Phone Numbers to Keep Handy

If an accident or emergency does occur, you must be ready to handle the situation calmly and wisely. Report every accident to your supervisor immediately. It is important to have emergency phone numbers written next to the phone. The list should include:

- Police department.

- Fire department.

- Responsible family member at work.

- Your supervisor.

- Patient's physician.

- Emergency number, if your city has one available.

- Nearest hospital.

- Ambulance service.

- Poison control center.

- If there is no phone in the home, arrange in advance to use a neighbor's phone in the case of an emergency.

SECTION 2: GERIATRIC CARE IN THE HOME

OBJECTIVES: WHAT YOU WILL LEARN

When you have completed this section, you will be able to:

- Describe the geriatric patient physically and emotionally.

- List and define common chronic conditions of geriatric patients.

- Describe nuring care for the geriatric patient in the home.

**KEY IDEAS:
THE GERIATRIC PATIENT**

The **geriatric patient** is an individual who will require physical care and emotional support. This person did not grow old at age 70 or 75. Aging is a gradual process that takes place during life. Each person ages and deteriorates at his own rate. Many geriatric persons are active and alert; however, some of them may have developed a condition that restricts them in one or many ways. You will note that some geriatric persons may have had a change of hair color, that their skin is dry and wrinkled, that some have had difficulty with their teeth and now wear dentures, that they talk loudly because their hearing is becoming impaired, that they complain of stiffness in some joints, that their bones are brittle and fractures are common, that many of them have frequency of urination due to loss of muscle tone, and that appetites may decrease.

Sometimes you will notice changes in behavior such as being repetitious in conversation; they may be forgetful, neglectful of personal care. They may be fussy, confused, fearful, and unable to sort out the environment. The geriatric person may have a different attitude about death than a young person because of his age or because he has watched many friends and family members grow ill and die. Many of them are lonely, and feel useless, unwanted, and a burden to their families. Some will give up in the struggle to recover and make no effort to get well. A patient in this mood may lose interest in other people, in his surroundings, in eating or taking care of his own activities of daily living.

Sometimes geriatric patients are confused for short or lengthy periods. The patient may not know where he is. He may be talking as if reliving experiences from his past. He may be speaking to people who are not in the room. Report these episodes of confusion to your supervisor. It may be caused by poor circulation of blood within the brain due to a narrowing of the blood vessels. Make an effort to orient this patient. Tell him the time and day and where he is. Tell him who you are and why you are there.

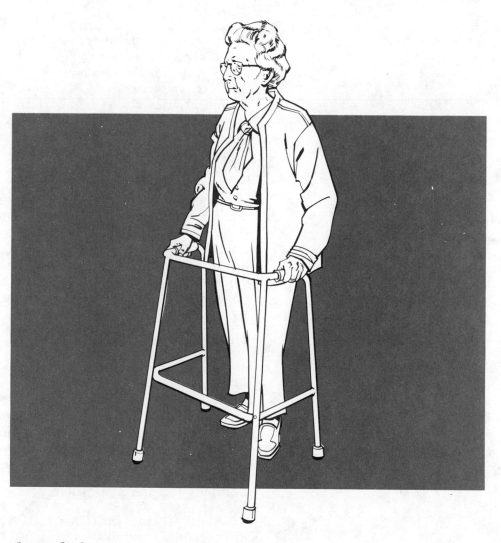

Physical Changes

As we grow older, many other physical changes take place that make functioning independently more and more difficult. The body's central nervous system may slow down. This could create problems in detecting heat, pain, and cold. Thought processes may be slow and memory may become poor. All the senses—hearing, sight, taste, touch, and smell—may not be as sharp as they once were. Muscle tone may be poor due to a lack of exercise. An inadequate sense of balance might make the patient unsteady on his feet or cause a change in his walking patterns. The bones tend to become brittle and break easily. Quick changes in position can cause the blood pressure to drop and, as a result, the patient will feel dizzy or faint.

Accident Prevention

It is for these reasons that you must be so diligent in your efforts to protect your patient from accidents. Every patient is an individual and has different needs. Some patients may need your assistance to get in and out of bed or to walk from room to room. If you notice that your patient is unsteady, report it to your supervisor. The unsteady patient may benefit from the use of a cane or a walker. A sturdy, hard chair, placed beside the patient's bed, will give him something to hold on to when he is getting up out of bed. Be sure the patient's clothing is not so long that he is likely to trip over it. If the height of the bed is adjustable, make sure it is in the lowest position.

Skin Care

The patient's skin may be extremely dry, flaky, and wrinkled. This may be due to the decreased amounts of oils being produced by the oil glands and by poor circulation. Dry skin may be less elastic and more sensitive than normal skin. Circulation tends to slow down in the older patient. This can happen because arteries harden, because fatty deposits build up in the blood vessels, or because of other medical reasons. Lack of frequent movement and exercise can contribute to problems. Difficulties concerning appetite, elimination, and sleeping are also related to lack of physical activity. These problems of aging skin and circulation make the geriatric patient especially susceptible to decubitus ulcers.

As a home health assistant, it is your responsibility to give thorough skin care frequently and to urge the patient to move about as often as he is able. Different patients will need varying amounts of assistance from you when changing position. If the patient is helpless or nonambulatory, you will need to turn him many times each day. Keep the principles of good body mechanics in mind and use a pull (turn) sheet to make the job easier. Sharpen your nursing skills concerning skin care by reviewing the section, Decubitus Ulcer Care, given earlier.

The Patient as a Person

You should be sensitive to both the physical and the emotional needs of your geriatric patient. If he is treated with kindness and respect, the older person will feel better about himself. Holding someone's hand and a few kind words will make most patients feel more secure and less worried. Take the time to talk to your patient, to get to know him, and to let him become accustomed to you. You should behave in ways that show you are interested and concerned about the patient as a person.

Common Chronic Conditions

Along with the normal body changes that occur as a person grows older, there are many chronic conditions that may occur. The various body parts grow old at different rates. That is, some body parts get old sooner than others. Some diseases and conditions are related directly to aging. Examples include the loss of vision because of cataracts in the eyes and hardening or softening of the bones and joints. The following is a list of some common medical conditions of the geriatric patient.

COMMON MEDICAL CONDITIONS/DISEASES	WHAT OCCURS AS A RESULT OF THESE CONDITIONS/DISEASES
Arthritis	Inflammation of the body joints causing pain and loss of movement.
Cataracts	Clouding of the lens of the eye causing decreased vision.
Parkinson's Disease	A disease of the central nervous system causing tremors in the body. This patient may shuffle his feet instead of taking steps.
Heart Disease	A number of different problems in the circulatory system sometimes causing pain, fatigue, and anxiety.
Cancer	A change in cell growth causing pain and loss of weight.
Cerebral Vascular Accident (C.V.A.)	Arterial changes in the brain possibly leading to stroke and paralysis.
Diabetes	A disturbance of the carbohydrate metabolism because of an imbalance of hormones (insulin).

KEY IDEAS: NURSING CARE FOR THE GERIATRIC PATIENT

Assisting the Patient to Follow Doctor's Orders

The home health assistant must help the patient by strictly following the supervisor's orders. If the patient is taking medications you may need to remind him to take them at the right time. You may need to help the patient read the labels on the medicine containers. The patient must take the correct medicine at the proper time. Write down the name of the medication and the time it was taken, so you can report accurately to your supervisor.

The Bed-bound Patient

When a patient is bed-bound he has the same needs as an ambulatory patient, but he will require more help from you in meeting these needs. Emotional support and encouragement can be very helpful. If family members are living in the home or visiting often, you can involve them in the care of the patient by permitting them to prepare the patient's favorite foods, to feed the patient, to shave the patient, to comb the patient's hair, or to do any similar tasks.

Proper positioning of the patient in bed will help make him comfortable. The back and joints should be supported to prevent unnecessary strain. Changing the patient's position at least every two hours will promote circulation and will help in preventing decubitus ulcers. Support the patient's arms and legs. Pillows can be used for support but never put the support behind the knees, unless you have specific instructions to do so.

For proper body alignment and good support, the mattress should be firm. The bed can be made firmer by sliding a plywood board, cut just to the size of the mattress, between the mattress and the box springs. Your supervisor must give you permission for making your patient's bed firmer. Protect the mattress with a plastic sheet. A large heavyweight plastic bag can be used for this purpose. Cover the plastic with a quilted cotton pad or a sheet. A draw sheet or a regular sheet that has been folded so that it is about three to four feet wide can be used over the plastic and bottom sheet. The sheets should be changed daily or more frequently when they become wet or soiled.

Activities of Daily Living for the Bed-bound Patient

Assisting with the activities of daily living will be a big part of your job when caring for the bed-bound patient. A daily bed bath will not only keep the patient clean, but it will also help him to feel relaxed and refreshed. Oral hygiene, back rubs, and care of the hair and nails, all help the patient look and feel better. The bed-bound patient may need less food than before his illness, due to a lack of physical activity. However, meals should be well balanced and served attractively.

SECTION 3: NEWBORN AND INFANT CARE IN THE HOME

OBJECTIVES: WHAT YOU WILL LEARN

When you have completed this section, you will be able to:

- Prepare infant formula.
- Sterilize water, bottles, nipples, and caps.
- Feed and burp an infant.
- Provide care for an infant's umbilical cord.
- Give an infant a bath.

Most infants are fed six times a day, every four hours, but many infants need to be fed more often that that. If the mother is breast-feeding her baby, you may bring the baby to her when it is time for a feeding. If the baby is being bottle-fed, you may need to prepare the formula. Discuss care of the newborn infant with the mother and your supervisor and follow their instructions.

Rules to Follow: Storing Formula

- Formula can be kept refrigerated for two days without spoiling.
- After two days it must be thrown away.
- If you are not sure how long formula has been in the refrigerator, discard it.
- Do not risk the baby's health by feeding him formula that might be spoiled.
- Formula will begin to spoil within two hours when it is left at room temperature.
- Keep the bottle refrigerated until ten minutes before the feeding.

Three Different Types of Formula:

- Ready to feed
- Powder
- Concentrated liquid

Ready-to-Feed Formula (Prepared Formula). Before opening the can or bottle the formula comes in from the store, it does not need to be refrigerated. Wash all cans and bottles before opening. This type of formula needs no preparation. Remember to shake it before opening. Open the can with a can opener that is clean (sterilized) and pour the contents into sterile (clean) bottles. Open bottles of ready to feed formula by unscrewing the cap. All you need to do now is screw a clean (sterilized) standard nipple right on the bottle the formula came in and feed the baby.

Powdered Formula. Powdered formula costs less per serving than ready-to-feed formula. Wash and dry all cans before opening. Use a clean (sterilized) can opener. Follow the instructions on the label carefully as to the amounts of powder and sterile water to mix together. Be sure to mix the powder with water that you have boiled (sterilized). Mix the powder and sterile water in sterile bottles, a clean pitcher, or clean pot. Once mixed, this formula must be kept refrigerated.

Concentrated Liquid Formula. Concentrated liquid is the least expensive type of formula. Shake and wash all cans before opening. Use a sterile (clean) can opener. To prepare this formula, mix one part concentrate to one part sterile (boiled) water (one can concentrate to one can sterile (boiled) water). You must sterilize (boil) the water before you mix the formula. Be sure to mix the formula in sterile (clean) bottles or a sterile (clean) pitcher. Once mixed, this formula must be kept refrigerated.

In certain areas, you will not be instructed to boil water or to sterilize bottles and nipples. Ask your supervisor for instructions for your area.

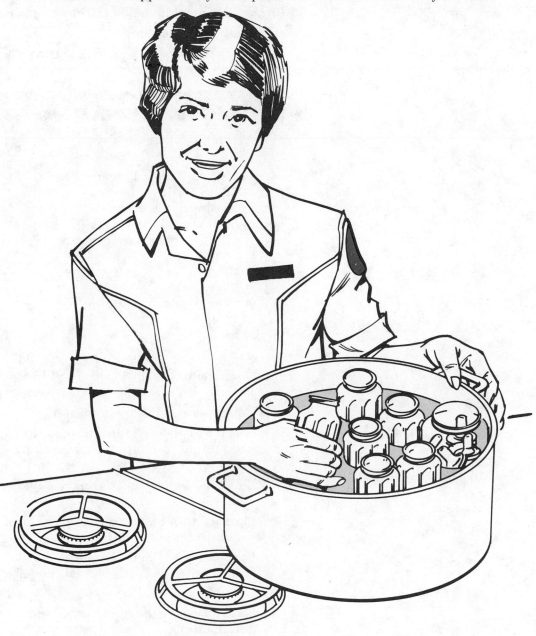

In certain areas you will not be instructed to sterilize bottles and nipples. Ask your supervisor for instructions for your area.

Procedure: Sterilizing Tap Water

1. Assemble your equipment:
   a) Saucepan
   b) Water
   c) Stove
   d) Timer, watch, or clock
2. Wash your hands.
3. Fill the saucepan ⅔ full with water.
4. Place the filled pan on the stove burner and turn on to high or full setting. Be sure the pan is covered.
5. When the water comes to a full boil, begin timing. Allow the water to remain at a full boil for 20 minutes in covered pan.
6. Turn off the burner.
7. Allow the water to cool before using it to mix the formula.
8. Wash your hands.

Procedure: Sterilizing Bottles

1. Assemble your equipment:
   a) Bottles
   b) Nipples, caps, and jar
   c) Bottle brush
   d) Dishwashing detergent
   e) Hot water from the tap
   f) Large pot with cover or a special sterilizing pot for baby bottles
   g) Small towel
   h) Tap water
   i) Stove
   j) Timer, watch, or clock
   k) Tongs
2. Wash your hands.
3. Scrub bottles, nipples, and caps with hot soapy water. Use the bottle brush to clean inside the bottles. Always squirt hot soapy water through the holes in the nipples to clean out any dried on formula.
4. Rinse thoroughly with hot water.
5. Fold the small towel to fit the bottom of the pot and lay it there. This will prevent the bottles from breaking. (This is done when you do not have a bottle rack.)
6. Stand the washed bottles on the towel in a circle around the inside of the pot.
7. Place the caps and nipples into the clean empty jar. Place into the pot at the center of the bottles.
8. Pour water into and around the bottles and into the jar with the nipples until ⅔ of each bottle is under water.
9. Cover the pot.
10. Place the pot on the stove burner and turn on the burner to the high or full setting.
11. When the water comes to a full boil, begin timing. Allow the water to remain at a full boil for 25 minutes.
12. Remove the nipples and caps in the jar 10 to 15 minutes after the full

(continued next page)

boil began. With the nipples still inside the jar, stand the jar on the table to cool.

13. Turn off the burner.

14. Take the cover off of the pot and allow it to cool.

15. Remove the sterile bottles from the pot with sterile tongs.

16. Empty the water out of the pot. The pot is now sterilized, so you can use it for mixing the formula.

17. Wash your hands.

KEY IDEAS:
BURPING THE INFANT

Most infants, especially those who are bottle-fed, swallow some air while drinking. Air in the gastro-intestinal tract can cause vomiting and abdominal pain. You can prevent a build-up of the air by feeding the infant slowly, stopping after every two ounces to burp the baby.

There are two methods for burping the baby:

METHOD A:

Cover your shoulder with a clean cloth. This could be a small towel or a cloth diaper. Hold the baby in a vertical position, so his head is resting on your shoulder. Gently rub and/or pat the infant's back until you hear the burp.

"METHOD A"

BURPING THE BABY

- Use a diaper or towel over your shoulder

- Press the baby against your shoulder

- Pat the baby gently on the back

METHOD B:

Sit the infant on your leg so his feet are dangling on your side. Put one of your hands on the infant's chest and lean the baby over so your hand is supporting him. Gently rub and pat the baby's back with your other hand until you hear the burp. (See the picture on the following page.)

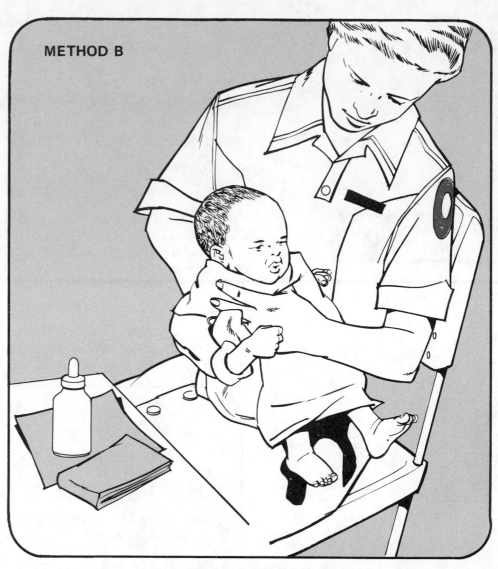

METHOD B

KEY IDEAS:
WHEN FEEDING THE BABY
FROM A BOTTLE

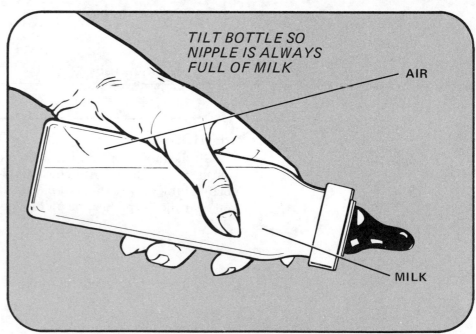

*TILT BOTTLE SO
NIPPLE IS ALWAYS
FULL OF MILK*

AIR

MILK

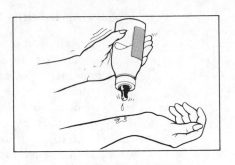

CHECK THE TEMPERATURE OF
THE FORMULA

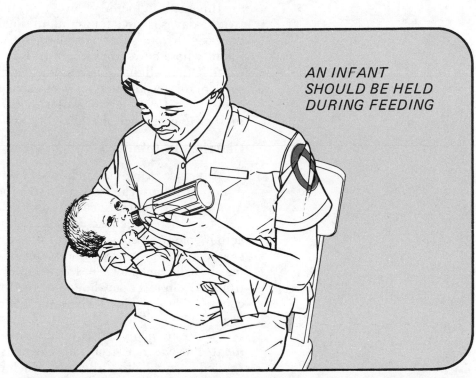

*AN INFANT
SHOULD BE HELD
DURING FEEDING*

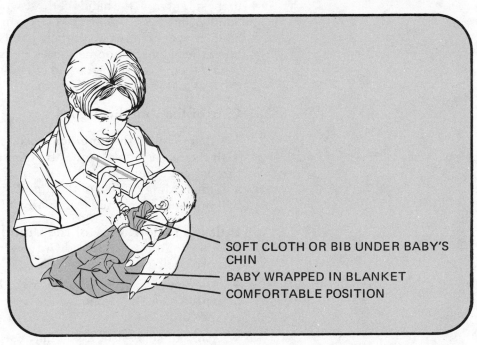

SOFT CLOTH OR BIB UNDER BABY'S
CHIN

BABY WRAPPED IN BLANKET

COMFORTABLE POSITION

Observing Infant's Stool

You will need to observe the infant's stool at each diaper change in order to detect constipation or diarrhea. When you observe a change from what has been normal for your patient, report your observations to your supervisor and to the mother.

The bottle-fed infant will have stools that are yellowish or mustard color. They will be lumpy, but soft. One to three bowel movements each day is normal for an infant that is bottle-fed every three to four hours.

The breast-fed infant will have stools that are yellowish or mustard color, but the color may change slightly and may appear to have a greenish tint, depending on the mother's diet. The stools will be looser and smoother than the stools of a bottle-fed infant. It is not unusual for the stools to look like there are tiny seeds in them. A bowel movement after every feeding or only once or twice a day is normal for an infant that is breast-fed every two to three hours. Check with your supervisor if you suspect that the infant is constipated. An infant whose bowel movement is dry and formed is considered to be constipated. Often, all that is necessary to correct this situation is to offer the infant some plain sterile water between each formula feeding. Usually the infant will drink ½ to 1½ ounces of water. If the constipation persists, encourage the mother to notify her physician or clinic and report this to your supervisor.

Diarrhea in Infants

Diarrhea in infants can be a very serious problem and requires immediate attention. Infants can loose all of their body fluids and chemicals very quickly. An infant with diarrhea can become dehydrated within two days. You will be able to see a noticeable change in the infant's elimination pattern and in the actual color and consistency of the stools when an infant has diarrhea. The stools may appear green and watery, running right out of the diaper. There may be a distinct odor. The frequency of the stools may increase to two or three times within just a few hours. At the first sign of diarrhea, ask the mother to contact the physician for specific instructions and/or report to your supervisor.

There are many causes for diarrhea in infants. It may be caused by equipment that was not sterilized (cleansed) properly, by carelessly prepared or spoiled formula, or by allergies. Much diarrhea is caused by passing bacteria to the infant from the hands of those who handle him. This is the reason proper handwashing is so essential when caring for an infant. Encourage anyone who handles the infant to wash their hands frequently and certainly before handling the baby or equipment used in his care. Be sure to explain why you are asking them to do this, to avoid offending anyone. Frequent handwashing can prevent and limit unnecessary diarrhea.

Care of the Umbilical Cord

Before birth, the **umbilical cord** serves as a lifeline, connecting the fetus with the mother's placenta. All nourishment is passed from mother to fetus through the umbilical cord. At the time of delivery the cord is clamped and cut and the healing process of the umbilicus begins. Within 5 to 10 days the cord will dry, turn black, and eventually fall off.

Rules to Follow: Care of the Umbilical Cord

- Keep the diaper folded down away from the cord. A wet diaper on top of the cord could cause an infection.

- At every diaper change, wash the cord with plain rubbing alcohol on a cotton ball. The alcohol will help speed up the drying process and will keep the cord clean.

- Ask your supervisor if you may use the alcohol. Follow her instructions.

- Never pull on the cord. Let it fall off by itself. Laying the infant on his abdomen will not hurt the cord. Binders or belly bands are not advised.

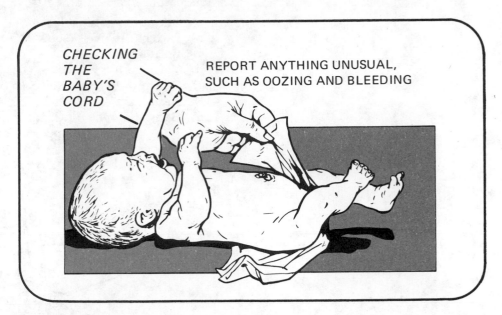

CHECKING THE BABY'S CORD

REPORT ANYTHING UNUSUAL, SUCH AS OOZING AND BLEEDING

Sponge Bathing the Infant

While the umbilical cord is still attached to the baby, he can be washed by giving him a sponge bath. A tub bath is not permitted until the cord has fallen off. The infant should receive a sponge bath at least once a day, usually in the morning. Bathe the infant more often, if it is necessary.

Sponge bathing an infant means gently washing each part of the baby's body with mild soap and warm water, but not submerging the infant in water. Safety of the infant is very important. Whenever in doubt about anything, call your supervisor. A safe table or counter is a convenient place to give a sponge bath. Clear off the counter and wash it well. Spread a towel on the counter to make a soft and warm place on which to place the baby. Prepare warm water, mild soap, washcloth, blankets, and towels before bringing the baby to the counter. Only one part of the body is washed at a time. Wash, rinse, and dry each body part or area very well. Then cover the body part right away with the bath blanket. If you do not have a bath blanket, use a towel.

Tub Bathing the Infant

After the cord has fallen off, the infant can be given a tub bath. You can use a large sink or a baby bath tub. If you are using a sink, be sure to clean the sink and counter. Scrub the sink with a cleanser and rinse it thoroughly. Assemble your equipment before you begin so you will not need to leave the room to get something that you may have forgotten. Lock the front door so no one can come in and distract you or the infant's mother. Taking the phone off the hook will prevent it from ringing during the bath, if the mother agrees. You cannot leave the infant in the tub or on the counter to answer the phone or the doorbell.

Bath time should be a pleasant and enjoyable time for mother and baby. Try to involve the mother as much as she is able and take the opportunity to teach her how to care for the baby. The infant's safety is your first responsibility. Keep your hands and eyes on the baby throughout the bath.

Procedure: Giving the Infant a Tub Bath

1. Assemble your equipment:
   a) Infant tub or sink
   b) Two bath towels (soft)
   c) Cotton balls
   d) Washcloth
   e) Warm water 100°F (37.8°C) (warm to the touch of the elbow)
   f) Baby soap
   g) Baby shampoo (optional)
   h) Baby powder, lotion, or cream
   i) Diaper
   j) Clean clothes

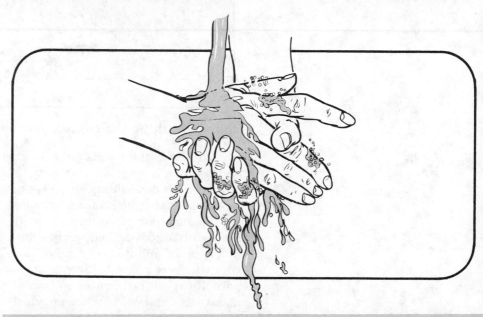

2. Wash your hands.
3. Wash the sink or tub with a disinfectant cleanser and rinse thoroughly.
4. Line the sink or tub with a bath towel.
5. Place a towel on the counter next to the sink or tub as you may want to lay the infant down to dry him.
6. Fill the tub or sink with 1 to 2 inches of warm water 100°F (37.8°C). This will be warm to the touch of the elbow.

(continued next page)

7. Undress the infant, wrap him in a towel or blanket, and bring him to the tub or sink.

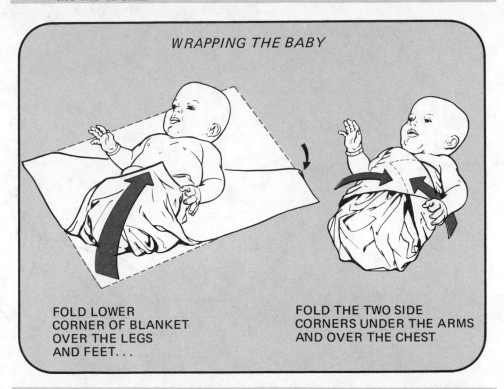

WRAPPING THE BABY

FOLD LOWER
CORNER OF BLANKET
OVER THE LEGS
AND FEET...

FOLD THE TWO SIDE
CORNERS UNDER THE ARMS
AND OVER THE CHEST

8. Using a cotton ball moistened with warm water and squeezed out, gently wipe the infant's eyes from the nose towards the ears. USE A CLEAN COTTON BALL FOR EACH EYE.

(continued next page)

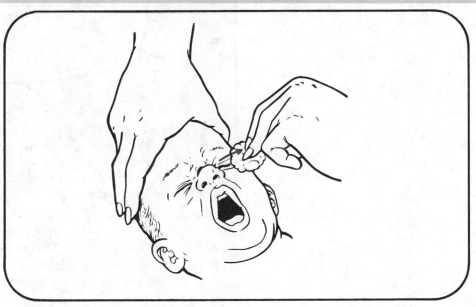

9. To wash the hair, hold the infant in the football hold, with the baby's head over the sink or tub. This will free your other arm to wet the hair, apply a small amount of shampoo, and rinse the hair.

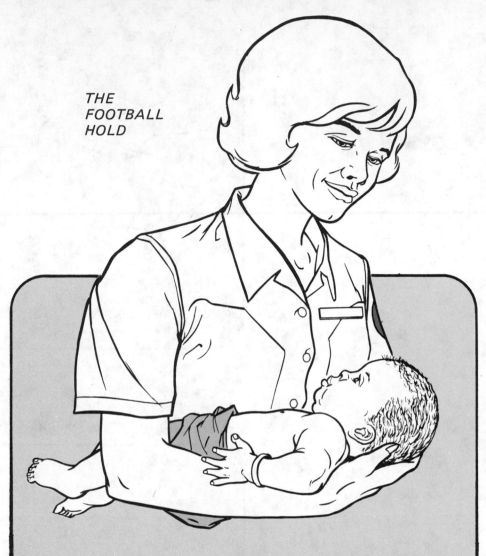

THE FOOTBALL HOLD

To use the football hold, support the baby's head in the palm of your left hand. The baby's back will be supported along your left forearm. His hips will be pressed against your waist by your left elbow, holding him securely in place. You may use either arm for this hold, as long as you support his head and back.

10. Dry the infant's head with a towel.

11. Unwrap the infant and gently place him on the towel in the sink or tub. One of your hands should always be holding the baby. Never let go, not even for a second.

(continued next page)

12. Wash the infant's body with the soap and the washcloth, being careful to wash between the folds (creases) of the skin.

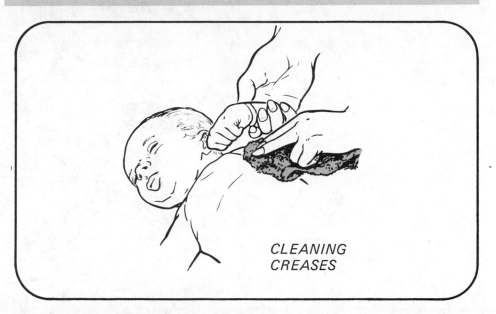

CLEANING
CREASES

13. If the infant is female, always wash the perineal area from front to back.

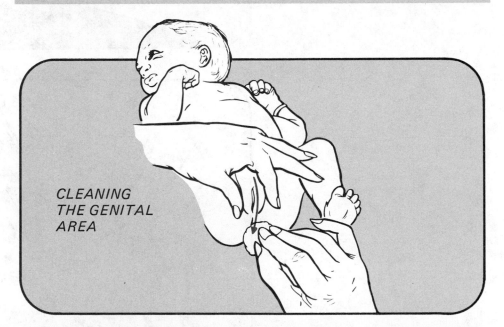

CLEANING
THE GENITAL
AREA

14. Rinse the infant thoroughly with warm water.
15. Lift the infant out of the water and onto the towel you laid out on the counter.
16. Dry the infant well, being careful to dry between the folds of skin.
17. Now you can apply powder, lotion, or cream to the infant, whichever the mother prefers or as instructed by your supervisor.

(continued next page)

18. Diaper and dress the infant.

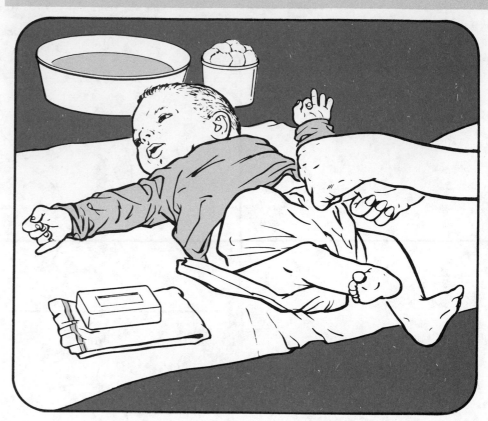

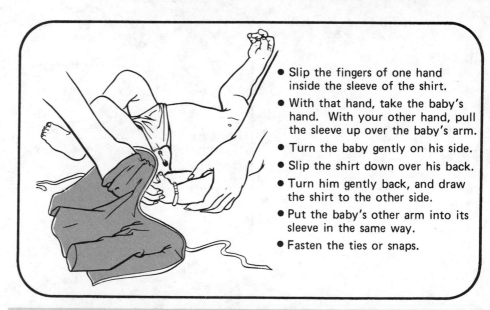

- Slip the fingers of one hand inside the sleeve of the shirt.
- With that hand, take the baby's hand. With your other hand, pull the sleeve up over the baby's arm.
- Turn the baby gently on his side.
- Slip the shirt down over his back.
- Turn him gently back, and draw the shirt to the other side.
- Put the baby's other arm into its sleeve in the same way.
- Fasten the ties or snaps.

(continued next page)

19. Place the infant in his crib or allow the mother to hold him. Show the mother how to hold the infant in either the upright position or the cradle position.

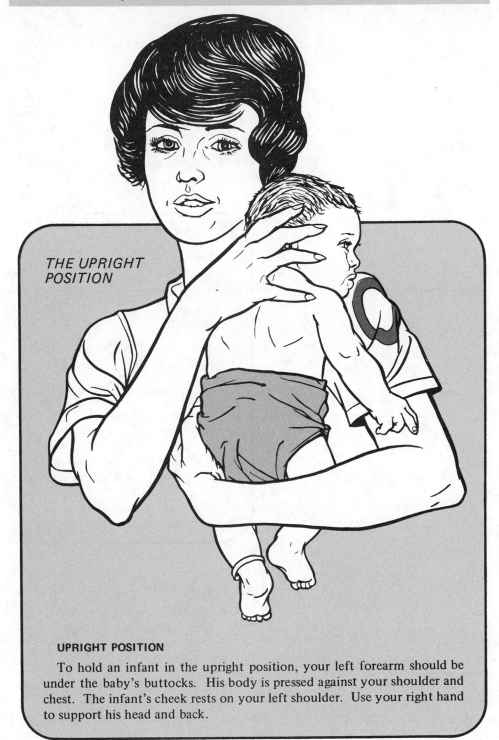

THE UPRIGHT POSITION

UPRIGHT POSITION

To hold an infant in the upright position, your left forearm should be under the baby's buttocks. His body is pressed against your shoulder and chest. The infant's cheek rests on your left shoulder. Use your right hand to support his head and back.

(continued next page)

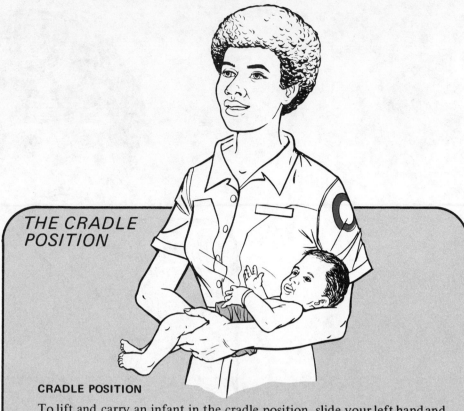

THE CRADLE POSITION

CRADLE POSITION

To lift and carry an infant in the cradle position, slide your left hand and arm under the baby's back. Use your left arm to support his head, back, and buttocks. Put your right hand under the baby's buttocks. Then move your left arm and hand up toward the infant's head before picking him up. You use your left arm and hand to give more support to the back, shoulders, and head while your right hand and arm support his buttocks, legs, and feet. Pick up the baby by cradling him in your arms, with his body against your chest.

20. Clean and return the equipment and supplies to their proper place.
21. Clean the area where the bath was given.
22. Wash your hands.

KEY IDEAS: INFANT SAFETY

When the patient is an infant, you must take special precautions to protect the baby from preventable accidents. Even if an infant has not yet learned to roll over he can wiggle and kick until he falls off beds, chairs, tables, or counters. *Never leave an infant unattended* on any of these surfaces. If you are far from the infant's crib and you must leave him unattended for a few seconds, put him on the floor. The safest place for an infant is in his crib, with the side rails up. Some people keep babies in a carriage or a drawer because they do not have a crib. Other things you can do to prevent accidents when caring for an infant include:

- Washing your hands before handling the infant or his supplies.
- Placing the infant on his side or belly after eating to prevent aspiration.

- Keeping the crib rails in the up position when the infant is sleeping or playing.
- Using only one to two inches of bath water and never leaving the infant alone in the water.
- Never placing the infant who is in an infant seat on tables, chairs, beds, or counters.
- Keeping all medications and cleaning solutions out of the reach of all children.

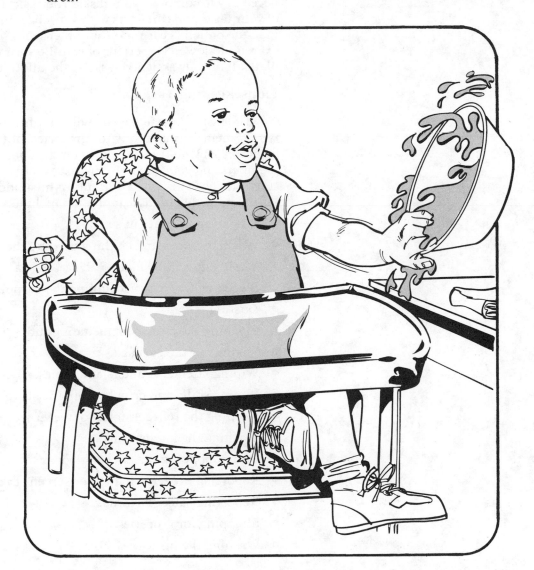

SECTION 4: HOUSEHOLD MANAGEMENT

OBJECTIVES: WHAT YOU WILL LEARN

When you have completed this section, you will be able to:

- Plan your time on the job.
- List housekeeping tasks expected of a home health assistant.
- Record your activities and those of the patient.

Preparing and serving meals and keeping the patient's home neat and clean are part of what is expected of you on the job. However, patient care and safety come first. All of the housekeeping tasks can be done between nursing tasks. Convenient times occur when the patient is sleeping, reading, watching television, or conversing with visitors.

Planning Your Time

Planning your schedule for the day can help you to minimize the time necessary to complete your tasks. The easiest way to organize is to make a list of your tasks and carry this with you, checking off each task as it is completed. Plan the patient's care and your other tasks so the patient will have periods of exercise followed by periods of rest. Be sure your plan will allow you to complete all of your assigned tasks in the allotted amount of time.

Housekeeping Tasks

The tasks expected of you will vary from home to home. In some homes a family member might buy the groceries, but in another home your employer (supervisor) would want you to do the shopping. It is best to ask the family members and your supervisor to list exactly what is expected of you before you start the job. This will avoid future misunderstandings. Housekeeping tasks for the home health assistant often include:

- Preparing the patient's meals.
- Washing linens and clothing used by the patient.
- Wiping up spilled food.
- Sweeping floors or vacuuming the carpets.
- Dusting.
- Cleaning the bathroom including tub, toilet, sink, floor, and mirror.
- Taking out the garbage.
- Wiping kitchen counters and tables.
- Wiping spills and crumbs from the stove.
- Keeping the refrigerator and freezer free of spoiled food.
- Washing the kitchen sink.
- Damp mopping the kitchen floor.
- Reporting broken windows or screens to avoid an insect problem.
- Reporting safety hazards.
- Shopping for groceries.
- Washing the dishes.

Infection Control

It is your responsibility to control the spread of microorganisms in the home by using proper handwashing technique and by doing sufficient housecleaning to maintain a clean environment for the patient. You should use hot water and ample amounts of detergent when washing dishes. Cleaning the bathroom frequently with a disinfectant detergent will help to eliminate odors and will cut down on the growth of bacteria. If there is more than one person using the bathroom, encourage them each to use their own towels. Laundry bleach is an inexpensive and effective disinfectant that can be found in most homes. If there are no supplies available, discuss this with your supervisor.

Equipment and Supplies

Check to see what cleaning supplies are already in the home and make a list of supplies needed. Submit your list to your employer or supervisor. In some homes, cleaning supplies and even patient care supplies may be limited. You will have to be flexible and improvise with what is available.

- If there is no toothpaste, substitute baking soda on a wet toothbrush or a solution of mouthwash and water.
- If there is no disinfectant cleaning liquid or powder, you can use a solution of liquid laundry bleach and water.
- If there is no ice cap (bag), improvise by taking a plastic bag or plastic glove and filling it half full of ice. Close the bag with a rubber band or a knot. Wrap this in a small towel before applying it to the patient's skin.

Food Service

Try to involve the patient and the family in meal planning. Ask about the patient's favorite foods and how to prepare them. Ask for the times that the patient prefers to have his meals. Inquire about food allergies and dislikes. Be sure to check with your supervisor to see if a special or therapeutic diet has been prescribed by the physician. If so, you must be sure the patient adheres to it strictly.

Make a list of needed foods and supplies as you plan the menus. If you are asked to buy the groceries, save all receipts to give to your employer. If a family member will be doing the marketing, you can show your menu plan and grocery list to him. After the food is purchased, it is your responsibility to see that it is stored properly to avoid health hazards. Be sure dairy products, partly used items, and leftovers are kept in the refrigerator.

The bed-bound patient's appetite may be small. Even if the meals are small they must be well balanced. The patient will have a more pleasant disposition and regain his strength more quickly if he is eating properly. Be sure the patient is taking enough fluids. Some geriatric patients have difficulty in chewing because dentures do not fit well or because their own teeth are in poor condition. If you notice this, report it to your supervisor and try to provide softer, more easily chewed foods.

Reporting and Recording

A written record of your activities and those of the patient must be kept carefully. Any medications taken by the patient and any treatments given should be recorded. The doctor and your supervisor may want a record of the patient's food intake, activity, vital signs, and sugar and acetone results when testing the urine.

Your supervisor may provide you with special forms for recording this information. If not, you may use a clean sheet of plain white paper. Be sure your handwriting is neat and legible. Write down each activity as soon as it is completed. *DO NOT* rely on your memory. If you are to report to your supervisor by phone, be sure this is done. If you follow the last step of every procedure in this book, it tells you exactly what to report or write down to tell your supervisor or the family member you are reporting to.

Activities of Daily Living—A Sample Daily Report

Home Health Assistant—Miss Jones   6-22-81
Patient's name—Doris Smith

8 a.m.   Arrived at patient's home. Greeted the patient, put laundry into washing machine, prepared breakfast.

8:15	Washed the patient's hands and face and assisted with oral hygiene.
8:30	Morning meal served (orange juice, dry cereal with milk, one slice of bacon, hot tea). The patient ate all of her breakfast.
8:50	Dishes washed. Prepared for patient's bath.
9:15	Partial bath given. Patient washed her own arms, chest, and perineal area. Small reddened area on patient's right buttock, the size of a dime, noted. Massaged area with lotion. Mouth care given and patient's hair combed. Linen changed.
10:00	Bathroom cleaned.
10:30	Mrs. Smith complained of slight headache in her forehead. Reported to supervisor.
11:00	Read to the patient from the newspaper.
11:30	Patient sleeping in bed. Vacuumed living room and prepared grocery list.
12:00 Noon	Mrs. Smith's son arrived to visit. He offered to buy the groceries. Laundry dried, folded and put away.
12:30 p.m.	Patient watching T.V. Lunch prepared and served. Patient ate ¾ of her meal which consisted of: small tuna salad with sliced tomato, a slice of toast with margarine, 8 oz. milk, crackers, and jello.
1:00	Mouth care given. Patient visiting with a neighbor who came here for ½ hour. Kitchen cleaned.
2:00	Patient resting in bed. Refrigerator cleaned.
2:30	Took the patient for a walk in front of the house. She walked for 10 minutes. The patient enjoyed the walk, her tolerance of this activity was good.
4:00	Supper prepared. Patient's daughter arrived. She will serve the meal and clean up the dishes. Son brought the groceries, and visited for 15 minutes. Groceries put away.
4:15	Daughter given a full report of the day's activities.
4:30	Patient appeared relaxed and comfortable. She stated she felt better. Headache is completely gone. She offers no complaints at this time. Left the patient's home at 4:35 p.m.

WHAT YOU HAVE LEARNED

As a home health assistant, you are an important part of the health care team. All the health care you deliver is given under a physician's orders and the direct supervision of a registered nurse. You will be caring for many different kinds of people in a variety of surroundings. Remember that all of the procedures and information given in this book can be adapted to your work in the home. As far as possible, nursing care is given in the home in the same way as it would be given in any health care institution. You will need to be flexible and understanding. Due to a lack of equipment, in many instances you will have to improvise. Because you will be working physically away from your supervisor, it is important for you to maintain frequent communication with her. Written records of your activities and those of the patient will help you report accurately to your supervisor.

19 CARE OF THE DYING PATIENT

1. The Dying Patient
2. Postmortem Care (PMC)

SECTION 1: THE DYING PATIENT

OBJECTIVES: WHAT YOU WILL LEARN

When you have completed this section, you will be able to:

- Make the dying patient as comfortable as possible.
- Help meet the emotional needs of the patient.
- Help meet the special needs of the patient's family.
- Identify signs of approaching death.

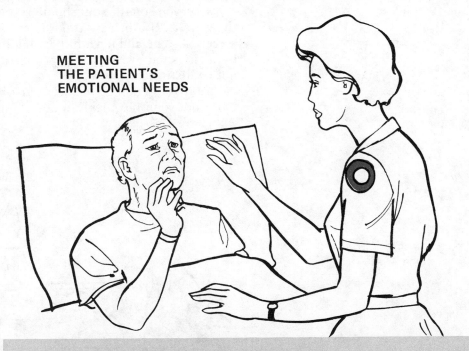

MEETING
THE PATIENT'S
EMOTIONAL NEEDS

WHEN A PATIENT SUSPECTS HE IS GOING TO DIE, HE MAY REACT IN VARIOUS WAYS:

- HE MAY ASK EVERYONE ABOUT HIS CHANCES FOR RECOVERY
- HE MAY BE AFRAID TO BE ALONE, AND WANT A LOT OF ATTENTION FROM YOU
- HE MAY ASK A LOT OF QUESTIONS
- HE MAY SEEM TO COMPLAIN CONSTANTLY
- HE MAY OFTEN SIGNAL MEMBERS OF THE STAFF
- HE MAY MAKE MANY APPARENTLY UNREASONABLE REQUESTS

Some patients who enter a health care institution are **terminally ill**, that is, dying. Sometimes death is sudden or unexpected. More often it is not. Your first responsibility is to help make the patient as comfortable as possible. Your second responsibility is to assist in meeting the emotional needs of the patient and his family.

The most important single fact to remember when you are caring for a dying patient is that he is just as important as the patient who is going to recover. You will not have the satisfaction of contributing to his recovery, but you will know that you have helped a human being to end his life in peace, comfort and dignity. Everyone must die. Surely we would all prefer to die in reassuring and comfortable surroundings.

Try to be very understanding. The patient may want to believe he will get well. He may want people around him to reassure him that he won't die. When a dying patient talks to you, listen. But don't give him false hopes. Don't tell him that he is getting better. If you did that, the patient, sooner or later, would know that you had lied to him. He might resent you for this.

People have different ideas about death and the hereafter. These ideas depend on the patient's beliefs and background. You must show respect for the patient's beliefs. Be careful not to impose your own beliefs on him or his family.

The Patient's Family

When it is known that death is approaching, the dying patient's family may want to spend a lot of time with him. This is usually permitted as much as possible.

Everyone on the staff should respect the family's need for privacy during their visits. If a private room is not available, the patient's area should be screened so he and his family will have the privacy they need. When the patient is visited by his pastor, priest, rabbi, or minister, assure them they will not be disturbed.

Don't stop doing your work just because the patient's family is present. Carry out your job quickly, quietly, and efficiently. Don't wait until the family

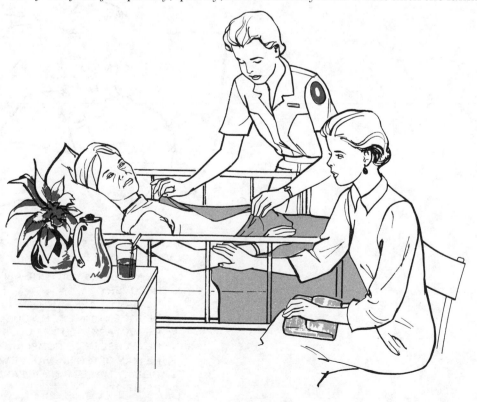

has gone before taking care of the patient. They might think that, because he is dying, he is being neglected by the hospital staff.

The patient's family may ask you many questions. Don't ignore their questions. Answer any you can. Also, do whatever is asked of you, if it is allowed.

There will be some questions that you can't answer. For example, you may be asked, "What did the doctor say today about his condition?" Refer the family to your head nurse or team leader.

Even if the patient becomes unconscious, the family may want to stay with him. Family members may continue to hope for his recovery. They will watch you perform your patient care procedures. They will want you to make the patient comfortable, even if you cannot help him recover.

Unconscious patients require as thorough care as those who are conscious. Their needs must still be met. Sometimes you must ask the family to leave the bedside while you are giving care to the patient. Explain this to the family. Tell them that you will let them know when you have finished.

Some visitors stay with the patient for many hours at a time. Be as helpful to them as you can. You might suggest that they have a cup of coffee. Tell them where the coffee shop is. Also, learn the policy in your institution on serving meals to visitors. You may be able to arrange for trays to be delivered to the patient's family at mealtimes. If this is not allowed, tell the visitors where they can find the cafeteria or a nearby restaurant. Make sure the visitors know the location of the washroom, lounge and telephones.

Remember at all times to be quietly courteous, understanding, sympathetic and willing to help. These are the marks of a competent nursing assistant. Don't feel helpless or guilty because you can't improve the patient's condition. You can help the patient and his family most by maintaining a concerned and efficient approach to your work.

Patient Care

A patient approaching death continues to be given routine personal care, such as baths and mouth care. That is, he is given the same care he would receive if he were expected to recover. Members of the nursing staff should

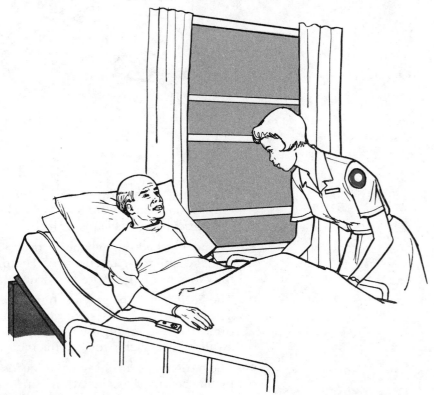

stay calm and sympathetic. This may help to relieve some of the patient's fears and make this time easier for him. As the patient becomes weaker and finally helpless, his condition may require more of your time. You will probably be doing many things for him that he had earlier taken care of himself.

Rules to Follow: Care of the Dying Patient

- Keep the room well ventilated and lighted as usual. Because the dying patient's eyesight is usually failing, a dark room may frighten him.

- The patient may be most comfortable lying on his back. He may have his head raised slightly and have a pillow under his knees for support. Change the patient's position at least every two hours to keep him comfortable and to prevent irritation of his skin.

- As long as the patient is conscious, speak to him in your normal voice. Even if he seems to be unconscious, use your normal voice when you are talking to someone else in the room.

- Don't say things you wouldn't want the patient to hear. The dying patient's hearing is usually one of the last senses to fail.

- Respect the patient's need for spiritual support. Learn the policy in your institution concerning religious observances and requirements at the time of death. For example, if a Roman Catholic patient wishes to see a priest or appears to be in danger of dying, a priest should be called. Because the body of an Orthodox Jewish patient should not be touched after death until the rabbi or proper religious authority arrives, it is important to straighten the patient's limbs before death occurs.

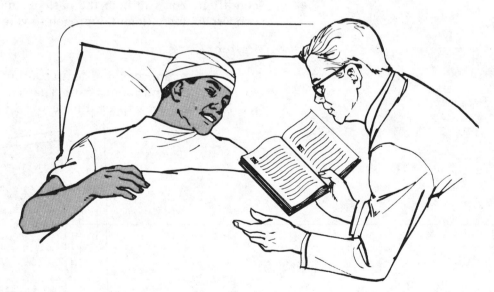

- The dying patient may be incontinent, that is, unable to control the elimination of urine or feces. He may soil the bed often. Your job is to keep the patient's body clean at all times.

- Change the bedding whenever necessary. This will keep the patient's skin from becoming irritated and will help to keep the patient comfortable. You may also be giving more back rubs than usual.

- The patient may be given softer food and in smaller amounts than usual. The amount and consistency of the food will depend on what the patient's digestive system can tolerate. He may be given liquids as long as he can swallow. This helps to keep his mouth moist.

- The patient approaching death needs special mouth care. His mouth may be dry because he is breathing through it. His mouth also may be dry because a nasogastric tube is being used. In this case, you might use an applicator with glycerine (or other lubricant) to swab the patient's mouth and lips. If the patient's mouth has a lot of secretions in it, tell the head nurse. She may use suction to remove the secreted material. If the patient has dentures, ask your head nurse or team leader if you should leave them in the patient's mouth or take them out. If you remove the dentures, place them in a denture cup with the patient's name on the cover.

- A patient may be receiving oxygen through a nasal catheter or mask. If so, check his nostrils from time to time. Tell your head nurse or team leader if the nostrils are dry and encrusted.

- A patient's nostrils also may become dry and encrusted because he has difficulty in breathing. If you notice dryness, with your head nurse's or team leader's permission, clean the nostrils with cotton swabs moistened slightly with glycerine (or other lubricant).

Signs of Approaching Death

Death comes in different ways. It may come quite suddenly after a patient has seemed to be recovering. Or it may come after a long period during which there has been a steady decline of body functions. Death also may result from complications during convalescence. Here are some signs showing that death may be near:

- Blood circulation slows down. The patient's hands and feet are cold to the touch.

- If the patient is conscious, he may complain that he is cold. Keep him well covered.

- The patient's face may become pale because of decreased circulation.

- His eyes may be staring blankly into space. There may be no eye movement when you move your hand across his line of vision.

- The patient may perspire heavily, even though his body is cold.

- The patient loses muscle tone, and his body becomes limp. His jaw may drop and his mouth may stay partly open.

- Respirations may become slower and more difficult.

- Mucus collecting in the patient's throat and bronchial tubes may cause a sound that is sometimes called the "death rattle."

- The pulse often is rapid, but it becomes weak and irregular.

- Just before death, respiration stops and the pulse gets very faint. You may not be able to feel the patient's pulse at all.

- Contrary to popular belief, a dying person is rarely in great pain. As the patient's condition gets worse, less blood may be flowing to the brain. Therefore the patient may feel little or no pain.

If you notice any of these signs or any change in the patient's condition, report to your head nurse or team leader immediately. Try to be with the patient as much as possible, even if you cannot do a lot. Just being there will often be comforting.

SECTION 2: POSTMORTEM CARE (PMC)

OBJECTIVES: WHAT YOU WILL LEARN

When you have completed this section, you will be able to:

- Give postmortem care gently and respectfully.
- Protect the patient's valuables.
- Remove the patient's body from the unit discreetly.

If you observe any signs of approaching death, tell your head nurse or team leader immediately. The nurse will examine the patient and confirm what you have found. Until you have received direct instructions from your head nurse or team leader, no postmortem care can be given to a patient. The word **postmortem** means after death.

In some health care institutions, the head nurse or team leader confirms that a patient has no pulse or has stopped breathing and she calls a "Code." Code, Code Blue, Cardiac Arrest, or whatever name is used for the code in your institution, is an emergency announcement to the entire staff. A pre-assigned team will come to help the patient within one minute. Then every means available to keep the patient alive is used. Only when the team fails to keep the patient alive is the patient declared to be dead by a physician.

After a patient has died, his body still must be treated with respect and must be given gentle care. If family members are present, they usually wait outside the room until the doctor has finished his examination. The patient's family will probably be allowed to view the body if they wish.

Sometimes the family is not present when the patient dies. In this case, the nurse calls the doctor and tells him the family is not there. Either the doctor or the nurse then notifies the family and finds out whether they wish to view the body before it is sent to the morgue. If so, the body stays in the room until the family arrives.

When the family is present, they are given the patient's personal belongings. These items are checked against the clothing list to be sure that everything is accounted for. You will learn the procedure in your health care institution for taking care of the deceased patient's clothes. If the members of the family do not wish to view the body, you will then proceed with the postmortem care.

Postmortem care should be done before rigor mortis sets in. **Rigor mortis** means that the body and limbs become stiff.

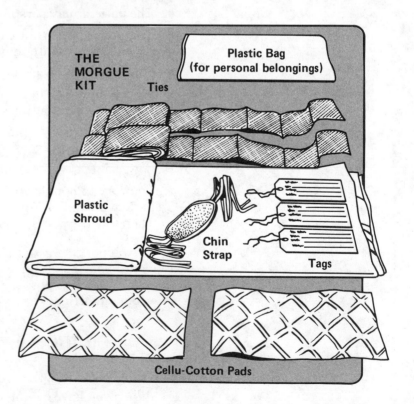

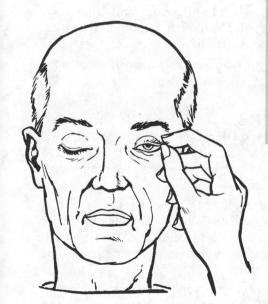

Procedure: Giving Postmortem Care

1. Assemble your equipment:
   a) Postmortem care kit from **CSR** (central supply room) containing:
      - Plastic shroud or sheet
      - Chin strap (if used in your institution)
      - Cellulose pads
      - Three identification tags, to be filled out by the head nurse, team leader, or ward clerk
      - Roll of 1-inch bandage or ties
      - Large bag for personal belongings
      - Laundry bag
      - Disposable bed protector
   b) Stretcher
   c) Equipment for bed bath:
      - Large towel
      - Wash basin with water at 115°F (46.1°C)
      - Washcloth

2. Wash your hands.

3. Identify the patient by checking the identification bracelet.

4. Ask visitors to step out of the room.

5. Pull the curtain around the bed for privacy.

6. Lower the backrest.

7. Remove all pillows except one, which is to be placed under the patient's head.

8. Place the patient's body in the supine or dorsal recumbent position, straightening the arms and legs. Move the body gently to avoid bruising.

9. Close the patient's eyes if they are open:
   a) Take the lashes and gently pull the eyelids over the eyes.
   b) Avoid touching the eyelids themselves. Pressure may give them an unnatural appearance.

(continued next page)

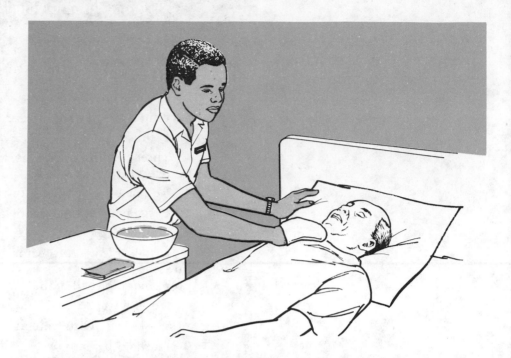

Procedure continued

10. Bathe the body, if necessary, to remove any discharges or secretions.

11. Replace dentures in the mouth. In some institutions the dentures are left in a denture cup labeled with the patient's name for the mortician to take. Follow the instructions of your head nurse or team leader regarding the dentures.

12. Close the patient's mouth. Do this by cupping your hand under his chin and applying slight pressure. If the mouth will not stay closed, roll up a towel and place it under the chin as a support.

13. Fasten the chin strap in place, protecting the face with a cellulose pad.

14. Comb the hair, if necessary.

15. Remove all soiled dressings, bandages, and tubes as per the instructions of your head nurse or team leader. Cover all wounds or open incisions with a fresh, small, clean dressing, using adhesive tape to hold them in place. Remove old marks from adhesive tape with adhesive remover.

16. Remove all jewelry and give to the head nurse or team leader. If rings cannot be removed because of swelling, they should be secured in place with a 1-inch bandage tied around them or a piece of tape. This must be reported to the head nurse or team leader so that a notation can be made on the patient's chart.

17. Fold the arms over the abdomen. Tie the wrists and ankles, loosely, with bandages or ties. Place cellulose pads under the bandages to prevent bruising.

18. Attach identification tags to the bandage on the wrist and to the right big toe. The tags are filled out by the head nurse, team leader, or ward clark with the patient's name, sex, identification number, room number, and age.

19. Place the deceased body on the shroud or sheet with a disposable bed protector under the buttocks.

(continued next page)

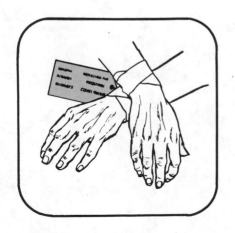

Procedure continued

20. Cover the body with the shroud, folding the shroud or sheet over the body, and tie it with bandages or ties at the waist, above the elbows, and below the knees.

21. Attach the third identification tag to the shroud at the waist bandage.

22. With the help of other nursing assistants, move the body onto a stretcher and cover it with a sheet.

23. Close the doors to all the patient's rooms and then move the stretcher to the morgue. Try to give the appearance of simply moving a patient to another place.

24. Every item belonging to the deceased patient is placed in a large bag. The bag is labeled with all needed information such as the patient's name, sex, age, room number, identification number, and date. Follow your institution's policy as to where you place this bag of personal belongings.

25. Strip all linen from the bed, placing it into the laundry bag, and then carry it to the dirty linen hamper.

26. Wash your hands.

27. Report to your head nurse or team leader:

    - That postmortem care was given.
    - That the body was taken to the morgue.
    - That the jewelry was given to the head nurse or team leader.
    - Where you placed the bag of personal belongings.
    - That the bed was stripped of dirty linen.
    - The date and time this was done.

WHAT YOU HAVE LEARNED

As a patient approaches death, you should treat him sympathetically and respectfully. Personal care should be given in the usual way. The dying patient and his family have strong emotional and physical needs. As a nursing assistant you should respond with understanding and quiet confidence. After death, the patient's body should be treated with gentleness and reverence. Special care should be taken to avoid bruises. Remember that throughout these procedures the patient's body must be handled gently and carefully.

20 INTRODUCTION TO MEDICAL TERMS

1. Introduction to Medical Terms and Abbreviations
2. Medical Specialties and Words to Remember

SECTION 1: INTRODUCTION TO MEDICAL TERMS AND ABBREVIATIONS

OBJECTIVES: WHAT YOU WILL LEARN

When you have completed this section, you will be able to:

- Recognize many abbreviations commonly used in health care institutions.
- Spell and pronounce various medical terms correctly.
- Divide words into their elements.
- Define the terms prefix, suffix, and root.
- Distinguish between similar word elements and to define them.
- Describe word elements and their meanings (prefixes, roots, and suffixes).
- Define terms and elements relating to anatomy and physiology, diseases and diagnoses, and surgical procedures.

KEY IDEAS: ABBREVIATIONS AND THEIR MEANINGS

Abbreviations are the shorthand of the medical and nursing professions. They are clear and efficient tools for the head nurse or team leader to tell you quickly what they want you to do. As a nursing assistant, you will use these abbreviations in your daily work. They will help you to understand instructions from your head nurse or team leader.

Abbreviations help you when you are receiving reports about your patients and in keeping your own notes on your daily assignments.

Abbreviations Used in Keeping Notes

ABBREVIATION	MEANING
aa	Of each, equal parts
ABR	Absolute bed rest
abd.	Abdomen
ac	Before meals
AD	Admitting diagnosis
A&D	Admission and discharge
ad lib	As desired, if the patient so desires
ADL	Activities of daily living
Adm.	Admission
Adm. Spec.	Admission urine specimen
A.M. or a.m. or am	Morning

Abbreviations Used in Keeping Notes (cont.)

ABBREVIATION	MEANING
amb.	Ambulation, walking, ambulatory, able to walk
amt.	Amount
AP or A.P.	Appendectomy
aqua	Water or H_2O
@	At
approx.	Approximately
B&B or b&b	Bowel and bladder training
bid or B.I.D. or b.i.d.	Twice a day
BM or B.M. or bm or b.m.	Bowel movement, feces
B.P. or BP	Blood pressure
BR or br or B.R. or b.r.	Bedrest
BRP or B.R.P. or brp	Bathroom privileges
BSC or bsc	Bedside commode
°C	Centigrade or Celsius degree
c̄ or c	With
Ca	Cancer
Cath.	Catheter
CBC or C.B.C.	Complete blood count
cc or c.c.	Cubic centimeter
CCU or C.C.U.	Cardiac care unit/coronary care unit
CBR or C.B.R. or cbr	Complete bed rest
CO	Carbon monoxide
C/O or c/o	Complains of
CO_2	Carbon dioxide
CS or cs or C.S. or c.s.	Central supply
CSD or csd or C.S.D.	Central service department
CSR or csr or C.S.R.	Central supply room
CVA or C.V.A.	Cerebrovascular accident or stroke
CPR or C.P.R.	Cardiopulmonary resuscitation
dc or d/c	Discontinue
Del. Rm. or d.r. or DR	Delivery room
Disch. or dish or D/C	Discharge
D. & C. or D&C	Dilatation and curettage
drsg.	Dressing
DOA or D.O.A.	Dead on arrival
Dr. or Dr	Doctor
DX	Diagnosis
ECG or EKG	Electrocardiogram
ED or E.D.	Emergency department
EEG or E.E.G.	Electroencephalogram
EENT or E.E.N.T.	Eyes, ears, nose, and throat
E. or E	Enema
ER or E.R.	Emergency room
°F	Fahrenheit degree

Abbreviations Used in Keeping Notes (cont.)

ABBREVIATION	MEANING
F. or Fe. or F or Fe	Female
FBS or F.B.S.	Fasting blood sugar
FF or F.F.	Forced feeding or forced fluids
ft	Foot
Fx	Fractional Urine or fracture
gal	Gallon
GI or G.I.	Gastrointestinal
gt	One drop
gtt	Two or more drops
Gtt or G.T.T.	Glucose tolerance test
GU or G.U.	Genitourinary
Gyn.	Gynecology
H_2O	Water or aqua
hr	Hour
HS or hs	Bedtime or hour of sleep
ht	Height
hyper	Above or high
hypo	Below or low
H.W.B. or hwb or HWB	Hot water bottle
ICU or I.C.U.	Intensive care unit
in. or in	Inch
I&O or I. & O.	Intake and output
irr	Irregular
Isol. or isol	Isolation
IV or I.V.	Intravenous
L	Liter
Lab. or lab	Laboratory
lb	Pound
Liq or liq.	Liquid, liquor
LPN or L.P.N.	Licensed practical nurse
LVN or L.V.N.	Licensed vocational nurse
M	Male
Mat	Maternity
MD or M.D.	Medical doctor
meas	Measure
mec	Meconium
med	Medicine
min	Minute
ml	Milliliter
Mn or mn or M/n	Midnight
N.A. or N/A	Nursing aide or nursing assistant
n/g or ng. or N.G.T.	Nasogastric tube
noct	At night
NP	Neuropsychiatric; or nursing procedure

Abbreviations Used in Keeping Notes (cont.)

ABBREVIATION	MEANING
NPO or **N.P.O.**	Nothing by mouth
Nsy	Nursery
O₂	Oxygen
OB or **O.B.**	Obstetrics
Obt or **obt**	Obtained
OJ or **O.J.**	Orange juice
Ord.	Orderly
OOB or **O.O.B.**	Out of bed
OPD or **O.P.D.**	Outpatient department
OR or **O.R.**	Operating room
Ortho	Orthopedics
OT or **O.T.**	Occupational therapy; or oral temperature
oz	Ounce
PAR or **P.A.R.**	Postanesthesia room
pc	After meals
Ped or **Peds**	Pediatrics
per	By, through
p.m. or **P.M.** or **pm** or **PM**	Afternoon
PMC or **P.M.C.**	Postmortem care
PN or **P.N.**	Pneumonia
po	By mouth
post or **p**	After
postop or **post op**	Postoperative
post op spec	After surgery urine specimen
PP	Postpartum (after delivery)
PPBS	Postprandial blood sugar
pre	Before
prn or **p.r.n.**	Whenever necessary, when required
preop or **pre op**	Before surgery
pre op spec	Urine specimen before surgery
prep	Prepare the patient for surgery by shaving the skin
Pt or **pt**	Patient, pint
PT or **P.T.**	Physical therapy
q	Every
qd	Every day
qh	Every hour
q2h	Every two hours
q3h	Every three hours
q4h	Every four hours
QHS or **qhs**	Every night at bedtime
qid or **Q.I.D.**	Four times a day
qam or **q am** or **q.a.m.**	Every morning
qod or **Q.O.D.**	Every other day
qs	Quantity sufficient; as much as required
qt	Quart

Abbreviations Used in Keeping Notes (cont.)

ABBREVIATION	MEANING
r or **R**	Rectal temperature
Rm or **rm**	Room
RN or **R.N.**	Registered nurse
rom or **R.O.M.**	Range of motion
RR or **R.Rm.**	Recovery room
Rx	Prescription or treatment ordered by a physician
s or **s̄**	Without
S&A	Sugar and acetone *A C Test*
S&A or **S.&A. Test**	Sugar and acetone test
S&K or **S. & K. Test**	Sugar and ketone test
SOB	Shortness of breath
sos	Whenever emergency arises; only if necessary
SPD	Special purchasing department
Spec or **spec**	Specimen
ss or **s̄s̄**	One-half
SSE or **S.S.E.**	Soapsuds enema
stat	At once, immediately
Surg	Surgery
tid or **T.I.D.**	Three times a day
TLC or **tlc**	Tender loving care
TPR	Temperature, pulse, respiration
U/a or **U/A** or **u/a**	Urine analysis
Ung.	Ointment; unguentine
V.D. or **vd**	Venereal disease
VDRL	Test for venereal disease
V.S. or **VS**	Vital signs
WBC or **W.B.C.**	White blood count
w/c	Wheelchair
wc or **W.C.**	Ward clerk
wt	Weight

Roman Numerals. The dots or "eyes" are used to eliminate a margin of error.

$$1 = \text{I or } \dot{\text{I}} \quad 2 = \text{II or } \ddot{\text{II}} \quad 3 = \text{III or } \dddot{\text{III}} \quad 4 = \text{IV or } \dot{\text{IV}} \quad 5 = \text{V or } \overline{\text{V}}$$

Guide to Pronunciation

New medical terms in this section are followed by simple guides to their pronunciation. Only long vowels are marked in the pronunciation guides. Pronunciation of other vowel sounds is shown only on words that are very difficult to pronounce correctly. As an exercise, and using rules given in the figure, pronounce each new word aloud.

Accents. The principle accent is written in capital letters. Example: DOC tor.

Syllables. Division between syllables is indicated by a slash (/). Example: gas/TRI/tis.

Vowels

Symbol	Name	Example
> ā	long a	> āle
> ă	short a	> ădd
> ē	long e	> ēve
> ĕ	short e	> ĕnd
> ī	long i	> īce
> ĭ	short i	> ĭll
> ō	long o	> ōld
> ŏ	short o	> ŏdd
> ū	long u	> c̄ube
> ŭ	short u	> ūp

Word Elements

Many medical terms are composed of several smaller, simpler words or word elements. This discussion describes and shows how to use three primary word elements that are combined frequently to form medical terms. These three word elements are the prefix, the root, and the suffix.

- The **root** is the body or main part of the word. It denotes the primary meaning of the word as a whole.

- The **prefix** is a word element combined with the root. It changes or adds to the meaning of the words. A prefix is always added to the beginning of a root.

- The **suffix** is also a word element used to change or add to the meaning of a root. It is always added to the end of the root.

The word elements of medical terms work very much like these examples. The main difference is that most medical word elements are derived from foreign languages, mostly Latin and Greek. So before you will be able to easily recognize the meanings of medical terms, you must learn the English meanings of the word elements in those terms. A list of common word elements in medical terms, with their meanings and guides to pronunciation, is given here. (The many anatomical terms and diseases that are named for their discoverer are not listed here.)

You may encounter a few special problems as you begin your study of medical terminology. First, a word that has been created from several word elements may leave out, change, or add certain letters so that it conforms to rules of spelling and pronunciation.

This chart shows some familiar English words that are composed of common word elements. These should give you an idea of what is meant by the term **word elements**.

Examples of Combining Word Elements

Prefix	Root	Suffix	Word
dis	agree	able	disagreeable
	war	like	warlike
un	pardon	able	unpardonable
inter	nation	al	international
speed (o)	meter		speedometer
	beauty	full	beautiful

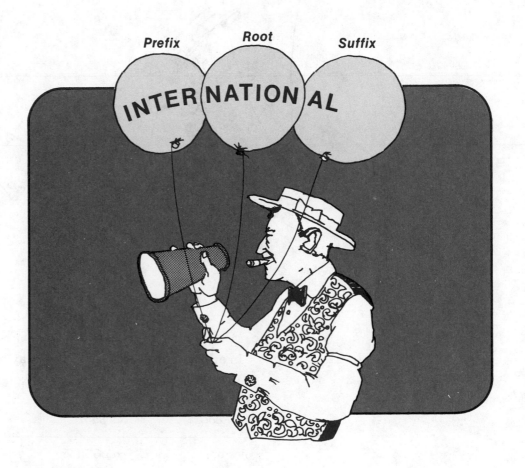

Combining Word Elements. Medical terms (like many English words) do not necessarily contain all three elements. The medical term may be a combination of a prefix and a root.

Examples of Prefixes and Roots

Prefix	+	Root	Prefix	Root
ectoderm		EC/to/derm	ecto	derm
retropubic		RE/tro/pu/bic	retro	pubic
endoskeleton		EN/do/skel/e/ton	endo	skeleton
hemiplegic		hem/i/PLE/gic	hemi	plegic
hypertension		hy/per/TEN/sion	hyper	tension

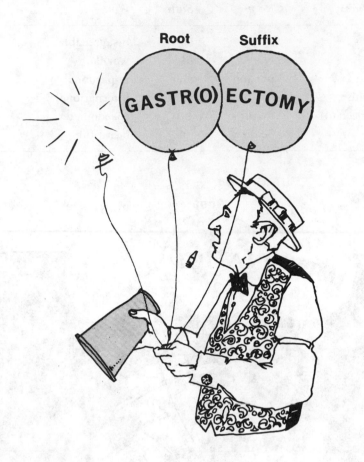
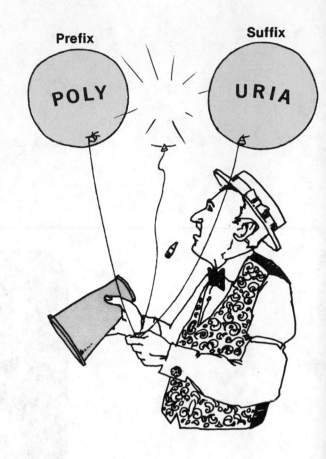

In other medical terms, the root may be combined with only a suffix.

Examples of Roots and Suffixes

Root	+	Suffix	Root	Suffix
colostomy		co/LOS/to/my	col(o)	ostomy
gastrectomy		gas/TREC/to/my	gastr(o)	ectomy
myasthenia		my/as/THE/ni/a	my(o)	asthenia
osteoma		os/te/O/ma	oste(o)	oma

Some medical terms may be formed by using prefixes and suffixes alone.

Examples of Terms Formed by Combining Prefixes and Suffixes

Prefix	+	Suffix	Prefix	Suffix
diarrhea		di/ar/RHE/a	dia	rrhea
endoscopy		en/DOS/co/py	end(o)	oscopy
excise		ex/CISE	ex	cise
epilepsy		EP/i/lep/sy	epi	lepsy
polyuria		pol/y/U/ri/a	poly	uria

Some medical terms are formed by combining two roots. The resulting word describes the disease or treatment more accurately.

Examples of Terms with Two Roots

Root	+	Root	First Root	Second Root
Bronchopneumonia		bron/cho/pneu/MO/ni/a	broncho	pneumo
gastroenteritis		gas/tro/en/ter/I/tis	gastro	enter (o)
osteoarthritis		os/te/o/ar/THRI/tis	osteo	arthr (o)
pyelonephritis		py/e/lo/neph/RI/tis	pyelo	nephr (o)

Examples of Spelling Variations

Prefix	Root	Suffix	Word	
em	pyo	ema	empyema	em/py/E/ma
endo	arterio	itis	endarteritis	end/ar/ter/I/tis
	neuro	ology	neurology	neu/ROL/o/gy
supre	renal		suprarenal	su/pra/RE/nal
	stomato	itis	stomatitis	sto/mat/I/tis

Second, many of the word elements you should be familiar with are similar in spelling but quite different in meaning. Here is a list of word elements that often present difficulties. Examine this list carefully.

Examples of Similarity Between Terms

Word Element	Example	Meaning
ante	*ante*febrile	*before* onset of fever
anti	*anti*febrile	used *against* fever
a	*a*dipsia	*absence* of thirst
ad	*ad*renal	*near* the kidney
a, an	*an*uria	*absence* of urine
ano	*ano*rectal	pertaining to *anus* and rectum
ad	*ad*oral	*near* the mouth
adeno	*aden*itis	*gland*ular inflammation
cyto	*cyto*genesis	production (origin) of the *cell*
cysto	*cysto*gram	x-ray record of the *bladder*
di	*di*atomic	containing *two* atoms
dia	*dia*gnosis	to know *through* (recognize) a disease
dis	*dis*sect	to cut *apart*
dys	*dys*menorrhea	*difficult* or painful menstruation
en	*en*cephalitis	inflammation *of* the brain
entero	*entero*plasty	operative revision of *intestines*
hema	*hem*angioma	angioma consisting of *blood* vessels
hemi	*hemi*analgesia	pain relief in *half* of body
hemo	*hemo*toxin	a *blood* cell poison
hyper	*hyper*tension	*high* blood pressure
hypo	*hypo*tension	*low* blood pressure

Word Element	Example	Meaning
ileo	*ileo*cecum	section of *small intestine*
ilio	*ilio*sacrum	part of hip *bone*
inter	*inter*stitial	lying *between* spaces
intra	*intra*cranial	*within* the skull
macro	*macro*scopy	seen *large*, as with the naked eye
micro	*micro*scopy	seen *small*, as by microscope
myo	*myo*logy	study of *muscle*
myelo	*myelo*ma	tumor of the *bone marrow*
necro	*necro*sis	state of tissue *death*
nephro	*nephro*sis	condition of the *kidneys*
neuro	*neuro*sis	*nervous* condition
osteo	*osteo*logy	study of *bone*
oto	*oto*logy	study of the *ear*
per	*per*cussion	a striking *through* the body
peri	*peri*cardial	*around* the heart
pre	*pre*clinical	*before* the onset of disease
pyo	*pyo*genic	*pus* producing
pyro	*pyro*genic	*fever* producing

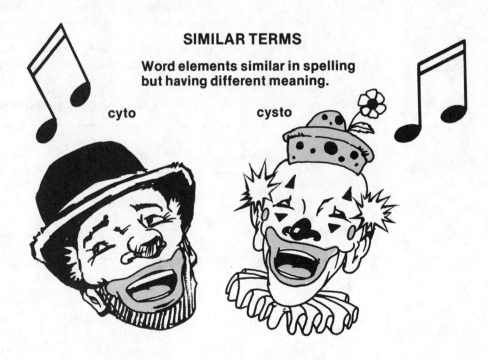

SIMILAR TERMS

Word elements similar in spelling but having different meaning.

cyto   cysto

Two groups of suffixes often contain quite similar word elements, each of which has a specific meaning.

-gram	electrocardiogram	*record* of heart action
-graph	electrocardiograph	*machine* that makes record
-graphy	electrocardiography	*process* of making record

Example: Electrocardio*graphy* is performed by a technician who connects parts of the patient's body to an electrocardio*graph*, which produces a record of the patient's heart action called an electrocardio*gram*.

-ectomy	gastrectomy	surgical *removal* of the stomach
-ostomy	gastrostomy	surgical *opening* into the stomach
-otomy	gastrotomy	surgical *incision* into the stomach

Example: An infant who swallowed a pin requires a gastr*otomy* to remove the pin from his stomach.

A patient unable to take food by mouth has a gastr*ostomy* performed and is fed by tube directly into the stomach.

The doctor performs a gastr*ectomy* on a patient with bleeding ulcers.

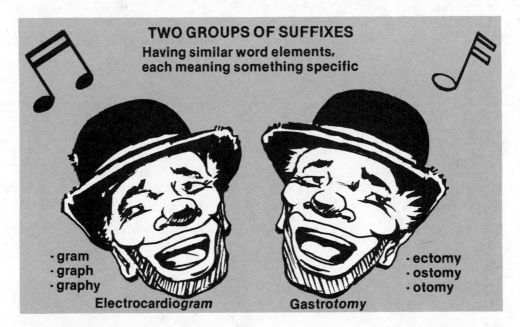

Glossary of Word Elements

The following list of word elements is arranged in alphabetical order. Word elements most often used as prefixes are followed by a hyphen (ambi-). Suffixes are preceded by a hyphen (-algia). Remember that sometimes a term changes its function (a prefix is used as a root, for example) when it is used in a different word.

1. Say out loud each word element and its meaning.
2. Pronounce the words given as examples.
3. Try to figure out the meaning of the sample word from the information given in the list. For example, the third word on the list is *adrenal.* Ad means *near* or *toward.* Now look up *renal.* You will find that it means *kidney.* Therefore adrenal means *near the kidney.*
4. Make flashcards for yourself. Write the new word on little cards with the meaning on the back. Look at the cards as often as you can.

Glossary of Word Elements

Word Element	Refers to or Means	Example	
A-, AN-	without, lack of, absent, deficient	asepsis a/SEP/sis	anorexia an/or/EX/i/a
AB-, ABS-	from, away	abnormal ab/NORM/AL	abscess ABS/cess
AD-	near, toward	adrenal	ad/REN/al
ADENO	gland	adenopathy	ad/en/OP/a/thy
AERO	air	anaerobe	an/A/er/obe
ALB	white	albumin	al/BU/min
-ALGIA, -ALGESIA	pain	analgesia	an/al/GE/si/a
AMBI-	both	ambidextrous	am/bi/DEX/trous
ANGIO	vessel (blood or lympth)	angioma	an/gi/O/ma
ANO	anus	anoscope	A/no/scope
ANTE-	before	antenatal	an/te/NA/tal
ANTI-	against	antiseptic	an/ti/SEP/tic
ARTERIO	artery	arteriosclerosis	ar/ter/i/o/scler/O/sis
ARTHRO	joint	arthroplasty	AR/thro/plas/ty
-ASTHENIA	weakness	myasthenia	my/as/THE/ni/a
AUTO-	self	autonomic	au/to/NOM/ic
BI-	two, twice	biweekly	bi/WEEK/ly
BRADY-	slow	bradycardia	bra/dy/CAR/di/a
BRONCHO	bronchus	bronchitis	bron/CHI/tis
CARDIO	heart	myocardium	my/o/CAR/di/um
-CELE	tumor, swelling, hernia, sac	enterocele	EN/ter/o/cele
-CENTESIS	puncture	thoracentesis	tho/ra/cen/TE/sis
CEPHALO	head	hydrocephaly	hy/dro/CEPH/a/ly
CHOLE	gall	cholelithiasis	cho/le/lith/I/a/sis
CHOLECYSTO	gallbladder	cholecystectomy	cho/le/cys/TECT/o/my
CHOLEDOCHO	common bile duct	choledochostomy	cho/led/o/CHOS/to/my
CHONDRO	cartilage	chondroma	chon/DRO/ma
-CIDE	kill	germicide	GERM/i/cide
CIRCUM-	around	circumcision	cir/cum/CI/sion
-CISE	cut	excise	ex/CISE
COLO	colon	colitis	co/LI/tis
COLPO	vagina	colporrhaphy	col/POR/rha/phy
CONTRA-	against	contraception	con/tra/CEP/tion
COSTO	rib	intercostal	in/ter/COS/tal
CRANIO	skull	craniotomy	cra/ni/OT/o/my
CYANO	blue	cyanotic	cy/an/OT/ic
CYSTO	urinary bladder	cystogram	CYS/to/gram

Word Element	Refers to or Means	Example	
CYTO	cell	monocyte	MON/o/cyte
DE-	down; from	decubitus	de/CU/bi/tus
DENTI	tooth	dentistry	DEN/tis/try
DERMO, DERMATO	skin	dermatology	derm/a/TOL/o/gy
DI-	two	diataxia	di/a/TAX/i/a
DIA-	through, between, across, apart	diarrhea	di/ar/RHE/a
DIS-	apart	dissect	dis/SECT
DYS-	painful, difficult, disordered	dysmenorrhea	dys/men/or/RHE/a
ECTO-	outer, on the outside	ectoparasite	ect/o/PAR/a/site
ECTOMY	surgical removal	prostatectomy	pros/ta/TEC/to/my
-EMESIS	vomiting	hematemesis	hem/at/EM/e/sis
-EMIA	blood	leukemia	leu/KE/mi/a
EN-	in, inside	encapsulated	en/CAP/su/la/ted
ENCEPHALO	brain	encephalitis	en/ceph/a/LI/tis
ENDO-	within, inner, on the inside	endometrium	en/do/ME/tri/um
ENTERO	intestine	enteritis	en/ter/I/tis
EPI-	above, over	epigastric	ep/i/GAS/tric
ERYTHRO	red	erythroblast	e/RYTH/ro/blast
-ESTHESIA	sensation	paresthesia	par/es/THE/si/a
EX-	out	excretion	ex/CRE/tion
FEBR	fever	afebrile	a/FEB/rile
FIBRO	connective tissue	fibroid	FI/broid
GASTRO	stomach	gastrointestinal	gas/tro-in/TEST/in/al
-GENE, -GENIC	production, origin	neurogenic	neu/ro/GEN/ic
GLOSSO	tongue	glossalgia	glos/SAL/gi/a
GLUCO, GLYCO	sugar, sweet	glycogen	GLY/co/gen
-GRAM	record	myelogram	MY/e/lo/gram
-GRAPH	machine	electroencephalograph	e/lec/tro/en/CEPH/al/o/graph
-GRAPHY	practice, process	ventriculography	ven/tri/cu/LOG/ra/phy
GYNE	woman	gynecology	gy/ne/COL/o/gy
HEMA, HER-MATO, HEMO	blood	hematology	hem/at/OL/o/gy
HEMI-	half	hemiplegia	hem/i/PLE/gi/a
HEPA, HEPATO	liver	hepatitis	hep/a/TI/tis
HERNI	rupture	herniation	her/ni/A/tion

Word Element	Refers to or Means	Example	
HISTO	tissue	histology	his/TOL/o/gy
HYDRO-	water	hydronephrosis	hy/dro/neph/RO/sis
HYPER-	over, above, increased, excessive	hypertension	hy/per/TEN/sion
HYPO-	under, beneath, decreased	hypotension	hy/po/TEN/sion
HYSTER	uterus	hysterectomy	hys/er/ECT/o/my
-IASIS	condition of	psoriasis	psor/I/a/sis
ICTERO	jaudice	iceterus	IC/ter/us
ILEO	ileum (part of small intestine	ileitis	il/e/I/tis
ILIO	ilium (bone)	iliosacrum	il/i/o/SA/crum
INTER-	between	intercellular	inter/CELL/u/lar
INTRA-	within	intramuscular	in/tra/MUS/cu/lar
-ITIS	inflammation of	appendicitis	ap/pen/di/CI/tis
LAPARO	abdomen	laparotomy	la/par/OT/o/my
-LEPSY	seizure, convulse	narcolepsy	NAR/co/lep/sy
LEUKO	white	leukorrhea	leu/kor/RHE/a
LIPO	fat	lipoma	lip/O/ma
LITH	stone, calculus	lithotomy	lith/OT/o/my
-LYSIS	loosen, dissolve	hemolysis	hem/OL/y/sis
MACRO-	large, long	macrocyte	MAC/ro/cyte
MAL-	bad, poor, disordered	maladjusted	mal/ad/JUST/ed
-MANIA	insanity	kleptomania	klep/to/MAN/ia
MAST	breast	mastectomy	mas/TEC/to/my
MEGA-	large	acromegaly	ac/ro/MEG/a/ly
MEN	month	mcnstruation	men/stru/A/tion
MESO-	middle	mesentery	MES/en/ter/y
-METER	measure	thermometer	ther/MOM/e/ter
METRO	uterus	metrorrhagia	met/ror/RHA/gia
MICRO-	small	microscope	MIC/ro/scope
MONO-	single, one	monocyte	MON/o/cyte
MUCO	mucous membrane	mucocutaneous	mu/co/cu/TA/ne/ous
MYELO	spinal cord, bone marrow	myelomeningocele	my/el/o/men/IN/go/cele
MYO	muscle	myopathy	my/OP/a/thy
NARCO	sleep	narcotic	nar/COT/ic
NASO	nose	nasopharynx	nas/o/PHA/rynx
NECRO	death	necropsy	NEC/rop/sy
NEO-	new	neoplasm	NE/o/plasm
NEPHRO	kidney	nephritis	ne/PHRI/tis

Word Element	Refers to or Means	Example	
NEURO	nerve	neuralgia	neu/RAL/gi/a
NON-	no, not	nontoxic	non/TOX/ic
OCULO	eye	oculist	O/cu/list
-OLOGY	study of	bacteriology	bac/ter/i/OL/o/gy
-OMA	tumor	carcinoma	car/ci/NO/ma
OOPHOR	ovary	oophorectomy	o/opho/REC/to/my
OPHTHALMO	eye	ophthalmoscope	oph/THAL/mo/scope
-OPIA	vision	diplopia	dip/LO/pi/a
ORCHI	testicle	orchipexy	ORCH/i/pex/y
-ORRHAPHY	to repair a defect	herniorrhaphy	her/ni/OR/raph/y
ORTHO-	straight	orthopedics	orth/o/PED/ics
-OSCOPY	look into, see	esophagoscopy	e/soph/a/GOS/co/py
OSIS	condition of	neurosis	neu/RO/sis
OSTEO	bone	osteoporosis	os/te/o/por/O/sis
-OSTOMY	surgical opening	colostomy	col/OST/o/my
OTO	ear	otolith	OT/o/lith
-OTOMY	incision, surgical cutting	gastrotomy	gas/TROT/o/my
PARA-	alongside of	paraplegia	par/a/PLE/gi/a
PATH	disease	pathology	pa/THOL/o/gy
PED (Latin)	foot	pedicure	PED/i/cure
PED (Greek)	child	pediatrics	pe/di/AT/rics
-PENIA	too few	leukopenia	leu/ko/PEN/i/a
PERI-	around, covering	pericarditis	pe/ri/car/DI/tis
-PEXY	to sew up in position	nephropexy	NEPH/ro/pex/y
PHARYNGO	throat	pharyngoplasty	pha/RYN/go/plas/ty
PHLEBO	vein	phlebitis	phle/BI/tis
-PHOBIA	fear, dread	photophobia	pho/to/PHO/bi/a
-PLASTY	operative revision	rhinoplasty	RHI/no/plas/ty
PLEGIA	paralysis	quadriplegia	qua/dri/PLE/gi/a
-PNEA	breathing	orthopnea	or/thop/NE/a
PNEUMO	air, lungs	pneumonia	pneu/MO/ni/a
POLY-	much, many	polyuria	po/ly/U/ri/a
POST	after	postpartum	post/PAR/tum
PRE-	before	preoperative	pre/OP/er/a/tive
PROCTO	rectum	proctoscopy	proc/TOS/co/py
-PTOSIS	falling	nephroptosis	neph/rop/TO/sis
PYELO	pelvis of kidney	pyelonephritis	py/el/o/neph/RI/tis
PYO	pus	empyema	em/py/E/ma
PYRO	heat, temperature	pyrexia	py/REX/i/a
RENAL	kidney	suprarenal	su/pra/RE/nal
RETRO-	behind, backward	retrosternal	ret/ro/STER/nal

Word Element	Refers to or Means		Example
-RHAGE	hemorrhage, flow	hemorrhage	HEM/or/rhage
-RHEA	flow	diarrhea	di/ar/RHE/a
RHINO	nose	rhinopathy	rhi/NOP/a/thy
SALPINGO	oviduct	salpingectomy	sal/pin/GEC/to/my
SEMI-	half	semicircular	sem/i/CIR/cu/lar
SEPTIC	poison, infection	septicemia	sep/ti/CEM/i/a
STOMATO	mouth	stomatitis	sto/ma/TI/tis
SUB-	under	subacute	sub/a/CUTE
SUPER	above	suprapubic	su/pra/PU/bic
-THERAPY	treatment	hydrotherapy	hy/dro/THER/a/py
-THERMY	heat	diathermy	DI/a/therm/y
THORACO	chest	thoracotomy	thor/a/COT/o/my
THROMBO	clot	thrombosis	throm/BO/sis
THYRO	thyroid gland	thyroxine	thy/ROX/ine
TRANS-	across	transfusion	trans/FU/sion
-URIA, -URIC	condition of, presence in urine	glycosuria	gly/co/SUR/i/a
URO	urine	uremia	u/RE/mi/a
UNI	one	unicellular	u/ni/CELL/u/lar
VASO	blood vessel	vasoconstriction	vas/o/con/STRIC/tion

Formulating Medical Terms

Many medical terms referring to parts of the body systems and functions come from Latin or Greek root elements. These roots should not be seen as synonyms for English equivalents. Rather, they should be understood as referring to the English terms. Careful study will increase your familiarity with Latin and Greek roots and the English words that come from them.

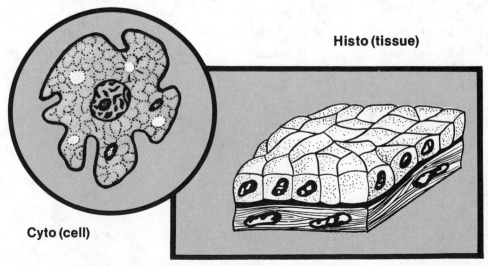

Histo (tissue)

Cyto (cell)

Word Element	*Refers to*
Integumentary system (skin)	
dermo, dermato	skin
muco	mucous membrane
Musculoskeletal system	
myo	muscle
myocardio	heart muscle
myocolpo	vaginal muscle
myometro	uterine muscle
osteo	bone
chondro	cartilage
fibro	connective tissue
arthro	joint
costo	rib
cranio	skull
ilio	hipbone, ilium
sacro	tailbone, sacrum
myelo	bone marrow
Respiratory system	
aero	air
naso, rhino	nose
pharyngo	throat
tracheo	windpipe
thoraco	chest
broncho	bronchus
pneumo	lung
Circulatory system	
cardio	heart
hema, hemato, hemo	blood
vaso	blood vessel
arterio	artery
phlebo	vein
lympho	lymphatic system
angio	blood and lymphatic vessels
erythro	red
leuko	white
cyano	blue
Digestive system	
stomato	mouth
denti	teeth
glosso	tongue
pharyngo	pharynx, throat
esophago	esophagus, food pipe
gastro	stomach
entero	small intestine
hepa, hepato	liver
cholecysto	gallbladder
chole	bile, gall
lipo	fat
choledocho	common bile duct
ileo	ileum
colo	large intestine
append	appendix
procto	rectum
ano	anus
laparo	abdomen
Nervous system	
encephalo	brain
myelo	spinal cord
neuro	nerve

Word Element	Refers to
oculo, ophthalmo	eye
oto	ear
Endocrine system	
adeno	gland
cephalo	head
thyro	thyroid
glyco, gluco	sugar
prostato	prostate
Urinary system	
nephro, renal	kidney
pyelo	kidney pelvis
hydro	water
uro	urine
uretero	ureter
cysto	urinary bladder
Reproductive system	
andro	man
gyne	woman
orchi, orchido	testicles
oophor	ovary
hyster, metro	uterus, womb
salpingo	oviduct
colpo	vagina
mast	breasts

Word Element: Path

When the word element **path** is found in a medical term, it always means *disease*. Examine the word **pathology.** The suffix **ology** means *the study of;* *pathology*, therefore, means the *study of disease*. Now use the word element *path* as a suffix to formulate a whole category of medical terms.

arterio*pathy*	any disease of the arteries
pneumono*pathy*	any disease of the lungs
uro*pathy*	any disease affecting the urinary tract

Word Element: Itis

The study of medical terminology can aid you in understanding the name of the specific disease for which the patient has been hospitalized. The word element **itis** means *inflammation of*. Almost every organ in the body is subject to infection by disease organisms that will cause an inflammatory reaction. The word to describe a diagnosis of this nature is formulated simply by adding the suffix **itis** to word for the body organ so affected.

appendic*itis*	inflammation of the appendix
dermat*itis*	inflammation of the skin
hepat*itis*	inflammation of liver tissue
rhin*itis*	inflammation of nasal mucosa
stomat*itis*	inflammation of the mouth

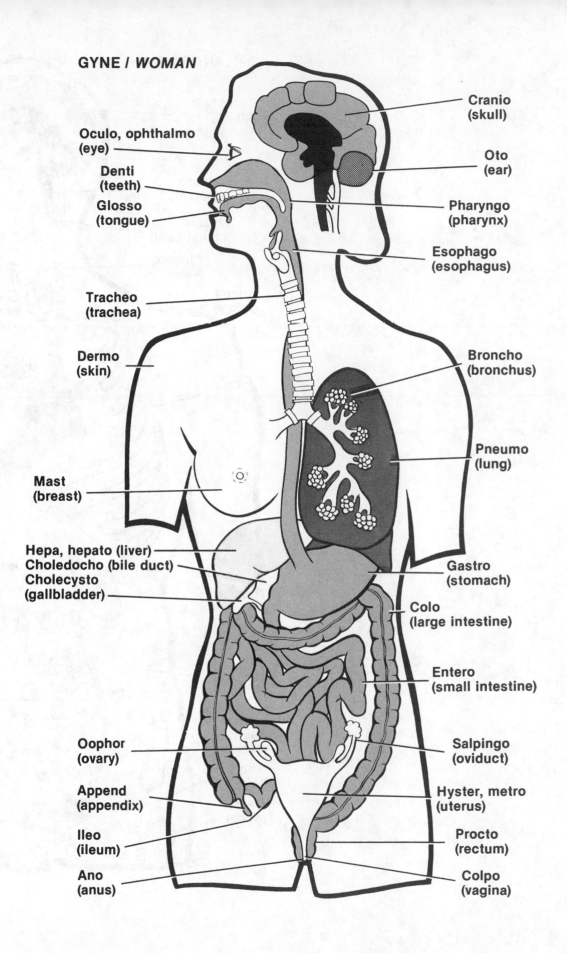

GYNE / WOMAN

Cranio
(skull)

Oculo, ophthalmo
(eye)

Oto
(ear)

Denti
(teeth)

Glosso
(tongue)

Pharyngo
(pharynx)

Esophago
(esophagus)

Tracheo
(trachea)

Dermo
(skin)

Broncho
(bronchus)

Pneumo
(lung)

Mast
(breast)

Hepa, hepato (liver)
Choledocho (bile duct)
Cholecysto
(gallbladder)

Gastro
(stomach)

Colo
(large intestine)

Entero
(small intestine)

Oophor
(ovary)

Salpingo
(oviduct)

Append
(appendix)

Hyster, metro
(uterus)

Ileo
(ileum)

Procto
(rectum)

Ano
(anus)

Colpo
(vagina)

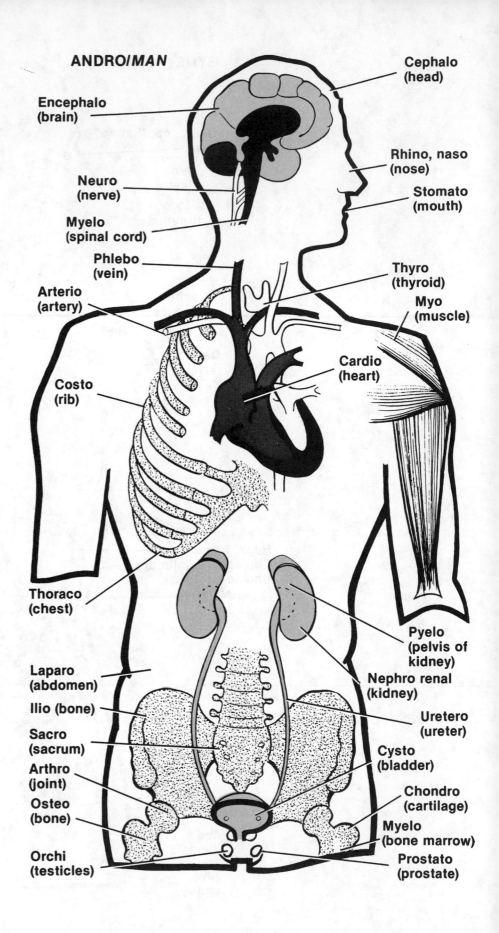

ANDRO/*MAN*

Cephalo
(head)

Encephalo
(brain)

Rhino, naso
(nose)

Neuro
(nerve)

Stomato
(mouth)

Myelo
(spinal cord)

Phlebo
(vein)

Thyro
(thyroid)

Arterio
(artery)

Myo
(muscle)

Cardio
(heart)

Costo
(rib)

Thoraco
(chest)

Pyelo
(pelvis of
kidney)

Laparo
(abdomen)

Nephro renal
(kidney)

Ilio (bone)

Ureter
(ureter)

Sacro
(sacrum)

Cysto
(bladder)

Arthro
(joint)

Chondro
(cartilage)

Osteo
(bone)

Myelo
(bone marrow)

Orchi
(testicles)

Prostato
(prostate)

Other Word Elements

Many terms concerned with a disease, its many symptoms, the tools and procedures used to diagnose it, and the diagnoses themselves are formulated in the manner described above. Study and learn the terms in common usage listed below.

Word Element	Example	Definition
algia	neur*algia*	*pain* along the nerves
centesis	thora*centesis*	*puncture* of chest wall to remove fluids
emia	ur*emia*	urinary wastes in the *blood*
febr	a*febr*ile	absence of *fever*
genic	pyo*genic*	*producing* pus
iasis	cholelith*iasis*	gallstone *condition*
lith	nephro*lith*	*stone* in the kidney
oma	lip*oma*	fatty *tumor*
oscopy	an*oscopy*	*visualization* of the anus
osis	nephr*osis*	disease *condition* of the kidney
plegia	hemi*plegia*	*paralysis* of one-half of the body
pnea	a*pnea*	absence of *breathing*
pyo	*pyo*derma	skin disease caused by *pus*-forming bacteria
therapy	hydro*therapy*	water used in *treatment* of disease
uria	poly*uria*	excessive *urine* production and urination

When you are working on a surgical floor, you will encounter another large group of medical terms. These describe surgical procedures. You will need to have some idea of the type of surgery done on a patient. For this you must learn the word elements used in the names for surgical procedures.

Word Element: Ectomy

The suffix *ectomy* means *surgical removal*. When used in combination with any word element denoting an organ or other body part, the term formed means that the organ or body part has been removed.

gastr*ectomy*	surgical removal of the stomach
thyroid*ectomy*	surgical removal of the thyroid gland
col*ectomy*	surgical removal of the large intestine

In many cases, an organ may be removed only partially. To indicate this procedure, other words are used to modify the medical term, for example:

subtotal thyroidectomy   *partial* cystectomy

Other modifying words may precede the medical term. This identifies the surgery performed even more accurately.

left salpingoophor*ectomy*	removal of the left ovary and oviduct
vaginal hyster*ectomy*	removal of uterus through the vagina
transurethral prostat*ectomy*	removal of the prostate through the urethra
total abdominal hyster*ectomy*	removal of the entire uterus through abdomen

Word Element	Example	Definition
orrhaphy	herni*orrhaphy*	*surgical repair* of a hernia
ostomy	ureter*ostomy*	*formation of an opening* for ureteral drainage
otomy	colp*otomy*	*surgical incision* into the vagina
pexy	cysto*pexy*	*fixation of bladder* to the abdominal wall
plasty	rhino*plasty*	*plastic surgery* of the nose

SECTION 2: MEDICAL SPECIALTIES AND WORDS TO REMEMBER

OBJECTIVES: WHAT YOU WILL LEARN

When you have completed this section, you will be able to:

- Describe medical specialties.
- Identify different physician's titles and to describe their meaning.
- Locate and define lists of words used in this book.

**KEY IDEAS:
MEDICAL SPECIALTIES**

Name	Physician's Title	Description
Allergy	Allergist	A subspecialty of internal medicine dealing with diagnosis and treatment of body reactions resulting from unusual sensitivity to foods, pollens, dust, medicines, or other substances
Anesthesiology	Anesthesiologist	Administration of various forms of anesthesia in operations or diagnosis to cause loss of feeling or sensation
Cardiovascular diseases; Cardiology	Cardiologist	A subspecialty of internal medicine involving the diagnosis and treatment of disease of the heart and blood vessels
Dermatology	Dermatologist	Diagnosis and treatment of diseases of the skin
Gastroenterology	Gastroenterologist	A subspecialty of internal medicine concerned with diagnosis and treatment of disorders of the digestive tract
General practice	General practitioner	The diagnosis and treatment of disease by medical and surgical methods, without limitation to organ systems or body regions, and without restriction as to age of patients
General surgery	Surgeon	The diagnosis and treatment of disease by surgical means, without limitation to special organ systems or body regions
Gynecology	Gynecologist	Diagnosis and treatment of diseases of the female reproductive organs

Word Element	Example	Definition
Internal medicine	Internist	The diagnosis and nonsurgical treatment of illnesses of adults
Neurological surgery	Neurosurgeon	Diagnosis and surgical treatment of brain, spinal cord, and nerve disorders
Neurology	Neurologist	Diagnosis and treatment of diseases of brain, spinal cord, and nerves
Obstetrics	Obstetrician	The care of women during pregnancy, childbirth, and the interval immediately following
Ophthalmology	Ophthalmologist	Diagnosis and treatment of diseases of the eye, including prescribing glasses
Orthopedics	Orthopedist	Diagnosis and treatment of disorders and diseases of the muscular and skeletal systems
Otolaryngology	Otolaryngologist	Diagnosis and treatment of diseases of the ear, nose, and throat
Pathology	Pathologist	Study and interpretation of changes in organs, tissues, cells, and alterations in body chemistry to aid in diagnosing disease and determining treatment
Pediatrics	Pediatrician	Prevention, diagnosis, and treatment of children's diseases
Physical medicine and rehabilitation	Physiatrist	Diagnosis of disease or injury in the various systems and areas of the body and treatment by means of physical procedures as well as treatment and restoration of the convalescent and physically handicapped patient
Plastic surgery	Plastic surgeon	Corrective or reparative surgery to restore deformed or mutilated parts of the body
Psychiatry	Psychiatrist	Diagnosis and treatment of mental disorders
Radiology	Radiologist	Use of radiant energy including x rays, radium, cobalt 60, etc., in the diagnosis of disease
Therapeutic radiology	Radiologist	The use of radiant energy, including x rays, radium, and other radioactive substances in the treatment of diseases
Thoracic surgery	Thoracic surgeon	Operative treatment of the lungs, heart, or the large blood vessels within the chest cavity
Urology	Urologist	Diagnosis and treatment of diseases or disorders of the kidneys, bladder, ureters, and urethra and of the male reproductive organs

**KEY IDEAS:
WORDS TO REMEMBER**

A   **abdomen**—the region of the body between the chest and the pelvis.

abdominal prep—the procedure for making the patient's abdomen ready for surgery. The preparation includes thorough cleansing of the skin and careful shaving of the body hair in the abdominal area.

abduction—to move an arm or leg away from the center of the body.

accuracy—the quality of being exact or correct, exact conformity to truth or rules, free from error or defects.

acute illness—comes on suddenly and runs its course within a few days.

adduction—to move an arm or leg toward the center of the body.

admission—the administrative procedures followed when a person enters the health care institution and becomes an inpatient. Admission covers the period from the time the patient enters the door of the hospital until he is settled in his room.

adrenal glands—two glands in the upper posterior dorsal area of the abdomen, near the kidneys.

alveoli—a microscopic air sac in the lung where oxygen passes into the blood.

ambulatory—able to walk about, not bedridden.

amputation—the cutting off of a body part by accident or through surgery.

anal—pertaining to the anus.

anatomical position—a person standing facing you, feet together, palms forward, head up.

anatomy—the study of the structure of an organism—such as a plant, an animal, or a human being—and any of its parts.

anesthesia—loss of feeling or sensation in a part or all of the body. Local anesthesia is the loss of sensation in a part of the body. General anesthesia is complete loss of sensation in the entire body.

anesthetic—a drug used to produce loss of feeling in a person. An anesthetic can be given orally, rectally, by injection, or by inhalation. A person who has been given an anesthetic is anesthetized.

antagonistic action—action that happens when two sets of structures are doing exactly the opposite thing. An example is antagonistic action of the biceps and triceps. One relaxes while the other contracts.

anterior—located in the front. The opposite of posterior.

antibiotic—a drug used in medical treatment that prevents disease-causing microorganisms from multiplying.

anus—the posterior opening in the body through which feces is excreted.

aorta—the name for the major artery that carries blood away from the heart.

artery—a blood vessel that carries blood away from the heart.

asepsis—the condition of being free of disease-causing organisms.

aspirate—to remove material from a body cavity by using a tube. Aspirate also means to draw material such as saliva, mucus, or food particles into the lungs from the mouth.

atrophy—muscles wasting away or decreasing in size.

auricles/atria—the two upper chambers of the heart. They are side by side. Each is known as an atrium, the left atrium or the right atrium.

autoclave—equipment used to sterilize instruments and other articles in the health care institution.

autonomic nervous system—the part of the nervous system that carries messages without conscious thought.

axillary—the area under the arms; the armpits.

B **bacteria**—sometimes called germs. A kind of microorganism. Many bacteria cause disease.

bassinet—a small crib made especially for newborn babies.

bed cradle—when in place over a body area such as a foot or arm, this equipment holds the bedclothes (sheets and blankets) away from the patient so that they do not touch that body part.

bedpan—a pan used by patients who must defecate or urinate while in bed.

bladder—a membranous sac that serves as a container within the body such as the urinary bladder which holds urine.

blood—the fluid that circulates through the heart, arteries, veins, and capillaries. It carries nourishment and oxygen to the tissues and takes away waste matter and carbon dioxide.

blood pressure—the force of the blood on the inner walls of the blood vessels as it flows through them.

body alignment—refers to the arrangement of the body in a straight line, the placing of portions of the body in correct anatomical position.

brain—the main organ of the central nervous system. It is the center of thought, movement, emotion, and speech and controls coordination of the nerves and responses from the sense organs.

bronchial tubes—branches of the trachea that lead into the lungs.

bursa—a sac found within a joint capsule. It is filled with synovial fluid, which helps to buffer the movement of the bones against one another.

C **calories**—units for measuring the energy produced when food is oxidized in the body.

cannula—a word used to mean any of the kinds of tubes that can be inserted into one of the body cavities. A cannula may be used to draw fluids out or to give oxygen.

capillaries—the very small blood vessels that carry blood to all parts of the body and the skin. Capillaries are a link between the ends of the arteries and the beginning of the veins.

carbohydrate—one of the basic kinds of food elements used by the body. It is composed of carbon, hydrogen, and oxygen. This includes sugars and starches.

cardiac—pertaining to the heart.

cartilage—a tough connective tissue that holds bones together.

catheter—a tube inserted in a body cavity, usually used to withdraw fluid.

catheterization—inserting a catheter into a body opening or cavity.

cell—the basic unit of living matter.

centigrade—a measurement of temperature using a scale divided into 100 units or degrees. In this system, the freezing temperature of water is 0° centigrade, written 0°C. Water boils at 100°C. Often referred to as Celsius.

central nervous system—the part of the nervous system made up of the brain, nerves, and the spinal cord.

cerebral—pertaining to the cerebrum, a part of the brain.

cerebrospinal fluid—fluid secreted by cells in cavities within the cerebrum. It circulates through the membranes that cover and protect the brain and spinal cord.

cervix—the narrow outer end of the uterus.

channel—path.

check and balance—a safeguard for health in which the systems of the body have built-in mechanisms that keep their activity in a state of balance.

chronic illness—continues over many years or a lifetime.

circulation—the continuous movement of blood through the heart and blood vessels to all parts of the body.

circulatory system—the heart, blood vessels, blood, and all the organs that pump and carry blood and other fluids throughout the body.

clean—a term used in health care institutions to refer to an object or area that is uncontaminated by harmful microorganisms.

colon—the large bowel. It extends from the large intestine to the anus.

coma—a state of deep unconsciousness often caused by disease, injury, or drugs.

communicable disease—a disease that is easily spread from one person to another.

complication—an unexpected condition, such as the development of another illness in a patient who is already sick.

compress—folded pieces of cloth or gauze used to apply pressure to a part of the patient's body. The compress may also be used to supply moisture, heat, cold, or medications to a specific part of the body.

congenital—born with, or from birth. It refers to a physical or mental characteristic present in a baby at birth. Sometimes referred to as a birth defect.

congestion—unusually large amounts of blood or fluid in a body part. It means an abnormal condition exists.

connective tissue—tissue that connects, supports, covers, ensheathes, lines, pads, or protects.

continuous—uninterrupted, without a stop.

contract—get smaller.

contracture—when muscle tissue becomes drawn together, bunched up, or shortened because of spasm or paralysis, either permanently or temporarily.

convalescent—getting well or recovering after an illness or surgery.

cooperate—to work or act together, to unite in producing an effect, or to share an activity for mutual benefit.

coronary (or cardiac) care unit—a special patient care unit where persons who have cardiac conditions receive intensive care; abbreviated CCU.

cyanosis—when the skin looks blue or has a gray color because there is not enough oxygen in the blood; often seen in the patient's lips and nailbeds, and in the skin under the fingernails. In a black patient, it may appear as a darkening of color.

D **death rattle**—a sound often made by a dying patient. It is caused by air passing through the mucus collected in the throat and bronchial tubes.

deceased—another word for dead.

decubitus ulcers—also called bedsores. These are areas of the skin that become broken and painful. They are caused by continuous pressure on a body part, and usually occur when a patient is kept in bed for a long period of time.

defecate—to have a bowel movement; to excrete waste matter from the bowels.

dehydration—a condition in which the body has less than the normal amount of fluid.

dentures—artificial teeth. Dentures may replace some or all of a person's teeth, and are described as being partial or complete, and upper or lower.

dependability—one who is dependable comes to work every day on time and does what is asked at the proper time and in the proper way.

diabetes—a condition that develops when the body cannot change its sugar into energy. When this sugar collects in the blood, the patient needs a special diet and may have to be given insulin.

diagnosis—finding out what kind of disease or medical condition a patient has. A medical diagnosis is always made by a physician.

diagnostic examination—an examination that helps the physician make a diagnosis. The physician talks to the patient, examines him, and may order tests and X rays taken.

diagnostic testing—tests done to help the doctor in the diagnosis of a patient.

diaphragm—the muscular partition between the chest cavity and the abdominal cavity.

diarrhea—an abnormally frequent discharge of fluid fecal material from the bowel.

diastolic blood pressure—in taking a patient's blood pressure, one records the bottom number as the reading for the diastolic pressure. This is the relaxing phase of the heartbeat.

digestive system—the group of body organs that carries out digestion. Digestion is the process in the body in which food is broken down mechanically and chemically, and is changed into forms that can enter the bloodstream and be used by the body.

dilates—gets bigger, expands.

dirty—a term used in the health care institution to refer to an object or area as being contaminated by harmful microorganisms.

disability—loss of the ability to use a part or parts of the body in a normal way.

discharge—this word has two special meanings. 1) When a patient is ready to leave the hospital, the hospital's business office helps him with his arrangements and with the checking out procedure. This process is called discharge. 2) The term used for unusual material coming out from some part of the body. For example, after a patient has had surgery, there may be a discharge of some kind of fluid coming out through the incision.

discoloration—change in color.

disinfection—the process of destroying most disease-causing organisms.

disposable equipment—equipment that is used one time only or for one patient only and then thrown away.

disposables—items used once and then thrown away. There are many kinds; they range from tissues and napkins to syringes and surgeon's gloves.

doctor—see physician.

dorsal—refers to the back or to the back part of an organ; the posterior part.

dorsiflexion—to bend backward.

drape—a covering used during an examination or an operation to cover the patient's body.

draping—covering a patient or parts of the patient's body with a sheet, blanket, bath blanket, or other material. Draping is usually done during physical examination of the patient, and during operations.

draw sheet—a small sheet made of plastic, rubber, or cotton. It is placed crosswise on the middle of the bed over the bottom sheet to help protect the bedding from a patient's discharges.

dry application—an application of warmth or cold in which no water touches the skin.

duodenum—the first part of the small intestine. Most digestion and most absorption of the end products of digestion occur in the duodenum.

E **edema**—abnormal swelling of a part of the body caused by fluid collecting in that area. Usually the swelling is in the ankles, legs, hands, or abdomen.

emaciation—a wasting away of the flesh, caused by disease and sometimes by lack of food. An emaciated person is extremely thin.

embryo—the name for a living human being during the first 8 weeks of its development in the uterus.

emergency department—an area in the hospital where people are brought because they have suddenly become ill or have had an accident.

emesis basin—a pan used for catching material that a patient spits out, vomits, or expectorates.

endocrine gland—a ductless gland in the body that secretes hormones, substances that affect the way some body systems do their work.

enema—a liquid that flows through a tube into the rectum to wash out its contents.

enzyme—a substance manufactured by living tissue that stimulates certain chemical changes in the body. For example, pancreatic enzymes cause complex food proteins to break down into simpler structures that can be absorbed by the intestines.

epithelium—the tissue cells composing the skin. Also the cells lining the passages of the hollow organs of the respiratory, digestive, and urinary systems.

esophagus—a muscular tube for the passage of food, which extends from the back of the throat (pharynx), down through the chest and diaphragm into the stomach.

ethical behavior—to keep promises and do what you ought to do, to act in accordance with the rules or standards for right conduct or practice.

evaporate—to pass off as vapor, as water evaporating into the air.

excreta—urine and feces; waste matter from the body.

excrete—to eliminate or expel waste matter from the body.

exhalation—the process of breathing out air in respiration.

expectoration—coughing up matter from the lungs, trachea, or bronchial tubes, and spitting it out.

extension—to straighten an arm or leg.

extremities—the arms, legs, hands, and feet.

F **Fahrenheit**—the name of a system for measuring temperature. In the Fahrenheit system the temperature of water at boiling is 212°. At freezing, it is 32°. These temperatures are usually written 212°F and 32°F.

fallopian tubes—the uterine tubes, one on either side of the uterus. These tubes are the passageways, also called the oviducts, through which the egg travels from the ovary to the uterus.

fanfold—a method of arranging bed linens so that the covers and spread are folded back out of the way, but still are on the bed and within easy reach.

feces—solid waste material discharged from the body through the rectum and anus. Other names for feces are stool, excreta, excrement, BM, bowel movement, and fecal matter.

fertilization—when a sperm cell and an egg cell meet, the two cells join, and the sperm cell is absorbed into the egg cell. This is also called "conception."

fetus—the name for the infant developing in the uterus, after the first 2 months.

fever—the term for a person's condition when his body temperature is above normal.

flatus—intestinal gas.

flex—to bend.

flexion—to bend a joint (elbow, wrist, knee).

fluid—applies to both liquid and gaseous substances.

fluid balance—the same amount of fluid that is taken in by the body is given out by the body.

fluid intake—the fluid taken into the body, from whatever source.

fluid output—the fluid given out of the body, no matter how.

force fluids—extra fluids to be taken in by a patient according to the doctor's orders.

Fowler's position—the patient's position when the head of the bed is at a 45° angle.

fracture—a break in a bone.

friction—the rubbing of one surface against another. Friction between the patient's body and his bedclothes often produces bedsores.

G **gastrointestinal**—the digestive system. Sometimes called the "GI system," an abbreviation for gastro (stomach) and intestinal.

gatch handle—a handle used on manually operated hospital beds to raise or lower the backrest and kneerest.

gavage—feeding a patient by putting a tube into his stomach. Nasogastric gavage is putting the tube through the patient's nostril and then through the esophagus into his stomach.

generalized application—one in which warmth or cold is applied to the entire body.

genital—refers to the external reproductive organs.

geriatric patients—those over 65 years of age.

germicide—a chemical compound used to destroy bacteria.

gestation—the time from conception until the birth of a baby. The gestation period for a human baby is about 280 days. Another word for gestation is pregnancy.

gland—an organ that manufactures a chemical that will be used elsewhere in the body.

graduate—a measuring cup marked along its side to show various amounts so the material placed in the cup can be measured accurately. The marks are called calibrations.

H **head nurse or team leader**—the person who supervises the nursing health care team, including the nursing assistant. It is the head nurse or team leader who will help you, the nursing assistant, and keep track of your performance.

health care institution—hospital, nursing home, convalescent home, extended care facility, or clinic, where health care services are provided both on an inpatient and outpatient basis.

heart—a four-chambered, hollow, muscular organ that lies in the chest cavity, pointing slightly to the left. It is the pump that circulates the blood through the lungs and into all parts of the body.

hemorrhage—excessive bleeding.

hereditary—characteristics passed down from parent to child. An example is the color of your eyes. Some diseases apparently are hereditary. An example is diabetes.

homeostasis—stability of all body functions at normal levels.

hormone—a protein substance secreted by an endocrine gland directly into the blood.

hospital—a building where sick and injured people are given medical treatment, services, and other kinds of health care. A hospital is one type of health care institution.

hygiene—the science that deals with the preservation of health. When used to describe an object or a person, it means clean and sanitary.

hyperextension—beyond the normal extension.

hypertension—high blood pressure.

hypotension—low blood pressure.

hypothalamus—a tiny structure at the base of the brain that has a lot of influence over all body activities, especially the activity of the pituitary gland.

I incident—any unusual event such as an accident or a condition that is likely to cause an accident.

incontinence—the inability to control one's bowels or bladder. An incontinent person cannot control oneself from urinating or defecating.

incubator—a special heated crib used in the care of premature babies.

infection—a condition in body tissue in which germs or pathogens have multiplied and destroyed many cells.

inflammation—a reaction of the tissues to disease or injury. There is usually pain, heat, redness, and swelling of the body part.

inhalation—the process of breathing in air in respiration.

insensible fluid loss—fluid that is lost from the body without being noticed, such as in perspiration or air breathed out.

insulin—a hormone produced naturally in the body by the pancreas. Insulin helps the body change sugar into energy. Insulin can be produced from animal pancreas, for use in the treatment of diabetes.

intensive care unit—an area in the health care institution for patients who need more intensive nursing care than ordinary patients.

intermittent—alternating; stopping and beginning again.

intracellular fluid—fluid within the cell.

intravenous—refers to the injection of fluids into a vein. Foods in liquid form and medications can be put into the patient's body in this way.

intravenous pole—also called IV pole or IV standard. A tall pole on rollers or casters used to hold the containers or tubes needed, for example, during a blood transfusion.

isolation gown—a special gown worn over a uniform when in the room of a patient with a communicable disease. The gown helps protect the uniform from being contaminated by harmful bacteria.

isolation procedures—special procedures used in caring for patients with communicable diseases to prevent the disease from spreading to other persons.

J   **job description**—the fundamental nursing tasks and procedures you, the nursing assistant, will be accountable for in your work will be found in the job description given to you by your employing health care institution or agency.

joint—a part of the body where two bones come together.

K   **kidney**—the organ lying in the upper posterior portion of the abdomen. It removes waste products and water from the bloodstream and excretes them as urine.

knee-chest position—a bent posture with the knees and chest touching the examining table. This position is sometimes used for examining the rectum. It is also used for women who have recently given birth, to get the uterus to fall forward into its normal position.

L   **lactation**—the body process of producing milk to feed a newborn baby.

licensed practical nurse (LPN) or licensed vocational nurse (LVN)—a member of the nursing health care team who is educated in a one-year course and licensed to give bedside nursing care and treatments. In some states, with additional training the LPN is permitted to dispense medications.

liquid—flowing freely, like water.

lithotomy position—the patient lies on her back with her legs spread apart and her knees bent. The position is used for performing a pelvic (vaginal) examination.

liver—the body's largest gland, located in the abdominal cavity. The liver has many functions in the chemistry and metabolism of the body and is essential to life.

localized application—one in which warmth or coldness is applied to a specific area or small part of the body.

lubricant—a substance such as petroleum jelly, glycerine, or cold cream that is used to make a surface smooth or moist.

lungs—the primary organs of breathing.

M   **medical asepsis**—special practices and procedures for cleanliness to decrease the chances for disease-causing bacteria to live and spread.

medical-surgical patients—those who have an acute or chronic illness that is treated with medication or surgery.

medication—a substance or preparation used in treating a disease. Medications can be in the form of pills, tablets, capsules, powders, syrups, liquids, suppositories, creams or lotions. Medications can be administered orally, rectally, vaginally, topically, intravenously, intramuscularly, or nasally (inhalation).

membrane—a thin layer of tissue. An example is the mucous membrane, as in the lining of the nose and throat.

meninges—the three membranes that protect the brain and spinal cord.

meniscus—a disc of cartilage found between two bones at a joint that acts to reduce wear and tear on the ends of the bones. The menisci found in the complicated knee joint are an example.

metabolism—the total of all the physical and chemical changes that take place in living organisms and cells.

metric system—a system of measurement based on the decimal system. Units are 10s, 100s, 1000s, and so forth.

microorganism—a living thing so small it cannot be seen with the naked eye, but only through a microscope.

mitered corner—a special way to fold the bedding at the corners when making a hospital bed. The mitered corner keeps the bedding neat and stretched tightly so that wrinkles are avoided.

modified—changed.

moist application—an application of warmth or cold in which water touches the skin.

mucus—a sticky substance secreted by mucous membranes, mainly in the lungs, nose, and parts of the rectal and genital areas.

muscle—tissue composed of fibers with the ability to elongate and shorten, causing bones and joints to move. Voluntary muscles are in body parts such as the neck, arms, fingers, and legs. Involuntary muscles are in organs such as the heart and intestines.

muscular system—the group of body organs that make it possible for the body and its parts to move.

N **negligence**—the commission of an act or failure to perform an act where the respective performance or nonperformance would deviate from that act which should have been done by a reasonably prudent person under the same or similar conditions.

nephron—the functional unit of the kidney that filters out those substances the body does not need, reabsorbing those it does need, and secreting those products that are harmful to the body. The result of this process is urine.

nerve impulse—a regular wave of negative electrical impulses that transmits information along the neuron from one part of the body to another.

nerves—bundles of neurons held together with connective tissue. They go to all parts of the body from the central nervous system, that is, from the brain and spinal cord.

nervous system—the group of body organs that control and regulate the activities of the body and the functioning of the other body systems.

neuron—a nerve, including the cell and the long fiber coming from the cell.

newborn—a baby in the first month of life.

nourishment—the process of taking food into the body to maintain life.

nurse—a person educated and trained to care for sick people and to help physicians and surgeons. Nurses are licensed as registered nurses (RNs) and licensed practical nurses (LPNs).

nursing assistant—a person who helps the registered nurse to care for patients. Nursing assistants usually work in hospitals, other health care institutions, or in the patient's home.

nutrients—food substances.

nutrition—the process by which the body takes in and uses food.

O **obese**—very fat.

objective reporting—reporting exactly what you observe.

objective symptoms—symptoms that can be observed and reported exactly as they are seen.

observation—gathering information about the patient by noticing any change.

obstetrical patients—women having babies.

omit—leave out.

ophthalmoscope—an instrument the doctor uses to look inside a patient's eye.

oral—anything to do with the mouth. Examples are eating and speaking.

oral hygiene—cleanliness of the mouth.

organ—a part of the body made of several types of tissue grouped together to perform a certain function. Examples are the heart, stomach, and lungs.

organism—a living thing.

orthopedics (orthopaedics)—the medical specialty that covers the treatment of broken bones, deformities, or diseases that attack the bones, joints, and muscles.

ostomy—a surgical procedure that provides the patient with an artificial opening, either temporary or permanent. The person's feces then can leave the body through this opening rather than through the rectum. The opening is usually made through the abdominal wall into a part of the large intestine.

otoscope—an instrument the doctor uses to look at the inside of a patient's ear.

ovary—one of a pair of organs in the female that produce mature eggs (ova) as well as producing the primary sex hormones of the female, estrogen and progesterone.

ovulation—the period of time in which the ovum is pushed out from the surface of the ovary and usually picked up by the oviduct. This usually occurs 14 days before the onset of the next menstrual period.

ovum—the egg in the female. After fertilization, it develops into a new organism of the same species.

oxidation—in the human body, this happens when food is combined with oxygen to create energy.

oxygen—a colorless, odorless gas making up about one-fifth of the volume of the air. It is essential for human life. Abbreviated as O_2.

oxygen tent—equipment used in the health care institution to provide large amounts of extra oxygen for a patient.

P **pancreas**—a large gland, 6 to 8 inches long, that secretes enzymes into the intestines for digestion of foods. It also manufactures insulin, which is secreted into the bloodstream.

paralysis—loss of the ability to move a part or all of the body.

paraplegia—paralysis of the legs and lower part of the body.

parenteral—refers to a method of bringing substances into the body by some way other than the mouth and intestines. An example is intravenous feedings.

pathogens—disease-causing microorganisms.

patient care unit—an area of the hospital set aside for patients who have similar conditions or illnesses.

patient lift—a mechanical device like a swinging seat used for lifting a patient into and out of such equipment as the hospital bed, bathtub, or wheelchair.

patient unit—the space for one patient including the hospital bed, bedside table, chair, and other equipment.

pediatric patients—children.

percussion hammer—an instrument used by the doctor to test a patient's reflexes by tapping the body at certain places.

perineum—the body area between the thighs. It includes the area of the anus and the external genital organs.

peristalsis—movement of the intestines that pushes the food along to the next part of the digestive system.

phagocytosis—a process in which a cell engulfs and destroys a foreign protein, such as a germ.

physician—a doctor. A person who is licensed to practice medicine.

physiology—the study of the functions of body tissues and organs.

pituitary gland—sometimes called the master gland. It is attached to the base of the brain and directs the flow of all hormones in the body.

placenta—the oval, spongy structure in the uterus through which the unborn baby receives its nourishment. Sometimes called afterbirth. The umbilical cord is attached to the placenta. The placenta is discharged from the mother's body soon after childbirth.

plasma—the liquid portion of blood, or blood from which the red and white cells and platelets have been removed.

pleural cavity—the chest cavity containing the lungs. The pleura is the membrane lining the chest cavity and covering the lungs.

posterior—located in the back or toward the rear.

postmortem—after death.

postoperative—after surgery.

postoperative bed—a standard hospital bed made up in a special way for a patient who is coming back to his unit after an operation. Sometimes called recovery bed, stretcher bed, or operating room bed.

postpartum—following childbirth.

premature birth—birth of a baby before the normal period of gestation (pregnancy) is over.

preoperative—before surgery.

prepuce—the foreskin of the penis. The foreskin is often removed in an operation called a circumcision.

professional registered nurse—a member of the nursing health care team who is educated for from two to four years and licensed to plan and carry out total patient care. The duties of the registered nurse may include dispensing medications, administering treatments, assisting physicians and supervising other members of the nursing health care team. The job of head nurse or team leader is an example of one important role filled by a professional registered nurse.

pronation—to bend downward.

prone—lying on one's stomach.

prostate—a male gland behind the outlet of the urinary bladder.

prosthesis—an artificial body part. There are prostheses (plural) for legs, arms, hands, feet, breasts, eyes, and teeth.

psychiatric patient—a patient who is being treated for a mental illness.

pulmonary—refers to the lungs.

pulse—the rhythmic expansion and contraction of the arteries caused by the beating of the heart. The expansion and contraction show how fast, how regular, and with what force the heart is beating.

Q **quadriplegia**—paralysis of both the upper and lower parts of the body.

R **radial pulse**—this is the pulse felt at a person's wrist at the radial artery.

range of motion (ROM)—These exercises move each muscle and joint through its full range of motion. Therefore, it assists the patient who is confined to exercise his muscles and joints.

rectal irrigation—washing out the rectum by injecting a stream of water; giving an enema.

rectum—the lower 8 to 10 inches of the colon. The anus is the body opening from the rectum.

recumbent position—lying down or reclining.

rehabilitation—the processes by which people who have been disabled by injury or sickness are helped to recover as much as possible of their original abilities for the activities of daily living.

reproductive system—the group of body organs that make possible the creation of new human life.

respiration—the body process of breathing; inhaling and exhaling air.

respiratory system—the group of body organs that carry on the body function of respiration. The system brings oxygen into the body and eliminates carbon dioxide.

restrict fluids—fluids that are limited to certain amounts.

reticuloendothelial system—the body system primarily responsible for our resistance to disease. The tissue is made up of cells from various systems all of which are capable of either producing antibodies or the process of phagocytosis.

reverse isolation—procedures used to prevent harmful organisms from coming into contact with the patient. See isolation procedure.

rigor mortis—stiffening of a person's body and limbs shortly after death.

rotation—to move a joint in a circular motion around its axis.
    —internal—to turn in towards the center.
    —external—to turn out away from the center.

S **saliva**—the secretion of the salivary glands into the mouth. Saliva moistens food and helps in swallowing. It also contains an enzyme (chemical) that helps digest starches.

scrotal prep—the procedures for making the genital area of a male patient ready for surgery. The preparation includes thoroughly cleansing the skin and carefully shaving hair in the area.

scrotum—a pouch below the penis that contains the testicles.

secrete—to produce a special substance and expel it. The salivary glands secrete saliva. The pancreas secretes insulin.

seizure—convulsion or paroxysms of involuntary muscular contractions and relaxations. Can be localized or generalized, with spasms either violent or quiet.

seminal vesicles—small glands in the male near the prostate and urethra where semen is stored before it is discharged.

sense organs—these organs make it possible for us to be aware of the outside world and ourselves through the senses of sight, hearing, smell, taste, and touch.

septicemia—a severe infection in the blood. Usually called blood poisoning.

shock—a state of collapse resulting from reduced blood volume and blood pressure, usually caused by severe injuries such as hemorrhage or burns on many parts of the body. Shock may also result from an emotional blow.

side lying—lying on one's side.

signs—objective evidence of disease. Signs can be observed by a trained person such as a doctor or nurse. Vital signs are special signals that doctors and nurses always look for. These are the patient's temperature, pulse, respiration, and blood pressure.

Sims' position—the patient lies on the left side with the right knee and thigh drawn up. This position permits a satisfactory rectal examination.

sitz bath—a bath in which the patient sits in a specially designed chair-tub or a regular bathtub with his hips and buttocks in water.

skeleton—the bony support of the body.

solution—liquid containing dissolved substances.

specimen—a sample of material taken from the patient's body. Examples are urine specimens, feces specimens, and sputum specimens.

sperm—a tiny tadpole-shaped cell from the male, capable of causing conception, or the beginning of a baby, if it fuses with a mature egg or ovum from the female.

sphincter—a ring-like muscle that controls the opening and closing of a body opening. An example is the anal sphincter.

sphygmomanometer—an apparatus for taking a patient's blood pressure.

spinal cord—one of the main organs of the nervous system. The spine is another name for the human backbone. The spinal cord carries messages from the brain to other parts of the body and from parts of the body back to the brain. The spinal cord is inside the spine (backbone).

spleen—an abdominal organ that manufactures blood cells during the life of the embryo.

splint—a thin piece of wood or other rigid material used to keep an injured part, such as a broken bone, in place.

spores—bacteria that have formed hard shells around themselves for protection. Spores can be destroyed only by sterilization.

sputum—waste material coughed up from the lungs or trachea.

staphylococcus—one type of bacteria that causes infection found in health care institutions. Antibiotic drugs are used to fight staphylococcus infections.

sterilization—the process of destroying all microorganisms including spores.

stethoscope—an instrument that allows one to listen to various sounds in the patient's body, such as the heartbeat or breathing sounds.

stimulus—a change in the external or internal environment that is strong enough to set up a nervous impulse.

stoma—an artificially made opening connecting a body passage with the outside, such as in a tracheotomy or colostomy.

stomach—the part of the digestive tract between the esophagus (food pipe) and the duodenum. The stomach churns food and starts the process of digestion.

stool—solid waste material discharged from the body through the rectum and anus. Other names include feces, excreta, excrement, bowel movement, and fecal matter.

stroke/hemiplegia—this may be due to hemorrhage, cerebral thrombosis, embolism, or a tumor of the cerebrum. Paralysis on only one half of the body is a result of this. The sudden apoplexy/hemiplegia is caused sometimes by hemorrhage, the result of rupture of a sclerosed or diseased blood vessel in the brain. Often associated with high blood pressure.

subjective reporting—giving your opinion about what you have observed.

suction—the action of, or capacity for, vacuuming up. This is accomplished by reducing the air pressure over part of the surface of a substance.

supination—to bend upward.

supine—lying on one's back.

suppository—a semisolid preparation (sometimes medicated) that is inserted into the vagina or the rectum.

surgical asepsis—when an area is made completely free of microorganisms. The area may be called surgically clean.

surgical procedure—the repair of an injury or a disease condition. In a surgical procedure, the surgeon usually makes an incision, that is, he cuts through the skin into the body.

symptom—evidence of a disease, disorder, or condition.

system—a group of organs acting together to carry out one or more body functions.

systolic blood pressure—the force with which blood is pumped when the heart muscle is contracting. When taking a patient's blood pressure, the top number is recorded as the systolic blood pressure.

T **taut**—pulled or drawn tight, not slack.

temperature—a measurement of the amount of heat in the body at a given time. The normal body temperature is 98.6°F (37°C).

tendons—tough cords of connective tissue that bind muscles to other bony parts.

testes—a pair of reproductive organs in the male that lie in the scrotum hanging from the perineal area, dorsal to the penis.

testicles—another word for testes.

therapeutic—refers mainly to the treatment of disease. Something that helps heal.

thermometer—an instrument used for measuring temperature.

thyroid—an endocrine gland, located in the front of the neck. It regulates body metabolism. This gland secretes a hormone known as thyroxine.

tissue—a group of cells of the same type.

tissue fluid—a watery environment around each cell that acts as a place of exchange for gases, food, and waste products between the cells and the blood.

tongue depressor—a flat blade-like instrument used to keep the patient's tongue flattened during an examination of the throat and mouth.

trachea—an organ of the respiratory system. It is located in the throat area. The trachea is commonly called the windpipe.

tracheotomy—a surgical procedure to make an artificial opening in a person's neck connecting his trachea with the outside. This surgery may be necessary when the person's trachea above the opening is blocked and he cannot breathe.

traction device—equipment for pulling and stretching parts of the patient's body by using pulleys and weights. Traction is used to keep broken bones properly lined up while they are healing.

transfer—moving a hospital patient from one unit to another.

trapeze—a metal bar suspended over the bed. It is used by a patient to help him raise or move his body more easily.

traumatic—refers to damage to the body caused by injury, wound, or shock. Sometimes used to refer to mental disturbances caused by emotional shock.

Trendelenburg's position—the bed or operating table is tilted so the patient's head is about a foot below the level of the knees. This position is used to get more blood to the head and prevent shock. Also called the shock position.

tumor—a growth in or on the body. There are two kinds: 1) benign tumors, which grow slowly and can usually be removed by surgery; 2) malignant tumors, which grow wildly and are sometimes called "cancer." They often are a threat to a person's life.

turning frames—reversible beds used in the care of patients with certain orthopedic conditions.

U **umbilical cord**—a rather long, flexible, rough organ that carries nourishment from the mother to the baby. It connects the umbilicus of the unborn baby in the mother's uterus to the placenta.

umbilicus—a small depression on the abdomen that marks the place where the umbilical cord was originally attached to the fetus. Another name for the umbilicus is the navel.

ureters—the tubes leading from the kidney to the urinary bladder.

urethra—the tube leading from the urinary bladder to the outside of the body.

urinal—a portable pan given to male patients in bed so they can urinate without getting out of bed.

urinalysis—a laboratory test of the patient's urine done for diagnostic purposes.

urinary system—the group of organs that have the function of making urine and discharging it from the body.

urinate—to discharge urine from the body. Other words used for this function are void and micturate.

uterus—an expandable female reproductive organ in which the fetus grows and is nourished by membranes called the placenta until it is time for the baby to be born.

V **vagina**—in the female, the birth canal leading from the vulva to the cervix of the uterus.

vaginal douche—a procedure by which a stream of water is sent into the patient's vaginal opening. The water may be plain or it may contain medication.

vaginal prep—the procedures for making the genital area of a female patient ready for surgery. The preparation includes thoroughly cleansing the skin and carefully shaving the pubic hair.

varicose veins—an abnormal swelling of veins, especially veins in the legs.

vas deferens—the tube carrying sperm from the testicles to the glands where they are stored in preparation for ejaculation.

vein—a blood vessel that carries blood from parts of the body back to the heart.

ventricles—the lower two chambers of the heart. They are side by side.

villus—a tiny fingerlike projection in the lining of the small intestine into which the end products of digestion are absorbed and carried to the bloodstream and then to the individual cells.

virus—the microscopic living parasitic agent that can cause infectious disease.

viscera—refers to the organs within the abdominal body cavity.

vital signs—temperature, pulse, respiration, and blood pressure.

void—to urinate, pass water.

vomiting—throwing up; the contents of the stomach are cast up and out of the mouth.

vomitus—vomited material; emesis.

W **ward clerk**(unit clerk)—a member of the nursing health care team who works at the desk of the nurses' station. The duties of the ward clerk include clerical work, answering the telephone, helping to direct traffic on the floor and filling out requisition slips.

well-balanced diet—a diet containing a variety of foods from each of the basic food groups.

WHAT YOU HAVE LEARNED

You must have a good working knowledge of medical terminology and abbreviations. This includes the ability to spell, define, and pronounce these terms accurately. Then you can communicate effectively with the other members of your health care team. Remember: learning medical terminology is similar to learning another language.

This chapter explains how medical terminology is related to body parts and functions. This includes anatomy, the various body systems, diseases and diagnoses, and surgical procedures.

When you begin the study of medical terminology, you should understand that medical terms are combinations of words or word roots. The information in this chapter should help you to recognize word elements and their meanings. Time, thought, and practice are needed before you can become really expert in the language of medicine. When you have mastered the meanings of the prefixes, roots, and suffixes given in this chapter, you will be able to apply what you have learned to the medical terms you see and hear on the job. Your efforts will help you reach the goal of all health care workers—the delivery of better patient care.

INDEX

W

Walker, 95
Ward clerk, responsibilities of, 4
Warm applications, 315
    dry, 332–333
    moist, 331–332
      procedure for applying, 325–326
    principle of, 316
    procedure for applying, 325
    purpose of, 315
    temperatures of, 316
Warm compresses, 340
    procedure for applying, 321–322

Warm soaks, 340
    procedure for applying, 325–326
Warm water bottles, 340
    procedure for applying, 326–328
Waste material, examination of, 217–218
Water, 58. *See also* Fluid
    drinking, passing to patient, 202
      procedure for, 202–203
    importance of, 205
    tap, sterilizing of, 402
Weighing of patient, 288, 289
Weight. *See* Body weight
Wheelchair, 95, 295
    transporting of patient by. *See*

Transporting of patient
White blood cells, 55
Windpipe. *See* Trachea
Womb. *See* Uterus
Word elements, 434, 446–449
    combining of, 435–437
    glossary of, 440–444
    similarity in terms, 437–439
    spelling variations, 437
    for surgical procedures, 449–450
    vowels, 434
Words, communication through, 27
Wound and skin precaution cards, 82
Wrist, exercise of, 147